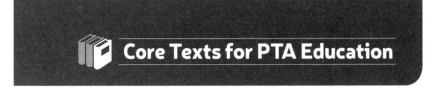

Core Texts for PTA Education

PROCEDURES AND PATIENT CARE
for the Physical Therapist Assistant

SERIES EDITOR

MIA L. ERICKSON, PT, EDD, CHT, ATC

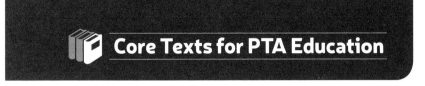

Core Texts for PTA Education

PROCEDURES AND PATIENT CARE
for the Physical Therapist Assistant

Jennifer Memolo, MA, PTA
Clarkson College
Omaha, Nebraska

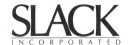

SLACK
INCORPORATED

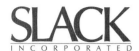

SLACK Incorporated
6900 Grove Road
Thorofare, NJ 08086 USA
856-848-1000   Fax: 856-848-6091
www.Healio.com/books
© 2019 by SLACK Incorporated

Senior Vice President: Stephanie Arasim Portnoy
Vice President, Editorial: Jennifer Kilpatrick
Vice President, Marketing: Michelle Gatt
Acquisitions Editor: Tony Schiavo
Managing Editor: Allegra Tiver
Creative Director: Thomas Cavallaro
Cover Artist: Katherine Christie
Project Editor: Erin O'Reilly

Procedures and Patient Care for the Physical Therapist Assistant includes ancillary materials specifically available for faculty use. Please visit http://www.efacultylounge.com to obtain access.

Library of Congress Cataloging-in-Publication Data
Names: Memolo, Jennifer, author.
Title: Procedures and patient care for the physical therapist assistant /
  Jennifer Memolo, .
Description: Thorofare, NJ : Slack Incorporated, [2019] | Series: Core texts
  for PTA education | Includes bibliographical references and index.
Identifiers: LCCN 2018058055 (print) | LCCN 2018058669 (ebook) | ISBN
  9781630914554 (Web) | ISBN 9781630914547 (Epub) | ISBN 9781630914530
  (paperback)
Subjects: | MESH: Physical Therapist Assistants | Patient Care--methods |
  Physical Therapy Modalities
Classification: LCC RM725 (ebook) | LCC RM725 (print) | NLM WB 460 | DDC
  615.8/2--dc23
LC record available at https://lccn.loc.gov/2018058055

Printed in the United States of America.

Last digit is print number: 10 9 8 7 6 5 4 3 2 1

DEDICATION

This book is dedicated to Sean, Morrissey, and Atticus, who inspire me every day.

CONTENTS

Procedures and Patient Care for the Physical Therapist Assistant includes ancillary materials specifically available for faculty use. Please visit http://www.efacultylounge.com to obtain access.

ACKNOWLEDGMENTS

I would like to thank the following faculty in the Clarkson College Physical Therapist Assistant Program: Caitlin, Michael, Jessica, Kim, Greta, and Karen for offering advice, support, and feedback, as well as patience while I wrote this book. Additional thanks goes to Clarkson College for allowing me access to labs and equipment, as well as LifeCare Center of Elkhorn, Kohll's Pharmacy, and Shannon Struby for letting me take and use pictures. Many thanks to my family for their support and feedback during this learning process. Thanks also to Tony Schiavo at SLACK Incorporated and Mia L. Erickson for their feedback and assistance as they guided me through this experience.

—Jennifer Memolo, MA, PTA

ABOUT THE AUTHOR

Jennifer Memolo, MA, PTA is from Alabama but currently lives in Omaha, Nebraska, where she teaches in the Physical Therapist Assistant program at Clarkson College. She received her BA in English at Birmingham-Southern College in Birmingham, Alabama, and went on to receive her MA in English/Creative Writing at East Carolina University in Greenville, North Carolina. She received her associate of science in a Physical Therapist Assistant program from Nash Community College in 2008 (Rocky Mount, North Carolina), at which time she moved to Omaha to work in inpatient rehabilitation and acute care. She has also worked in a skilled nursing facility, has served as Rehabilitation Director, and has worked for home health. In addition to teaching in the Physical Therapist Assistant associate of science and bachelor of science programs, she also teaches graduate level writing classes for nursing students at Clarkson College.

INTRODUCTION

This book, as indicated by its title, is for physical therapist assistants and provides detailed concepts regarding patient care specific to the discipline of physical therapy. While other health care practitioners could certainly use this text to learn about patient care techniques, this text is specifically written for the physical therapist assistant and attempts to address patient care methods that apply to that scope of practice. The hope is that this text will be useful to physical therapist assistant students as they learn about and prepare for patient care; however, it is additionally hoped that this text will become a reference and resource for physical therapist assistants as they graduate, study for the board examination, and practice as health care providers. Each chapter includes objectives, key terms, common abbreviations (with the understanding that abbreviations may differ from clinic to clinic and from state to state), and review questions at the end of each chapter to assist with retention and understanding. Also in each chapter is information adhering to the current best practice and an understanding of red flags a physical therapist assistant should know and report to supervising physical therapists or other health care providers. In addition to the textbook, an instructor's manual, including answers to the review questions, case studies, and recommended lab activities, as well as PowerPoint presentations have been added to assist with course creation.

Chapter 1

Preparation for Patient Care

KEY TERMS Communication | Comorbidities | Dermatomes | Documentation | Evaluation/assessment | Informed consent | Mobility | Modality | Orthostatic hypotension | Plan of care | Pressure injuries | State practice act

KEY ABBREVIATIONS APTA | CAPTE | HIPAA | ICF | ID | OCR | PICO | POC | POS | SOAP

Chapter Objectives

1. Analyze the relationship between a physical therapist assistant and a physical therapist, including delegation of tasks and how a physical therapist assistant makes changes within a plan of care (POC).
2. Describe the role of professionalism in the success of a physical therapist assistant's career.
3. Explain why adherence to the Health Insurance Portability and Accountability Act (HIPAA) is important, and provide examples of how to avoid infractions.
4. List reasons why documentation is important and necessary.
5. Identify information that would be categorized as Subjective, Objective, Assessment, or Plan (SOAP), and sort information into the correct area.
6. Identify reasons that informed consent is necessary.
7. List ways to improve communication with a patient.
8. Discuss evidence-based practice, and explain why it is important.

Introduction

The role of the physical therapist assistant is always changing, meaning that a dedicated practitioner will continue to learn and grow even after he or she has graduated from a Physical Therapist Assistant educational program. Your job as a physical therapist assistant is to educate and support your patients while helping them safely and efficiently progress with their therapy interventions. This book is meant to address specific areas of patient care of the physical therapist assistant, including legal and ethical concerns, as well as documentation and best-practice issues. In this ever-changing world and profession, maintaining professionalism is becoming more important than ever. A professional physical therapist assistant will be able to understand a physical therapist's evaluation and a POC, and will be able to make adjustments within a POC or know what actions to take if a POC must be altered. Additionally, a physical therapist assistant should be able to work with their supervising physical therapist and other therapists or health care providers, as patient care is always a team effort.

The Physical Therapist/Physical Therapist Assistant Relationship

Roles

A 2010 article noted that "education of PTs and PTAs about the appropriate utilization of PTAs and their preferred relationship is inadequate."[1(p51)] The American Physical Therapy Association (APTA) website (www.apta.org) includes information on the roles of physical thera-

Memolo J.
Procedures and Patient Care for the Physical Therapist Assistant
(pp 1-15). © 2019 SLACK Incorporated.

Box 1-1

Tasks a Physical Therapist Assistant Can and Cannot Do

- Cannot evaluate a patient
- Can observe and measure a patient's status after he or she is initially evaluated by the physical therapist
- Can treat within the scope of practice and POC
- Can change/modify interventions within the POC (with discussion with physical therapist)
- Can treat a patient per the state scope of practice

pists and physical therapist assistants, and it is important that both understand their roles in the team dynamic.[2,3] A physical therapist is expected to evaluate and diagnose individuals, and then to develop a POC for the patient's treatment. The physical therapist also conducts regular reevaluations, modifies the POC as needed, and creates and implements discharge plans.

Your role as a physical therapist assistant is to work with your supervising physical therapist to implement components of the POC. The physical therapist assistant can perform most tests and measures to collect data related to the therapy interventions to help show progress toward set goals. The physical therapist assistant cannot evaluate, reevaluate, or discharge a patient, nor can the physical therapist assistant change the POC established by the physical therapist; however, the physical therapist assistant can make observations about the patient's progress and report these findings to the physical therapist, which may result in changes to the POC.[1] In many cases, the physical therapist assistant is the practitioner seeing the patient on a regular, sometimes daily basis. This means the physical therapist assistant is the best person to recognize patient status changes and red flags. The physical therapist relies on the physical therapist assistant to provide accurate, valid data on the patient's progress to determine if goals are being met. Box 1-1 lists the tasks a physical therapist assistant can and cannot do.

Evaluations

A physical therapist is responsible for performing an initial evaluation, as well as regular reevaluations to assess patient progress toward set goals. It is an examination that includes taking a patient's history, reviewing the patient's body systems, and performing selected tests and measures to determine a physical therapy diagnosis. All evaluations have similar components, but they will also each be tailored for the individual's needs. For example, a patient coming to see a physical therapist after a knee replacement surgery will be asked about pain, will be tested for knee range of motion, and will be tested for strength in quadriceps and hamstrings.[4] This would differ from specific tests and measures for a patient seeking therapy after a car accident causing neck pain. Figure 1-1 shows a sample evaluation.

How Does a Physical Therapist Delegate to a Physical Therapist Assistant?

The physical therapist and physical therapist assistant are a team, and the physical therapist must determine if the patient being seen is eligible to also be seen by the physical therapist assistant. Remember, the physical therapist is responsible for the physical therapist assistant and patient management. The physical therapist must consider several aspects when delegating to the physical therapist assistant. The APTA *Code of Ethics for the Physical Therapist* states in Principle 5B that "physical therapists shall have primary responsibility for supervision of physical therapist assistants and support personnel."[5(p14)] This means that the physical therapist is responsible and culpable for the successes and mistakes a physical therapist assistant makes.

The state practice act for the state in which the physical therapist assistant is working will often dictate what he or she can do. These acts vary from state to state, so it is imperative that both the physical therapist and the physical therapist assistant are knowledgeable about what the state practice act includes. For example, in some states physical therapist assistants can perform sharp debridement of wounds; in other states, only physical therapists can perform this task. Additionally, the APTA and the Commission on Accreditation in Physical Therapy Education (CAPTE) have certain perspectives on what a physical therapist assistant can or cannot do. The APTA, for example, states in Procedural Interventions Exclusively Performed by Physical Therapists that only physical therapists should perform interventions that require "immediate and continuous examination and evaluation throughout the intervention," including spinal and peripheral joint mobilizations and sharp selective debridement of wounds.[6(p2)]

Clarkson College Outpatient Physical Therapy Clinic

Initial Evaluation and Treatment Plan- Ankle/Foot Evaluation

DOB: 10/17/1996
Ht: 6'3", Wt: 205

Date of Eval: 4/1/2018   Date of Onset: March 2018

Diagnosis: (L) ankle instability

History/Mechanism of Injury: pt is a 21 y.o. collegiate b-ball player with onset (L) ankle pain. pt states he has had multiple (L) sprained ankles over course of career, one so significant it was a season-ender. c/o unsteadiness while playing (wears lateral support brace) and then pain following activity. No pain or hx (R) ankle issues.

Psychosocial/Functional Deficits: pt feels he is unable to play b-ball 2° instability, unable to participate in off-season training. Worried about career impact.

PMH: (+) for (R) patellar tendonitis (resolved) 2016, hx (L) clavicle fx, hx (R) radial fracture (both as children). No other pertinent PMH.

Current Medications: ibuprofen (advil) prn for pain

Symptomology: Constant ____   Intermittent ✓   Variable ✓   Unchanging ____   Daily ✓

(↑) or ↓ symptoms with activities exercise, b-ball

Pain Pattern/Intensity (0-10 scale): Rest 5   Activity 6-7

Comments: ankle feels "loose" and occasionally "grindy" when playing. c/o "deep ache" in ankle following games/practice. Rest & ibuprofen help. pt does NOT like ice.

Observation/Inspection: no swelling/bruising noted. Visible dip inferior to (L) lat malleolus 2° ↓ ligamentous integrity.

Gait: (L) femoral IR @ HS, ↓(B) hip ext through TS, ↑ pronation (B), (L)>(R)

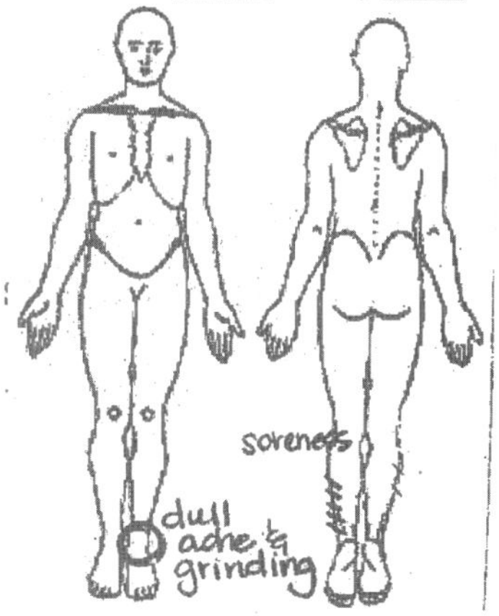

Proprioception/Somatosensory: (L) ankle hyposensitivity

SLS (R) 30", SLS (L) 14" prior to LOB (L) to recover from LOB), lumbar scan clear

+ = pain	AROM L	AROM R	PROM L	PROM R	Strength L	Strength R
Ankle DF	full	full	full	full	4+	4+
Ankle PF	AROM	AROM	PROM	PROM	5	5
Ankle INV	WNL	WNL	WNL	WNL	4-	4+
Ankle EVER					3+	4
Great Toe Flex					4+	4+
Great Toe Ext					4	4
Toe II-V Flex					4	4
Toe II-V Ext					4-	4-

Palpation: TTP to peroneal muscle bodies & post to (L) lat malleolus. TTP to plantar surface (L) foot including base 5th MT, (L) tibial tuberosity TTP & with OP into knee flexion.

Joint Play Assessment: (L) ankle severely hypermobile in all planes, (L) patellar hypomobility med/lat, (L) hip hypomobility w/ AP & OP, lumbar segmental mobility WNL.

Special Tests: (+)(L) TALAR TILT, (+)(L) ANTERIOR DRAWER, (+)(L) OBER'S, (+)(L) ELY'S w/ PAIN, (+) THOMAS TEST (B). JUMP MECHANICS: ↓ HIP EXT (B), ↑ IR & VALGUS WITH LANDING. (L) ANKLE LANDS IN SUPINATION FOLLOWED BY HYPER-PRONATION. 6 meter timed-hop test; (R) 6 sec, (L) 14 sec c̄ pain.

(diagram labels) soreness · dull ache & grinding

Figure 1-1. A sample evaluation. *(continued)*

HEP/Patient Education: educated pt on nature of diagnosis, causation and POC. Gave pt 4 way ankle ex c̄ RTB 3x10reps, 5x/wk. Intrinsic foot strengthening also prescribed at same rep/duration, frequency. Pt demos proper form & understanding of HEP.

ASSESSMENT: pt demonstrates s/s of chronic ankle instability on (L) c̄ (L) hip & knee biomechanical involvement (dysfunction). pt req. strengthening & stabilization to avoid Brostrom and return to peak athletic performance.
Problems/Physical Findings: ↓ (L) ankle stability, ↓ balance, generalized weakness, faulty joint mechanics, pain affecting functional mobility, altered resting muscle length

TREATMENT PLAN:
Patient will be seen __3__ x/wk for __8__ wks or __24__ visits for therapeutic exercise, neuro re-ed, gait/stair training, therapeutic activities, manual therapy, pt/caregiver education, and modalities prn.

GOALS		BY
1.)	pt will ↑ (L) SLS to 30 sec c̄ EC to ↑ (I) c̄ SLS activity and demo ↑ proprioceptive capacity.	4 wks
2.)	pt will ↑ (L) ankle strength (DF, inv, ev) to 5/5 to ↑ power c̄ sport related activity.	6 wks
3.)	pt will be (I) c̄ HEP.	1 wk (ongoing)
4.)	pt will ↓ pain complaints following activity to no more than 1/10.	8 wks
5.)	pt will ↓ 6m hop test to be equal to unaffected limb for ↑ sport performance.	8 wks

Barriers to achieving treatment goals? ☐ Yes ☑ No (potentially too aggressive c̄ progress)
Family/patient involved in and verbalized understanding of goals? ☑ Yes ☐ No _____
Patient was instructed in ankle/foot model as it pertains to the injury? ☑ Yes ☐ No _____

Clinician _____ PT, DPT

Figure 1-1 (continued). A sample evaluation.

The physical therapist assistant's education and experience also play a role in what the physical therapist will delegate. The physical therapist should be aware of what entry level means for the physical therapist assistant and should also consider where the physical therapist assistant has worked and what experience he or she has had. It would not be prudent, for example, for the physical therapist to delegate a patient that required myofascial release to a physical therapist assistant who has never performed this task before. Additionally, the physical therapist assistant bears some responsibility in this matter. The Standards of Ethical Conduct for the Physical Therapist Assistant states in Standard 3C that "physical therapist assistants shall make decisions based upon their level of competence and consistent with patient/client values."[5(p14)] This means that even if a physical therapist delegates a task to the physical therapist assistant, if the assistant does not feel comfortable or competent performing the task, he or she should communicate that to the physical therapist and not perform the task.

Finally, payer regulations related to physical therapist assistants may influence whether a patient will be delegated to a physical therapist assistant. Unfortunately, some payers have specific requirements regarding supervision, and some pay less or nothing for physical therapist assistant interventions.[7] Until recently, TRICARE, the health insurance affiliated with the US Department of Defense, did not recognize physical therapist assistants as TRICARE-authorized providers, meaning TRICARE would not pay for their services.[8] Only recently (as of November 2017) did verbiage in legislation change to potentially agree to cover physical therapist assistants. That bill is currently awaiting the President's signature, but the change would allow physical therapist assistants and certified occupational therapy assistants to treat TRICARE patients and be reimbursed.[9] Prior to that, a claim submitted for a physical therapist assistant's intervention could, in fact, be penalized under the False Claims Act.[8]

How Does a Physical Therapist Assistant Make Modifications Within the Plan of Care?

As mentioned earlier, the physical therapist assistant is often the person who sees the patient the most. This means the physical therapist assistant is sometimes the best person to recognize changes in the patient's status. A patient may respond well to the interventions provided; he or she does all the exercises and excels. The patient is able to complete many of the tasks with ease. How does the physical therapist assistant address this? The first thing to remember is that the physical therapist assistant cannot change the POC. If the goal is for the patient to walk 100 feet with a walker standby assist and the patient achieves this goal, the physical therapist assistant cannot make a new goal for the patient to walk 200 feet with the walker modified independent.

However, the physical therapist assistant can speak with the supervising physical therapist, notifying him or her of the goal achievement, and the physical therapist can change the POC. However, that does not mean that the physical therapist assistant does not have some autonomy within the POC to make adjustments to treatments. The key is still communication, but changes within the POC are common. For example, there is a patient who is having a great deal of pain in her lower back, and the physical therapist wrote in the POC "Treat pain with modalities." This means that the physical therapist assistant may try a moist hot pack first, but if this is not helpful, the physical therapist assistant could try another modality, such as electrical stimulation, to address the pain. This is not making a change to the POC. The physical therapist assistant should still communicate with the supervising physical therapist that a different modality was begun. (Note: it would be a change if the supervising physical therapist wrote "Treat pain with moist hot pack." Then, the physical therapist assistant would need to get a change from the physical therapist in the POC to initiate electrical stimulation.)

Another example might be that the physical therapist wrote in the evaluation for the patient to receive therapeutic exercise for right knee weakness. The assistant starts the patient off with 3 sets of 10 repetitions with a 1-pound (lb) cuff weight performing leg extensions, hamstring curls, and seated marching. If the patient performs these with no trouble or improves quickly, the assistant can make changes to the types of exercises (make the patient stand and perform marches), to the resistance (increase cuff weight to 3 lbs), to the frequency (3 sets of 15 repetitions), or to all 3 areas. This is not changing the POC, but it does progress the patient. Again, it is still important to communicate with the supervising physical therapist that changes are being made. This allows the physical therapist to stay informed and will help him or her perform reevaluations or prepare patients for discharge.

In a similar vein, what should the physical therapist assistant do if he or she notices negative changes in the patient status? If the patient with lower back pain receives electrical stimulation for her pain but complains of discomfort while receiving the treatment, it is the assistant's responsibility to make changes to the treatment: decrease the intensity, change the location of the electrodes, or adjust the waveform of the stimulation. These are not changes to the POC, but they are changes that respond to the patient's feedback. Likewise, if the patient performing leg exercises complains of chest pain with increased exercise intensity, the assistant should stop therapy immediately and monitor the patient's vital signs while also alerting the nursing staff.

If a patient responds to an intervention in a seriously negative way, such as the previously mentioned chest pain example, the supervising physical therapist should be notified. Sometimes during treatment sessions there are true emergencies. A patient may suffer a heart attack, stroke, or seizure during therapy. The physical therapist assistant

Box 1-2

When to Contact the Supervising Physical Therapist

- Patient is not reaching goals.
- Patient has met established goals.
- Patient has a new medical status.
- Physical therapist assistant has questions/concerns with POC.
- Physical therapist needs to change/update the POC.
- Patient needs to be discharged.

should understand basic first aid procedures, know the signs and symptoms of common diseases, and be able to contact help immediately. If the therapist works in home health care, calling 911 is the best choice. If the patient is in the hospital already, pulling the staff emergency button or cord will get help to the patient quickly. More will be discussed Chapter 12 about emergencies. Also, the assistant may notice that yesterday the patient spoke clearly, was not confused, and was able to follow all directions, while today, he or she is very confused and agitated, unable to follow commands, and hard to understand. The physical therapist assistant would recognize that this patient has had a change in status, and before therapy is continued, nursing staff or the patient's physician should be contacted. The supervising physical therapist would also need to be notified. Box 1-2 includes a list of when a physical therapist assistant should contact the supervising physical therapist regarding patient care.

Co-Treating With Other Health Care Providers

Just as the physical therapist and the physical therapist assistant are a team, they are also teammates with other health care providers. Especially in acute care, inpatient rehabilitation, or skilled nursing settings, patients often receive care from a variety of providers, including occupational therapists, speech therapists, social workers, psychologists, nurses, and physicians. Each person plays a specific role, and a physical therapist assistant should understand those roles and be able to work with other professions to provide a well-rounded, consistent plan for recovery. Occupational therapists often work with patients on activities of daily living, such as dressing, hygiene, cooking, cleaning, or driving. They may also assist the patient with preparing to return to work. Speech-language pathologists, as the name implies, help patients with recovering and improving speech; however, they also assist with swallowing and memory or cognition. Care for patients is

often coordinated among the various therapists seeing the patient. Also, just as it is important to communicate with the supervising physical therapist regarding patient status and changes, so is it important to communicate these changes with the other therapists, nursing staff, and physicians. If a patient needs to be on a positioning schedule to avoid pressure injuries, the nursing staff need to know as much as the other therapists do, in order to be consistent with care across the team. Sometimes, a simple positioning sign posted in the patient's room and reinforcement via verbal communication is all that is needed. In other cases, the patient status change may be potentially life threatening. If a patient demonstrates a sudden or concerning change in blood pressure, for example, everyone on the team should be aware. If the physical therapist assistant is the one to observe this change, therapy is stopped, vitals are taken, and nursing staff are notified immediately. Following this, the rest of the therapy staff should be contacted; this will help avoid patient injury. Written documentation is necessary, but often a quick word with the patient's nurse and other therapists can be beneficial.

In some cases, co-treating with therapists is an effective, efficient, and sometimes necessary method to treat patients. If the patient has suffered a traumatic brain injury, for example, and is not fully conscious all the time, it will be necessary for multiple team members to treat the patient at the same time to effectively treat that patient. One can assist with bed mobility and sitting the patient upright, while the other can work on arousal and orientation. Each therapist can then work on his or her own POC agenda, but can do so in cooperation with the other therapist. Goals and outcomes can be achieved together, and there are 2 people to help treat and move the patient as needed.

Professional Considerations and Patient Care

There are several topics a physical therapist assistant should keep in mind when performing patient care, including aspects of confidentiality, consent, and professionalism. The following sections will discuss these topics in detail.

Professionalism

There was once a student in a Physical Therapist Assistant program who, by all accounts, performed well academically. She received high grades on her tests and papers, as well as her practical examinations. However, this student was chronically late or just barely on time for classes and labs. She was equally late for outside service and learning activities. Although this student received good grades, the negative impression she made upon her peers and instructors as a result of her tardiness affected the professional component of her grade. Additionally, the instructors called the student in for discussions regarding her lack of punctuality, explaining that this would not serve her well in her career. The therapy world is relatively small, and she did not want to gain a reputation that would cause her to not get or maintain a job after graduation. Neither would her lack of timeliness impress her future patients or other coworkers. This was a problem that needed to be addressed quickly.

In all aspects of your career as a therapist, you must consider and maintain professionalism. But what does that mean? The APTA has a link to the Values-Based Behaviors for the Physical Therapist Assistant document, which specifies that the physical therapist assistant should demonstrate altruism, caring and compassion, continuing competence, duty, integrity, physical therapist/physical therapist assistant collaboration, responsibility, and social responsibility.[10] This document is a follow-up to the document created for physical therapists (The Professionalism in Physical Therapy: Core Values document to reflect the *Vision 2020 Strategic Plan*).[10]

The document lists examples of how a physical therapist assistant can demonstrate each quality. For example, altruism can be reflected in creating patient-centered interventions, offering to assist the physical therapist, providing enough time to meet the patient's needs, and placing the patient's needs ahead of one's own. Caring and compassion are demonstrated through listening to the patient actively; demonstrating respect for others; considering all aspects of a patient's situation, including social, emotional, cultural, or environmental influences; and refraining from acting on one's own biases. Continuing competence means that the physical therapist assistant is pursuing lifelong learning, documenting such learning via self-assessment, and attending continuing education courses. Duty is described as the "commitment to meeting one's obligations to provide effective physical therapy services," as well as to serve the profession.[10(p4)] Examples of integrity include adhering to the physical therapist assistant scope of practice and billing practices, as well as demonstrating honesty and ethical behavior. The document defines physical therapist/physical therapist assistant collaboration as the physical therapist/physical therapist assistant team working together, including educating the physical therapist on the roles and responsibilities of the physical therapist assistant, promoting a positive working relationship with the physical therapist, and seeking opportunities to collaborate with the physical therapist. Finally, responsibility and social responsibility reflect the need for the physical therapist assistant to accept his or her role and obligations as a physical therapist assistant; to communicate with patients, family members, and the physical therapist; to advocate for patients' needs in the clinic; to promote healthy lifestyles; and to advocate for changes in laws and regulations that positively affect physical therapy.[10] While this document and its lists are not exhaustive, the goal is to ensure the physical therapist assistant has a series of guidelines to facilitate professional and ethical behaviors in the clinic.

Everyone has his or her own ideas of what professionalism might entail, including everything from how a person dresses or styles his or her hair, to how to address each other in the classroom or clinic, to our involvement and interactions with the community and professional associations. The term *profession* can describe both an occupation and the standards and codes by which practice is evaluated.[11] Professionalism is being taught and graded in the classroom; many professions have integrated professionalism as an accreditation standard, including CAPTE.[11] This may mean that a student can be graded on dress, hair color, or tattoos, as well as how they address instructors (eg, Mrs. So-and-so instead of Jenny) and whether they attend professional meetings or continuing education courses. Additionally, the Clinical Performance Instrument, which is the tool clinical instructors use to grade students on clinical rotations, provides an area to assess students on professionalism. Regardless of how it is defined, professionalism will be a topic discussed both in the classroom and the clinic, and it is important in how people convey themselves as representatives of the profession. Being a professional in every sense of the word often influences patient rapport and employment, so it is worth consideration well beyond the graded classroom or clinical rotation experience.

Health Insurance Portability and Accountability Act

The HIPAA of 1996 can be found at www.hhs.gov/hipaa. The HIPAA is a set of federal standards aimed to protect the privacy of patients' medical records and other health information. It also provides patients with access to their medical records. Covered entities include health care providers, such as doctors, clinics, dentists, nursing homes, and pharmacies; health plans, including health insurance companies, health maintenance organizations, and government programs such as Medicare/Medicaid; and entities that process nonstandard health information they receive from other entities, such as electronic data, including those that help doctors get paid, companies that administer health plans, lawyers, IT specialists, and companies that store and destroy medical records. This law stipulates that covered entities must place safeguards that protect health information and ensure the prevention of disclosure. They must also limit use and disclosure of health information to that which is necessary (a need-to-know basis), and they must have procedures in place to limit who can see and access health information.

If a violation is made, a patient can file a complaint to the Office for Civil Rights (OCR). Once the complaint is received, the OCR will notify the person who filed the complaint and the person/entity named in the complaint. The complainant and the covered entity will be required to present information about the incident in question. The OCR reviews the information and may refer the case to the Department of Justice or may determine there was no violation. If there was a violation, the OCR takes measures to resolve the case via voluntary compliance from the entity, corrective action, and/or resolution agreement.[12] In this world of electronic medical charts, it has become increasingly difficult for hospitals and companies to protect patient information. It is important for you to be aware of your facility's or employers HIPAA safeguards and to follow these carefully to avoid unnecessary disclosure of patient information.

Your role with the HIPAA comes in the form of not talking about patients in public areas, using specific and private information, to people who do not need to know the information. Health information should be disseminated only on a need-to-know basis; talking with a patient's nurse or physician or with your supervising physical therapist about the patient is appropriate. For example, a patient's neighbor comes to visit him or her in the hospital. Outside the patient's room, the neighbor asks about the patient's prognosis. The neighbor may think he or she needs to know this information, but he or she does not. You should direct the neighbor to ask the patient because you cannot share that information. Let's also imagine you are in an elevator talking with your friend who is a nurse. You both have been working with a patient, so talking about his or her status with each other is not a problem. However, talking about the patient's status to each other in a full elevator is a problem. The other people in that elevator do not need to know that patient's information.

The key is to try speaking with only those who need to know the information and to do so in a private area. If you are documenting, make sure your notes are closed down or put away once you finish and you do not leave patient papers out in the open for anyone to read or inspect. Employers take the HIPAA very seriously, and you will be trained on HIPAA regulations at every clinical location, as well as every employer you go to for the rest of your career. Follow the rules, and you will be okay.

Documentation

The purposes of documentation are to allow for accurate replication of a treatment session, to reflect the patient's progress or lack of it, to protect the therapist in case of patient complaint or injury, and to provide necessary information to payer sources to allow for proper and fast payment. An article in *PT in Motion* detailed what a payer source wants to see in a physical therapy note, including the patient diagnosis, the POC, and goals.[13] These goals include the patient's prognosis, the skilled care provided by the physical therapist or physical therapist assistant, what measurable progress was made, what the outcomes of therapy were, and what was the patient status as of discharge.[13]

The classic framework for documentation is a SOAP note, which is an acronym for Subjective, Objective, Assessment, and Plan. The SOAP note is a type of problem-oriented medical record, developed by Lawrence Weed in the 1960s.[14] Many facilities and clinics have migrated to electronic data collection and documentation, which do not necessarily come in the form of a SOAP note; however, the SOAP note components are still present in electronic documentation, and the acronym still allows for complete documentation of the patient intervention. The APTA offers a Defensible Documentation guideline, which includes a list of basic elements that should be included in all documentation; this is very handy for students and clinicians.[15]

In the case of electronic documentation, the software is a great time-saving tool; however, some patients are more complex than the standard electronic form allows. Often these electronic tools still offer a free-writing space to write a detailed narrative of the patient scenario and care. It is worth noting that with the advent of electronic documentation, point of service (POS) documentation has become popular. This is a method for employers to get better productivity from their therapists, and it requires the therapist to document about the patient during the therapy session. The facility may provide the therapist with an iPad or laptop that is portable and easily available. The challenge is to thoroughly document while also being present and available for the patient during treatment time; some patients and therapists have complained that POS documentation makes the therapist more distracted during the therapy session.

Therapists should strive to document (or finish documentation) as soon as possible after the patient intervention. With POS documentation, most if not all of the documentation may be done at the time of intervention. In some outpatient clinics, documentation is done orally through a dictation service, and this is done at the end of the work day.

Each component of a SOAP note represents different information. Whether you are writing a true SOAP note or including the information into an electronic form, the type of information that correlates to each section does not change. Box 1-3 includes a list of SOAP note components broken down by section.

The S in SOAP stands for Subjective, and this reflects anything the patient reports or that the therapist is told by health care staff or that is read from the chart. This includes the patient history, patient complaints of pain or reports of nausea/vomiting, ambulation, degree of difficulty with tasks, or medicines administered.

The O stands for Objective, and this includes anything the therapist witnessed or performed during the therapy session, such as how far the patient ambulated and level of assist; patient behaviors, such as agitation, confusion, compliance, or facial expressions; wounds noted and affiliated measurements; and exercises performed with number of repetitions and sets. Any additional data collected, such as manual muscle testing, goniometric measurements, pain scales, or sensory testing, would be included in this section.

Box 1-3
SOAP Note Components

- S: Subjective data, or information gained through direct conversing with the patient or the patient's caregivers. Includes the patient's pain rating, the patient's perceptions (eg, "I'm feeling less stiff today"), the patient's functional abilities (eg, the patient reports he or she is able to walk the dog now), the patient's reported cognitive or emotional status, the patient's informed consent, the patient's response to interventions, any new patient problems or complaints, and any other relevant information (eg, medical history or home situation).

- O: Objective data, or information obtained through measurements and testing, as well as interventions conducted. Includes patient education, interventions (eg, transfers or exercises), data collected (eg, manual muscle testing or range of motion), description of the patient's functioning (eg, levels of assist required), and any other observable information (eg, wounds or shortness of breath).

- A: Assessment, or the place to indicate the patient's change in status as a result of interventions provided. Changes in pain, range of motion, muscle strength, levels of assist required, or functional abilities are noted here. This information should directly relate to data provided in the Subjective and Objective sections. Here is also the place to note progress toward short- and long-term goals.

- P: Plan. Here the intention for future sessions is documented. This includes communication with the patient or caregivers, including home exercise instructions, as well as any communication planned with the physical therapist or other health care providers. Additionally, this section includes specific plans for the next session, such as "will continue LE exercises for strengthening," and can also include modifications to the plan, such as "will increase reps to 12x next session."

The *A* stands for Assessment, and although we are careful to distinguish assessment from evaluation, as the physical therapist assistant cannot evaluate a patient, the physical therapist assistant is always assessing the patient and collecting data to report back to the physical therapist. Any objective data collected (and noted in the Objective section) can be assessed here. If the patient's pain decreased, include that in the Assessment section; if his or her strength increased, note that here. In this way the therapist highlights any patient changes, either of improvement or lack of it. Assistants should connect progress or lack of it to the physical therapist's POC and short- or long-term goals. If the patient is making progress toward goals or has met goals, the therapist can denote that here; likewise, if the patient status has declined, the therapist can indicate that as well.

The *P* stands for Plan and indicates what the therapist intends to work on for the next session. Some therapists get into the habit of writing "continue with plan of care" in this section, but health care payer sources are becoming increasingly specific about wanting more detailed information. If the intention is to increase repetitions, to change the wound care dressing, or to speak with the supervising physical therapist about updating goals, this should be specifically indicated in the Plan section.

Patient Identification and Informed Consent

In health care it is important to gain the patient's consent to treat. Typically, upon entering the patient's room or meeting the patient, the therapist will introduce him- or herself, confirm that the patient is who the therapist is supposed to treat, and ask the patient for consent to treat at that time. Confirmation of patient identity can be done by asking the patient's name, checking his or her identification (ID) bracelet, asking for date of birth, or checking the medical ID number; it is best practice to check 2 forms of ID. A therapist can also confirm diagnosis to confirm identity. It is important to ensure the correct patient is being treated, and it is easier than one would think to grab the wrong person. For example, imagine a physical therapist assistant entered a patient's room that was shared with another person. The physical therapist assistant asked the patient, "are you Mrs. Smith?" and the patient nodded. Off they went to the therapy gym, and the patient received 30 minutes of therapy. Only at the close of the intervention did the physical therapist assistant realize that he or she had the wrong patient, and the patient he or she had worked with had been too confused to answer such a leading question correctly. No harm had been done in this situation; however, if the physical therapist assistant had checked the patient's identity in a more thorough manner, the mistake likely would not have been made.

Informed consent also implies that the therapist educated the patient beforehand about the intended treatment, checked for precautions or contraindications for the treatment, and allowed the patient to ask questions about the planned interventions. The World Confederation of Physical Therapy's Declaration of Principle on Informed Consent states that "a competent adult" should be provided information about the proposed or planned treatment, the risks associated with the treatment, the benefits of the treatment, the time frame of the intervention, the costs of the treatment, and the alternatives to the proposed treatment.[16(p38)] Informed consent is communication

Box 1-4

Protocol for Gaining Patient Consent

- Introduce yourself and title/profession (if you are a student, identify this also and your school).
- Verify who you are treating (using at least 2 patient identifiers such as name, date of birth, medical ID number).
- Speak with the patient about current status or to gain relevant information.
- Educate patient on intended interventions and goals for the day.
- Gain permission to perform said interventions (can be written or oral).

between the therapist and the patient, establishing trust and allowing the patient to be autonomous in his or her health care decisions. Informed consent should be considered both a legal and ethical form of communication, and should be documented with every session. This both establishes the trust relationship between therapist and patient, and it also protects the therapist from legal action should the patient register a complaint or file a lawsuit. Lawson et al[17(p269)] asserted that "proceeding with treatment [without informed consent] constitutes a battery or non-consensual touching," so it is important to gain informed consent. Box 1-4 includes protocol for gaining consent.

Communication

It has already been discussed that the physical therapist assistant is a member of a team and that communication within that team is essential for effective and consistent care. It is equally important to practice effective communication with patients and their families or support systems, which is not always easy. Some patients have cognitive deficits or difficulty with arousal or attention. Some patients do not speak English, are deaf, hard of hearing, are unable to speak, or are visually impaired. Some patients come from cultures or ethnicities that present challenges to typical health care interventions. Some patients come with family members with whom the therapist must also communicate and interact. Some patients will say their pain is a 2/10 on the pain scale, yet their facial expressions are telling you that the pain is worse than that; some will say their pain is a 10/10 while calmly sipping a cup of coffee. These all can be challenges to quality or effective communication.

As a therapist, you are interacting with your patient not just as a diagnosis, but as a whole person. You must be a good listener and pay attention to nonverbal communication as much as what the patient says. The more your patient sees you as an involved, attentive therapist, the better your therapy sessions will progress. If you note a

communication barrier, you must determine how to work around it. Is the patient a visual learner? Perhaps a chart or diagram will better educate that person about his or her home exercise program. Try to avoid using medical terms such as *flex* (use *bend* instead) or *CVA* (refer to it as a *stroke*). Use concise directions and phrases, like "stand up" or "bend your knee" rather than "First we're going to work on standing from your chair." If the patient has cognitive deficits, to-the-point and step-by-step directions will work better than trying to describe the entire therapy plan in one breath. This also includes written as well as verbal directions. Encourage patients to bring in a family member or friend to help with at-home instructions or activities. If providing a written home exercise program, ensure your language is equally as clear and nonmedical. You will also need to make sure that the patient understands and can perform the home exercise plan prior to the patient leaving the facility; have the patient demonstrate reading and following the directions you provide and make adjustments if necessary. If a caregiver is assisting with the exercises, make sure he or she is also participating in the education.

If the patient is deaf or speaks another language, there are language boards, dry-erase boards, and interpreters to improve communication; if the patient speaks another language, there are also translator programs that facilities can use, as well as communication boards that use pictures rather than words (such as the Wong-Baker Faces Pain Rating Scale). Figure 1-2 shows examples of different communication methods. If the patient is from a culture that frowns on women being alone with men or that has stipulations about a woman's state of undress, see if there is a private treatment room available or if a therapist of the same sex can treat the patient. It is important that you practice cultural competence, as language may not be the only barrier. Box 1-5 offers definitions regarding cultural awareness.

In some cases, the environment can also affect communication. Perhaps you are treating a patient in a busy, noisy therapy gym. If the patient cannot hear you or is easily distracted, it might be better to move to a private treatment area to facilitate better communication.

Monitor the patient's response and make changes to the communication method used if the patient does not seem to understand. After explaining a procedure or plan, asking the patient "do you understand?" is not sufficient, because patients will often indicate that they do understand even if they do not. Instead, ask the patient to demonstrate or teach back the skills you are covering. Many educators and therapists promote the system of first telling the patient what you want him or her to do, then showing the patient what you want him or her to do, and finally having the patient demonstrate what you want him or her to do. This ensures that the patient has understood what is being taught and has a better chance of accurately repeating the skills at home. Encourage the patient to repeat the skills more than once, as repetition enhances learning.

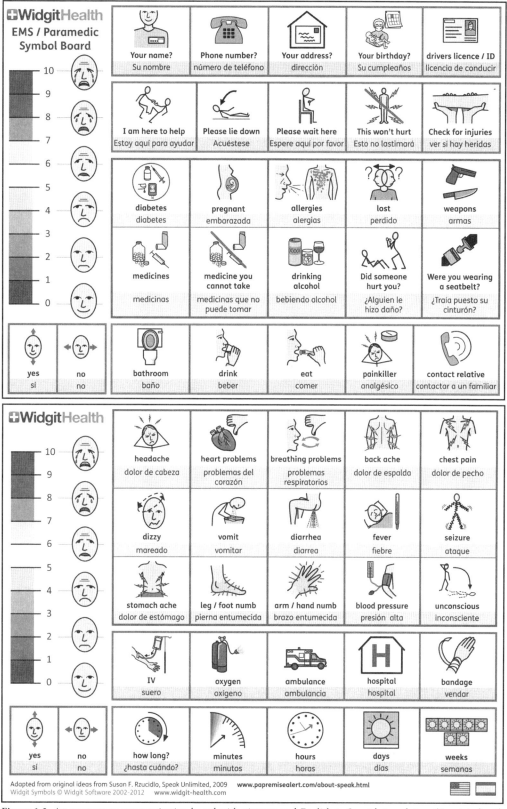

Figure 1-2. An emergency communication board with pictures and English to Spanish translation. (Reprinted with permission from Widgit Software.)

Box 1-5
Cultural Awareness Terms

- Culture: shared values, norms, traditions, art, history, and institutions of a group of people
- Cultural competence: skills that allow individuals to appreciate and understand cultural differences and similarities
- Cultural diversity: differences in race, ethnicity, language, nationality, and religion among groups within a community
- Cultural sensitivity: awareness of one's own and others' cultures
- Culturally appropriate: ability to demonstrate sensitivity to cultural differences and similarities in communication
- Ethnic: belonging to a common group often connected by race, nationality, and language with a common heritage
- Race: population defined by physical characteristics that are genetically transmitted

Box 1-7
Good Communication Skills

- Provide clear, direct instructions (written or verbal).
- Use touch in a therapeutic, directive, or guiding manner.
- Use language the patient can understand (layperson's terms vs medical terms).
- Listen actively to the patient, and observe facial expressions, gestures, or posture.
- Ensure the patient understands instructions by having the patient teach back or demonstrate the skills.
- Reduce or eliminate environmental distractions, such as noise and lights.
- Accommodate if patient has a language barrier.

Box 1-6
Examples of Nonverbal Communication

- Appearance: dress, cleanliness
- Pantomime: demonstrating the activity
- Posture: slouching, rigid, arms crossed
- Gestures: using hands or arms; thumbs up or OK sign
- Facial expressions: smiling, grimacing, frowning
- Touch: hold hands, pat on the back

A patient may say one thing and then communicate another with his or her nonverbal expressions. Let's say you are performing passive range of motion on a patient's hip. If you ask the patient "how does that feel?" he or she may report that it is not painful; however, you note that every time you reach the end range, his or her face contorts into a grimace. What the patient says does not match what his or her face reports. As a therapist, your job is to pay attention to these nonverbal expressions, so you can adjust your treatment session accordingly. You must speak to your patient and look at his or her body language to get the whole story. Explain that "no pain, no gain" is not the goal in therapy and that he or she must be honest with you to achieve the best outcomes.

The therapist's nonverbal messages are also important. Box 1-6 includes examples on nonverbal communication. Consider facial expressions; a smile or thumbs-up conveys a great deal even if the person does not otherwise understand. Avoid grimacing or showing negative facial or postural gestures.

A therapist's touch can convey much when verbal communication fails. A pat on the back or a squeeze of the hand can demonstrate care and encouragement. It is important to avoid potentially improper or misinterpreted gestures or touches. Be careful to avoid touching areas considered sexualized, such as buttocks, upper thighs, or breast tissue, unless the intervention calls for it, and then communicate clearly with the patient what is being done and why before he or she is touched. Be aware of patient modesty and drape all sensitive areas or use a private treatment room to additionally make the patient comfortable.

Give patients time to speak and answer questions, and listen carefully while also paying attention to nonverbal communication. Doing so will increase the rapport between the therapist and the patient and will make for easier interactions. Some patients who have had a stroke find it difficult to verbalize what they want to say quickly. These patients also may have delayed responses to the directions you provide. Be patient and wait to let the person first process what you have said and then to formulate his or her response. Box 1-7 includes a list of how to be an effective communicator with your patients.

International Classification of Functioning, Disability and Health

The *International Classification of Functioning, Disability and Health* (ICF) was created by the World Health Organization, and its goal is for physical therapy to minimize the effects of disability while maximizing a patient's function.[18] Prior to the ICF, there was the Nagi

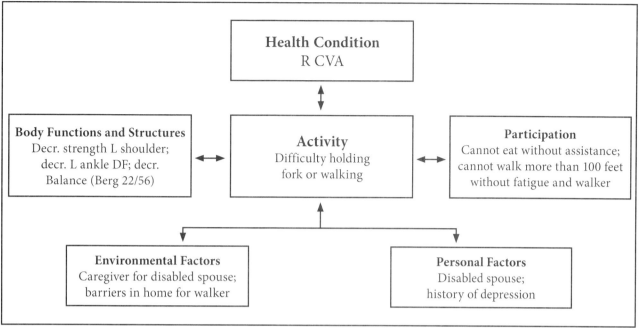

Figure 1-3. The World Health Organization's ICF model applied to the specific diagnosis of an R CVA.

Disablement Model from the 1960s, which used terms like *pathology, impairment, functional limitation*, and *disability*. Whereas Nagi spoke of disability in terms of when health ended, the ICF attempts to focus on health and function rather than dysfunction. Additionally, the ICF attempts to acknowledge that 2 persons with the same pathology can and often do have very different outcomes. The World Health Organization stated they wanted to measure function and use the model as a tool. The ICF uses terms like *health condition* (instead of pathology), *body functions* and *structure* (instead of impairment), *participation* (instead of disability), and *activity* (instead of functional limitation), and the ICF also takes into consideration environmental and personal factors and the roles these play in a person's health (which the Nagi model does not do). The ultimate goal of the ICF is to assist with planning and communication across the government and other sectors, to provide common language and terms, to give an organized data structure, and to serve multiple purposes.[18] Tempest and Jefferson[19] discussed several ways to use the model in rehabilitation, including as a means of goal setting, as a common language in notes, and as a guide for clinical decision making. Research is still ongoing on how best to utilize the ICF, though common consensus is that the model is a stronger way of looking at health and function. The APTA endorsed the ICF model in 2008, citing that the model allows physical therapists to "more accurately record and consider the many factors that contribute to a patient's treatment and recovery."[20] APTA's intention was to incorporate the language of the ICF into all publications and documents. This shows that the ICF model will become an integral part of clinical practice. This textbook attempts

to frame discussions of various diagnoses and outcomes within the context of the ICF model. Figure 1-3 shows the ICF model applied to a specific diagnosis.

Evidence-Based Practice

It has always been important to keep up with the latest research in order to provide the best and most up-to-date interventions in physical therapy. It has become increasingly important, however, to provide evidence-based practice, and both educators and practicing clinicians focus more on this in school and the clinic. Condon et al[21] provided the following 5 steps to best adhere to scientific evidence:
1. Create questions to ask about the intervention
2. Track down evidence to answer those questions
3. Appraise the evidence
4. Apply the evidence to patient treatment
5. Evaluate the effectiveness of steps 1 through 4 and review patient outcomes

Some clinicians and educators also use or endorse the creation of a PICO, which stands for Patient (the patient population involved), Intervention (an intervention used), Comparison (a comparative intervention), and Outcome (the outcome of each). A PICO helps a practitioner create clinical questions and also to attempt to answer or research those questions.

The EBRO classification system was created by the Dutch Cochrane Center and the Dutch Institute for Healthcare Improvement. The classification of study results and recommendations are according to the level of evidence. The basis for this classification came from EBRO recommendations, grading evidence from A1, which includes meta-

Table 1-1
EBRO Recommendations

A1	Meta-analyses (systematic reviews), which include at least some, randomized clinical trials at quality level A2 that show consistent results between studies
A2	Randomized clinical trials of a good methodological quality (randomized, double-blind, and controlled studies) with sufficient power and consistency
B	Randomized clinical trials of a moderate methodological quality or with insufficient power, or other nonrandomized, cohort or patient-control group study designs that involve intergroup comparisons
C	Patient series
D	Expert opinion

Table 1-2
EBRO Practice Recommendations

1	Supported by one systematic review at quality level A1 or at least two independent trials at quality level A2
2	Supported by at least two independent trials at quality level B
3	Supported by one trial at quality level A2 or B, or research at quality level C
4	Based on the expert opinion (eg, of working group members)

analyses and some randomized clinical trials, to D, which includes expert opinion. The practice recommendations that resulted are scored from 1 to 4, with 1 being that the practice is supported by one systematic review at level A1 or two trials at A2, and 4 being the practice is supported by expert opinion. Tables 1-1 and 1-2 provide the evidence and practice recommendation classifications.

Condon et al[21] indicated that utilizing evidence-based practice was difficult, and they compared it to learning a skill, like manual therapy. The study showed that many therapists do not utilize evidence-based practice. Instead, they showed that therapists use peers and social groups to gather information.[21] The University of North Carolina Health Sciences Library (Chapel Hill, North Carolina) includes a hierarchy of evidence, ranked from most reliable to least. Highest on the pyramid are meta-analyses or systematic reviews; lowest on the pyramid include surveys and case studies.[22] One might also include peers and traditions in that lowest of categories. It is advisable, then, to utilize evidence in meta-analyses and systematic reviews rather than rely only on the information gathered from clinical instructors, supervising physical therapists, and seasoned physical therapist assistants. Evidence-based practice has a good reputation and is generally associated with better patient outcomes. Although it may be more time consum-

ing, therapists should spend the effort keeping up with the most recent research as it applies to their interventions, especially studies with good reliability and validity. Health care is always changing, which means that new studies are being done all the time that either support or invalidate certain treatments. Reliability in a study means that the way by which a treatment is measured is dependable and can be replicated. A valid study means that the tests or measures are actually measuring what they say they will. Furthermore, new techniques or machines are coming out all the time, and they must be vetted before being accepted.

The APTA website offers clinical summaries for therapists, which synthesize evidence on how to treat or manage specific conditions/diagnoses. For example, patients at high risk for falls (specifically "community-dwelling elders") are recommended to have gait training and correction of environmental hazards, based on Level 1 evidence.[23] Specifically, dual-task training or dynamic gait training is recommended.[23] The summary includes recommendations for evaluations, tests and measures, interventions, as well as medical management. Physical therapists and physical therapist assistants can both benefit from reviewing these summaries to ensure they are providing the best (and most supported by evidence) treatments to their patients.

REVIEW QUESTIONS

1. How can a physical therapist assistant make changes to a patient's treatment without changing the POC?

2. What does the HIPAA state in relation to patient information?

3. When should a physical therapist assistant communicate with his or her supervising physical therapist or other health care staff? Give specific examples.

4. Why is documentation so important?

5. What is documented in the Assessment section of a SOAP note?

6. What does informed consent mean? Why is it important?

7. Find an evidence-based article that supports (or does not support) a therapeutic treatment. What is it about this article that makes it evidence based and how can that be useful to the field?

8. Name 3 ways to improve communication with a patient.

9. Think of a time you worked with someone who was not professional. What are some specific things that person said or did that made you view him or her as unprofessional? How could he or she have been more professional?

REFERENCES

1. Mathews H, Smith S, Hussey J, Plack M. Investigation of the Preferred PT-PTA Relationship in 2:2 Clinical Education Model. *J Phys Ther Educ.* 2010;24(3):50-61.

2. Role of a physical therapist assistant (PTA). *APTA.* http://www.apta.org/PTACareers/RoleofaPTA/. Updated 2018. Accessed August 22, 2018.

3. Role of a physical therapist (PT). *APTA.* http://www.apta.org/PTCareers/RoleofaPT/. Updated 2018. Accessed August 22, 2018.

4. Physical therapist examination and evaluation: focus on tests and measures. *Guide to Physical Therapist Practice. APTA.* http://guidetoptpractice.apta.org/content/1/SEC4.extract. Published 2014. Accessed August 22, 2018.

5. Kirsch NR. A delegate balance (ethics in practice). *PT in Motion.* 2016;8(6):12-15.

6. Physical therapists and direction of mobilization/manipulation: an educational resource paper. *APTA.* https://www.apta.org/StateIssues/Manipulation/PTsDirectionofMobilizationManipulation/. Published September 2013. Accessed August 22, 2018.

7. The physical therapist-physical therapist assistant team: a tool kit. *APTA.* http://www.apta.org/PTPTATeamToolkit/. Published 2014. Accessed August 23, 2018.

8. Levin K. TRICARE: The US military's health care program. *PT in Motion.* 2017;8(11):6-8.

9. Bill allowing PTAs in TRICARE ready for President's signature. *PT in Motion News.* 2017. http://www.apta.org/PTinMotion/News/2017/11/17/TRICAREPassesHouseAndSenate/. Published November 17, 2017. Accessed August 23, 2018.

10. Values-based behaviors for the physical therapist assistant. *APTA.* www.apta.org/ValuesBasedBehaviors/. Published January 2011. Updated January 2018. Accessed August 23, 2018.

11. McGinnis P, Guenther LA, Wainwright S. Development and integration of professional core values among practicing clinicians. *Phys Ther.* 2016;96(9):1417-1429.

12. How OCR enforces the HIPAA privacy & security rules. *US Department of Health and Human Services.* https://www.hhs.gov/hipaa/for-professionals/compliance-enforcement/examples/how-OCR-enforces-the-HIPAA-privacy-and-security-rules/index.html. Updated June 7, 2017. Accessed August 23, 2018.

13. Evans W. The keys to effective documentation. *PT in Motion.* 2016;8(7):8-12.

14. Grimes W. Dr. Lawrence Weed, pioneer in recording patient data, dies at 93. *New York Times.* June 21, 2017:B16. https://www.nytimes.com/2017/06/21/science/obituary-lawrence-weed-dead-patient-information.html. Accessed August 23, 2018.

15. Defensible documentation for patient/client management. *APTA.* http://www.apta.org/Documentation/DefensibleDocumentation/ChecklistSample/. Updated 2017. Accessed August 23, 2018.

16. Bennett J. Informed consent: tips and caveats for PTs. *PT: Magazine of Physical Therapy.* 2007;15(12):38-40.

17. Lawson D, Revelino K, Owen D. Clinical pathways to improve patient outcomes. *Physical Therapy Review.* 2006;11(4):269-272.

18. World Health Organization. How to use the ICF: A practical manual for using the *International Classification of Functioning, Disability and Health* (ICF). *World Health Organization.* http://www.who.int/classifications/draft-icfpracticalmanual2.pdf?ua=1. Published October 2013. Accessed August 23, 2018.

19. Tempest S, Jefferson R. Engaging with clinicians to implement and evaluate the ICF in neurorehabilitation practice. *NeuroRehabilitation.* 2015;36(1):11-15. Doi: 10.3233/NRE-141185.

20. ATPA endorses World Health Organization ICF Model. *APTA.* http://www.apta.org/Media/Releases/APTA/2008/7/8/. Updated August 13, 2012. Accessed August 23, 2018.

21. Condon C, McGrane N, Mockler D, Stokes E. Ability of physiotherapists to undertake evidence-based practice steps: a scoping review. *Physiotherapy.* 2016;102(1):10-19.

22. Evidence based physical therapy. *UNC Health Sciences Library.* http://guides.lib.unc.edu/ebpt-home/ebpt-5steps. Updated July 27, 2018. Accessed August 23, 2018.

23. Hartley G, Kirk-Sanchez N. Fall Risk in Community-Dwelling Elders. *PT Now.* http://ptnow.org/clinical-summaries-detail/fall-risk-in-communitydwelling-elders#Intervention. Published January 1, 2013. Updated June 22, 2017. Accessed August 23, 2018.

Chapter 2

Body Mechanics

KEY TERMS Body mechanics | Ergonomics | Flat back | Friction | Frontal plane | Genu recurvatum | Genu valgum | Genu varum | Gravity | Kyphosis | Kyphosis-lordosis | Lordosis | Pelvic tilt | Pes planus | Sagittal plane | Scoliosis | Sway back

KEY ABBREVIATIONS BOS | COG | MHP | VGL

CHAPTER OBJECTIVES

1. Describe the proper body mechanics for pushing, pulling, reaching, lifting, and carrying objects.
2. Demonstrate proper body mechanics and posture with patient care.
3. Explain the rationale for good body mechanics and posture.
4. Discern good from bad posture, and understand how posture connects to pain.
5. Teach another how to maintain proper body mechanics or posture.

INTRODUCTION

Have you ever closely looked at the spine on a skeleton? What do you notice? Although people may think of it like a straight beam in a house, the spine is actually curved, and for good reason. These curves are best observed from the sagittal plane. Why is the spine curved? The spine can withstand 10 times more forces with curves than if it were straight, and the spine is more flexible with curvatures. These curves, and the maintenance of them while performing daily tasks (both professional and otherwise), will allow you to be safe as a physical therapist assistant and will help you educate your patients to avoid injury also.

As you learn about how to be a physical therapist assistant, the 2 things that will thread through all interventions and activities you do are proper body mechanics and posture. You will learn about these topics early on in your education, and they are extremely important in both what you educate your patient about and how you protect yourself. In all areas of physical therapy, it is essential that you demonstrate proper body mechanics. You will be educating your patients on body mechanics, but keep in mind that you are a role model for your patients as well. They will be watching what you do and how you do it, so you must practice what you preach.

You must also keep your own safety in mind. Repeatedly lifting, carrying, transferring, or moving people or items while using incorrect the body mechanics will eventually injure you, causing you to miss work and possibly need surgery or therapy interventions yourself. Holder et al[1] conducted a study of occupational injuries in physical therapists and physical therapist assistants and found that both complained of muscle strains (69% and 78% respectively) within the first 4 years of practice. Furthermore, these complaints were connected to transferring patients or responding to unanticipated or sudden movements by patients (such as falls). Almost half of these injuries resulted in the therapist seeking medical attention from physicians, and one-quarter of those injuries resulted in the therapist missing work. Lorenz et al[2] reported that the risk of injury

Memolo J.
Procedures and Patient Care for the Physical Therapist Assistant
(pp 17-30). © 2019 SLACK Incorporated.

Box 2-1

Why Body Mechanics Are Important

- Energy efficient
- Reduces stress on joints, ligaments, and tendons
- Improves cardiac and respiratory function
- Encourages proper body control and balance
- Promotes safe movements

increased exponentially with the increase of spinal loads, especially when that was coupled with bending. They also found that although caregivers were educated in body mechanics and proper lifting techniques, many did not follow through in clinical practice.[2] Therefore, it is vitally important that you protect your own body to avoid injuries, so you can have a long and satisfying career.

Interestingly, more and more health care locations (eg, hospitals, outpatient clinics, skilled nursing facilities) are discouraging health care workers from performing repetitive lifting tasks in an effort to protect them from injury. Many health care locations now require the use of mechanical lifts to avoid excessive lifting or moving of patients, citing the fact that work-related musculoskeletal disorders are not prevented by good body mechanics alone.[3] These mechanical tools include, but are not limited to, body-weight supported treadmills, sit-to-stand assistive devices, and Hoyer lifts.[4] Even the use of nonmechanical tools, such as nonfriction sheets, reportedly improved therapist safety.[3] These machines are all powered by battery (rather than cranks) and have been shown to improve both the safety of patients and health care workers.[4] Indeed, the Darragh et al[3(p49)] study showed that with specific parameters (such as not transferring patients requiring more than 25% assistance) and the use of assistive equipment, "therapists reported that they were able to do more for their patients."

Many facilities have also implemented a no-lift policy. The Occupational Safety and Health Administration recommends that manual lifting of patients "be minimized in all cases and eliminated when feasible."[5] This may manifest in a mechanical lift policy at the facility, or, in the case of some facilities, staff are totally prohibited from lifting patients (often those who require lifts from the floor or are bariatric). In these cases, the local fire department is contacted to do the lifting. For example, there was a bariatric patient who lived at a skilled nursing facility, and she often fell on purpose, just so those "nice boys" from the fire department could help her. Unfortunately, the facility was charged for every visit from the fire department.

Although these recent studies have shown that in some cases body mechanics cannot prevent injury, there are other valuable uses to maintaining proper body mechanics. Energy conservation, balance, and improved respiration are additional reasons why good body mechanics are necessary. Box 2-1 includes reasons why body mechanics are important.

PRINCIPLES OF PROPER BODY MECHANICS

It is a common story: your patient states that he was just lifting a small bag of groceries from the trunk of the car when suddenly his back went out. Why is that so? The bag was not that heavy.

It is your job to recognize the true story. The patient did not suddenly harm himself lifting that bag of groceries. Rather, he has been lifting and moving incorrectly for years, causing micro-injuries along the way, which finally manifested in a sudden painful injury while lifting the groceries. The problem was not with the bag of groceries; his problem was his incorrect lifting and body mechanics.

Any time a person lifts, carries, pushes, or pulls something, he or she is working against gravity and friction. These forces add resistance to the task being attempted, and so it is important to use methods to reduce these forces or that are the most efficient and effective. One consideration is the center of gravity (COG). Normally, an adult's COG is located between the symphysis pubis and the umbilicus. The lower the COG, and the closer the COG is to the object or person being moved, the easier time a person will having lifting, transferring, pushing, or pulling something. When transferring a person, for example, the goal is to get low and close to the person. You and the patient must be comfortable with close quarters. This shortens the lever arm required to lift, and it reduces the amount of energy required to transfer the person. Try this at home: pick up a textbook or dictionary. Hold it out at arm's length. How long can you hold that book before your arms fatigue, or before your posture changes and you use other muscles to compensate? Now hold the book close to your chest. Is it easier to do this? Why?

Something else to consider is your base of support (BOS). The wider your BOS, the more stable you will be and the easier time you will have lifting or moving the object or person. Again, in a transfer scenario, you will not only get low and close to the person being transferred, but you will also widen your BOS to make yourself more stable. You do not want to lose your balance when attempting to move a person. Your vertical gravity line (VGL) is an imaginary line that bisects your body in the sagittal plane; it must stay within your BOS in order to maintain balance. Think about this: you are standing upright, but you slowly begin to lean forward at the hips. How far can you go before you must take a step, or else fall over? When you feel the need to take a step (or fall), you have reached the limit of how far your VGL can go beyond your BOS. If the VGL exceeds your BOS, you are no longer stable or balanced.

Whenever you intend to move an item or person, you should plan ahead. Consider who or what you are moving and to what location you are moving it. Consider and remove obstacles that might be in the way. Position yourself close to the item being moved and get your COG low; this will help shorten your lever arm. Keep a wide BOS and maintain your VGL within the BOS. Position your feet in the direction you plan to move to avoid unnecessary twisting or reaching. Avoid simultaneously twisting and flexing the trunk to prevent injury; instead, move your feet and pivot. Attempt to maintain normal lumbar lordosis in the spine; this will increase stability and reduce stress on the spine. Tighten your core muscles as you perform the movement, and use large muscle groups (leg muscles) instead of small muscle groups (back muscles) to lift. If possible, roll, push, or pull the item as it is easier and safer. If you have been immobile for a while, stretch and move around before attempting to lift something; more back injuries occur after attempting lifts or transfers in the morning (after being in bed all night in one position) than in the afternoon. Take your time when lifting. If you feel you cannot perform the lift on your own, get assistance; there is no need to injure your body to avoid injuring your pride. If you are lifting with another person, be sure you are both clear on what is happening, how, and when in order to avoid injury (Box 2-2). Although some of these rules require advanced planning and may seem time consuming, they are worth it to avoid an injury that could plague you for the rest of your life. Therapists must also remember the safety of their patients; if they attempt to lift or transfer a patient improperly, they could drop or injure that patient.

POSTURE

Correct Posture and Purpose

Correct posture involves the maintenance of normal lumbar lordosis, but there is more to it than that. First, one must be familiar with the planes of movement. The sagittal plane (Figure 2-1) bisects the body into left and right symmetrical sides. The frontal plane (Figure 2-2) divides the body into front and back. The transverse plane (Figure 2-3) splits the body into top and bottom halves. When considering and assessing posture, one must look at a person's body in all planes to get a full picture of what is going on.

Why is proper posture important? Let's say you have a patient come to the clinic complaining of knee pain. All scans and x-rays of the knee show no deterioration at the knee joint. Why, then, is the knee hurting?

Box 2-2
Principles of Body Mechanics

- Plan movements ahead of time.
- Shorten the lever arm (keep the item being moved/lifted close to COG).
- Lower COG and widen stance.
- Avoid trunk rotation and flexion simultaneously.
- Pushing/pulling is preferable to lifting.
- Maintain normal lumbar lordosis when lifting.
- Avoid lifting after prolonged inactivity (sitting, sleeping).
- Do not attempt to lift something beyond your capability (know when to ask for help).

A quick postural assessment may show that the person's posture is to blame. A 2011 study by Gross et al[6] showed that flat foot (pes planus) is the cause of frequent knee pain. Poor posture in one area, then, can affect the entire body. In another study, Franke[7] noted that both movement in the sacroiliac joint and the pelvic girdle result in lower back pain in patients. Franke[7] commented that stability in these areas led to less pain and that the muscles and fascia supporting the pelvic girdle allowed for transition of force to the lower extremities. A lack of stabilization causes poor posture, and that, in turn, is often caused by muscle weakness or fatigue. Being able to assess a patient's posture, see what is wrong, and then make the necessary changes through tactile cues and exercises or stretches can improve that patient's knee pain without the need for opioids or surgical intervention.

There are several things that can affect or change a person's posture. As mentioned earlier, weakness can be one. Other things that can affect posture are body deformities, lax ligaments (such as during pregnancy), soft tissue tightness, abnormal muscle tone (such as resulting from a cerebrovascular accident), and abnormal pelvic angles or joint positions. Additionally, postural deviations can be acquired from environmental sources, such as the child who carries her backpack only on one shoulder, or the new mother who only carries the baby on one side.

Just like with body mechanics, your posture is also important. If you are treating a patient, consider your posture and change your position to maintain proper posture. You will likely be doing a great deal of standing and holding certain postures while performing interventions.

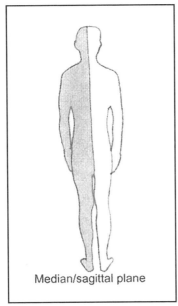

Median/sagittal plane

Figure 2-1. Sagittal plane.

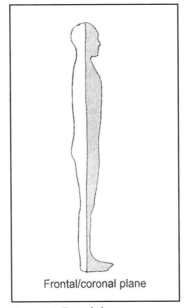

Frontal/coronal plane

Figure 2-2. Frontal plane.

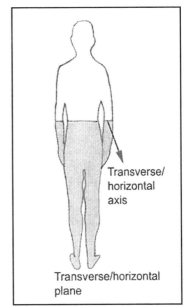

Transverse/
horizontal
axis

Transverse/horizontal
plane

Figure 2-3. Transverse plane.

Postural Assessment

A plumb line is an effective way to view a person's body to assess posture (Figures 2-4 and 2-5). The patient can stand in front of or to the side of the line to give the therapist a good baseline of what is proper posture and what is not.

In the sagittal plane, a plumb line should bisect the patient's ear, the midline of the acromion, the midline of the greater trochanter, just anterior to the knee, and just anterior to the malleolus. Possible deviations of the spine are flat back (Figure 2-6), sway back (Figure 2-7), and kyphosis-lordosis (Figure 2-8). From this position, you can also note genu recurvatum (hyperextension), forward head, or pes planus.

From the frontal plane, one could note raised shoulders, uneven nipples (in men), or uneven iliac crests. One could also observe genu valgus or varus, uneven anterior superior iliac spine, and ankle eversion/inversion or supination/pronation. Scoliosis can also be observed in the posterior frontal plane, especially if you have the patient bend forward.

When assessing a patient's posture, it is ideal to get the person to relax. Have them take a few marching steps to relax into their normal posture; patients will attempt to adopt the posture they think you are looking for, which may not be their normal day-to-day posture. Sometimes you can conduct a postural assessment without the patient being aware. It is also necessary to palpate the patient's body to completely discern postural deviations. Be familiar and comfortable with touching your patient, and know the bony landmarks used to determine postural deviations. Table 2-1 includes a list of postural deviations noted in each plane.

ERGONOMICS

Addressing ergonomics is a component of physical therapy not often considered. Physical therapists and physical therapist assistants often address complaints of pain or dysfunction from patients; however, when ergonomics are involved, prevention is the key. A patient may not yet have pain or injuries, but the goal is to ensure the patient stays healthy and functional.[8] An ergonomic assessment, whether it involves a cubicle or factory, can go a long way toward preventing injury in the future.

Standing

Standing for prolonged periods of time, just like sitting, should be avoided. Educate your patients about using cushioned mats and supportive shoes for jobs that require excessive standing time. Your patients should attempt to maintain normal lumbar lordosis, and they should take breaks whenever possible

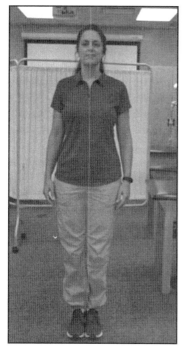

Figure 2-4. A plumb line in the frontal plane.

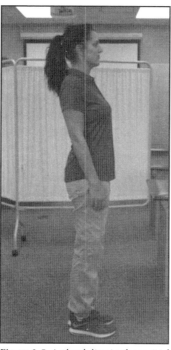

Figure 2-5. A plumb line in the sagittal plane.

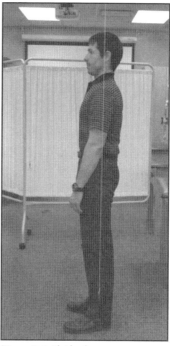

Figure 2-6. Flat back.

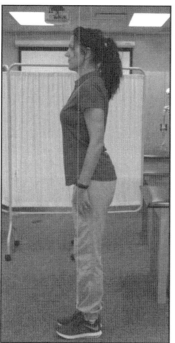

Figure 2-7. Sway back.

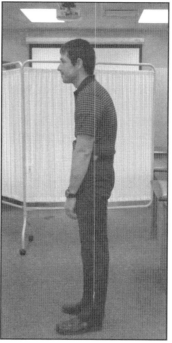

Figure 2-8. Kyphosis/lordosis.

Table 2-1
Postural Deviations Noted in Each Plane

Frontal anterior	Head tilt, nipples, sternum, umbilicus, anterior superior iliac spine, facial symmetry, shoulders, knees/feet
Frontal posterior	Head tilt, shoulders, scapulae, scoliosis, waist folds, posterior superior iliac spine, iliac crests, gluteal and popliteal folds, knees, calcaneus, medial arch
Sagittal	VGL (spinal curves, shoulders), hips (pelvic tilt), knees (hyperextension), ankles, trunk rotation, spine

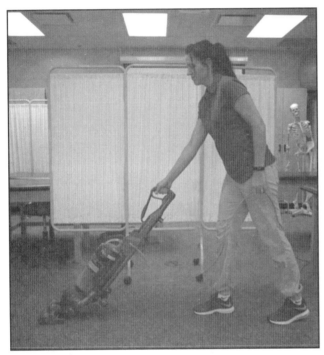

Figure 2-9. The correct way to vacuum.

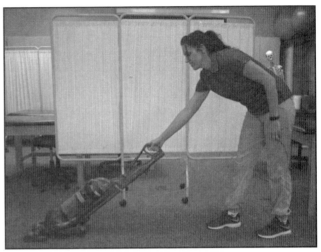

Figure 2-10. The incorrect way to vacuum.

Ask also about chores and daily home tasks. If the patient vacuums, does he or she walk with the vacuum cleaner or just push it out and in, bending at the waist? When the patient stands to wash dishes, does he or she raise a foot up on a step stool to take pressure off her lower back? When the patient bends over the sink to wash his or her face, does he or she bend at the hips and knees to maintain lumbar lordosis? When getting out of the car, does he or she swing his or her legs out first or simply twist and stand up? Nearly every task a person does at home is a test of body mechanics and posture, from picking up a toy on the floor to emptying the washer or dryer (Figures 2-9 through 2-12).

People do not often consider these daily tasks as culprits for pain, but they add up. Encourage your patients to adopt better postures or body mechanics, and to balance activity with rest, to avoid overuse or injury. Even better, adopt these practices yourself. You will be a better role model for your patients, and you will have a healthier back and posture to boot.

If you must stand, and you will often, put one foot up on a step stool to take pressure off your lower back, switching feet regularly (Figure 2-13). If you are able, treat a patient on a high-low mat or table; this will allow you to raise or lower the height of the treatment surface so you can reach the appropriate area while not adopting improper

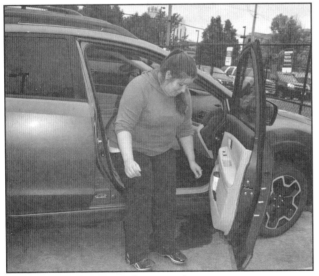

Figure 2-11. How to get out of car correctly.

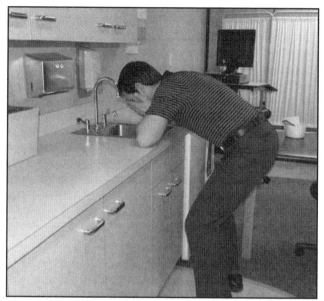

Figure 2-12. Washing the face correctly.

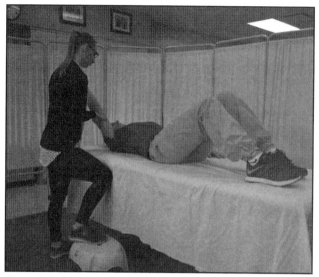

Figure 2-13. A treatment with a foot on a step.

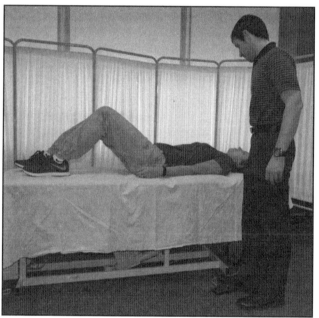

Figure 2-14. Raising/lowering the bed.

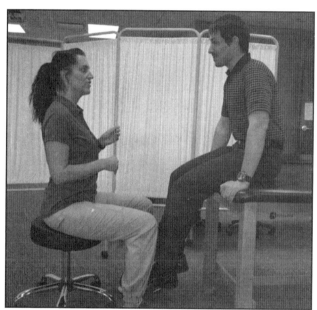

Figure 2-15. Sitting on a stool to treat.

body mechanics. Performing an ultrasound treatment to a patient's lower back can quickly become uncomfortable and potentially injurious if you do not have the patient at the appropriate height. If you are unable to raise or lower the height of the treatment area, using a footstool to raise yourself up or sitting in a chair to lower yourself down will make things much more comfortable (Figures 2-14 and 2-15).

If you note postural deviations in your patient (or yourself), there are some simple things you can do to help. Chin tucks, scapular squeezes, pectoral stretches in the doorway, posterior pelvic tilts in hook lying, hamstring stretches, mini-abdominal crunches, and wall slides are all excellent ways to encourage and improve standing or seated posture (Figures 2-16, 2-17, and 2-18). Generally, if there is a postural deviation, the source is often tightness in one muscle group and weakness in the opposite muscle group (such as tight pectoral muscles and weak rhomboids in a patient with rounded shoulders). Ultimately, your goal will be to determine, with your supervising physical therapist, what caused the postural deviation in the first place. Once you know the cause, you and your physical therapist are better equipped to fix or help the patient adapt to the situation.

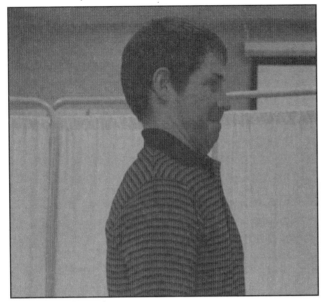

Figure 2-16. Chin tucks.

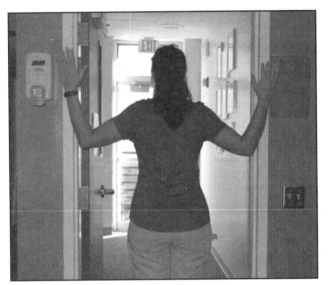

Figure 2-18. Pectoral stretches.

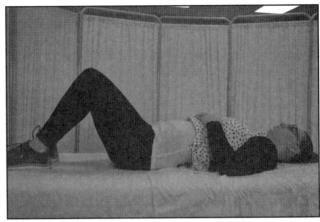

Figure 2-17. Pelvic tilts.

Seated

Pynt et al[9] noted that 75% of work is done while seated, and much research has been done regarding the effects of prolonged sitting on posture and health. Although the recommendation is that a person stands frequently throughout the day (at least once an hour), it is unreasonable to think your patient will not need to sit. A properly fitting chair should ideally have armrests, back support, and should be at a height that maintains 90 degrees of flexion in the hips and knees; feet should be able to touch the floor and remain flat.

Assess the desk at which your patient sits all day. Is the computer at eye level? Is the keyboard able to roll out and is it at the correct height so his or her feet are flat on the floor? Does the patient complain of neck or back pain? It may be a result of leaning forward at his or her desk. Do they get up and move around every so often? Kagen and Pencek[10] observed that when sitting for too long, the intervertebral disc pressure in the spine is twice as high as when standing and that the lower lumbar spine flattens by 30 degrees. Additionally, they noted that frequent breaks from sitting can be beneficial, including burning more calories, and even more importantly, preventing poor posture from sitting for too long.[10]

You can also talk to your patients about their home activities. Most people come home from work and sit—often all afternoon or evening. For example, Pynt et al[9] observed that 87% of Australians over the age of 15 years old watch television 3 or more hours a day, which involves a great deal of sitting. Encourage your patient to take standing breaks at home and to sit in supportive chairs when they must sit. Remind patients that sitting in the car counts too. Patients driving for long distances should take breaks every hour or so to get out and walk around; this will mitigate the postural issues that could result from prolonged sitting. The same rule applies for flying on a plane; passengers should get up and walk around as long as it is permitted. When seated in a car, truck, or van, educate your patient that the seat should be close enough for the driver to touch the pedals, and the seat should allow knees to be at the same level as the hips.

You should consider your own sitting habits and support surfaces. Consider both your posture and your body mechanics when treating patients; sitting in a chair is often a better choice for your posture when treating a patient also seated or on a low surface. Sitting on an unsupported chair (such as the ubiquitous rolling stool in therapy clinics) requires maintenance of normal lumbar lordosis and good, upright posture (Figure 2-19). It is also quickly fatiguing, and therapists are prone to adopting poor sitting posture when using an unsupportive stool for prolonged periods of time. Sitting in a supported chair is better for back support, but you still need upright posture while sitting (eg, while documenting; Figure 2-20).

PT 143 - Lab 6 - Gait Training

Activity 1

Part 1: Complete the following activities for EACH scenario:

- Correctly fit your partner for the assistive device.
- Educate your partner on appropriate gait pattern and weight bearing status.
- Educate your partner on proper ascending/descending of stairs while maintaining weight bearing status.

Patient 1: Dx: (R) hip fracture, PWB 50%, good UE strength, min (A). POC indicates gait training with rolling walker. *Mod 3-point*

Patient 2: Dx: (L) ankle fracture, NWB, good balance, CGA. POC indicates gait training with axillary crutches. *3-Point*

Patient 3: Dx: (L) TKR 4 weeks ago, WBAT, CGA. POC indicates gait training with straight cane. *Mod-2 point*

Patient 4: Dx: (L) hip fracture, TTWB, mod (A). POC indicates gait training with PUW. *Mod 3-point*

Patient 5: Dx: Spinal cord injury L3-L4, FWB, min (A). POC indicates gait training with forearm crutches. *2-point*

Patient 6: Dx: (L) CVA with (R) hemiplegia, FWB, mod (A). POC indicates gait training with hemi-walker and (R) sling. *Mod. 2 point*

Patient 7: Dx: (L) humeral fracture after fall due to decreased balance, (L) UE NWB, (B) LE FWB, min (A). POC indicates gait training with quad cane and (L) sling. *Mod 2 point*

Part 2: You will be assigned **ONE** of the above patients to answer the following (no more than 2 sentences).

1. Document gait training performed with the patient in an objective statement. (5pts)

2. Explain why you chose the gait pattern performed. (2pts)
   2 separate devices, easier gait pattern than mod 4

3. Explain what qualifications would need to be met in order to progress assistive device for the patient. (2 pts)
   Decrease Assist Level

4. What device would you progress patient to once the qualifications were met? Explain your choice. (1pt) *LBQC quad cane 1 cane   2→1 device   it is the still enough stability for gait momentum use*

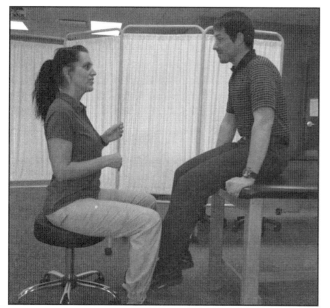

Figure 2-19. Unsupported sitting posture.

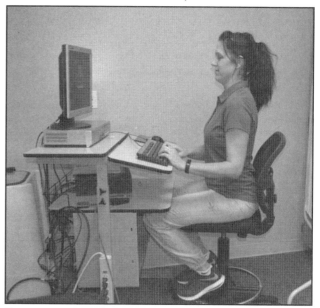

Figure 2-20. Supported sitting posture.

LIFTING TECHNIQUES

There are several ways to lift items and maintain your safety. Patient transfers will be discussed in detail in a later chapter; here, we will discuss general lifting, pushing, pulling, and reaching techniques for nonhuman objects. However, similar principles apply whether you are lifting a human or a box of supplies: get close to the object, lower your COG, widen your BOS, keep your VGL within your BOS, maintain lumbar lordosis, avoid twisting and flexing the spine, bend at the hips rather than the waist, and use large muscle groups rather than small muscle groups. Additionally, you should always plan for what you are moving, how much it weighs, your own physical strength, and where you are moving the object to. If someone else is assisting with the lift, make sure you are all on the same page when it comes to timing. Someone should be the leader and direct the lift ("one, two, three, lift" for example).

As stated before, pushing or pulling is easier than lifting and should be done if possible instead of lifting an item. However, sometimes that is not possible, and you must lift an object to move it to another area. The following sections discuss different types of lifts.

Deep Squat

A deep squat requires the lifter to lower his or her hips below the level of his or her knees. The lifter's feet are positioned parallel to each other and straddle the object being lifted. The lifter grasps the object, pulls it close to the body, and then stands, all while maintaining normal lumbar lordosis (Figure 2-21).

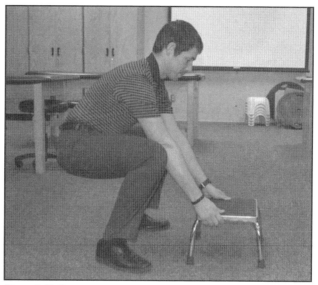

Figure 2-21. Deep squat.

Power Lift

A power lift is similar to a deep squat, except that the lifter does not squat so low that the hips go below the knees. The feet are still parallel but are behind the object rather than straddling it. The lifter grasps the object with both hands, pulls it close to the body, and stands up, again maintaining normal lumbar lordosis (Figure 2-22).

Straight Leg Lift

A straight leg lift is sometimes called a *waiter's bow*, since one may look like a bowing waiter at a fancy restaurant when performing this lift. The lifter's knees are only slightly flexed, and the lower extremities are parallel to each other. This lift is useful for getting items from the

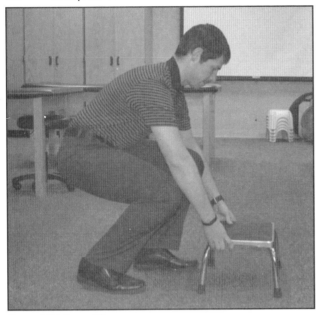

Figure 2-22. Power lift.

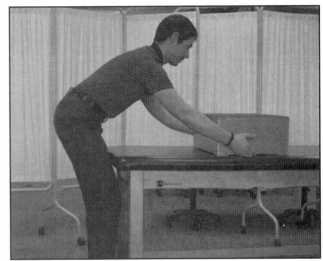

Figure 2-23. Straight leg lift.

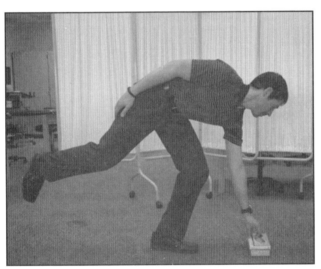

Figure 2-24. Single leg stance lift.

trunk of a car or back of a truck, as it does not require squatting low. Patients with painful knees may find this lift technique easier to perform. The lifter should maintain lower lumbar lordosis and bend at the hips rather than the waist. The object should be pulled close to the body before moving it (Figure 2-23).

Single Leg Stance Lift

The single leg stance lift is often called the *golfer's lift* due to the appearance of a golfer bending to retrieve a golf ball from a tee or cup. This lift is for lightweight items only, such as socks, pens, or other small items. The lifter shifts their weight to one leg, with knee and hip slightly flexed, while the other leg is kicked behind them, keeping that knee straight. The lifted leg acts as a counterbalance to the forward movement of the trunk. The lifter flexes forward

at the hips and uses one upper extremity (often the opposite upper extremity from the lower extremity being kicked back to maintain balance) to reach for and retrieve the item before coming back to vertical (Figure 2-24).

Half-Kneeling Lift

A half-kneeling lift requires the lifter to lower down to one knee while the other knee and hip are flexed at 90 degrees. This resembles the position of someone proposing marriage. The item being lifted is in front of the lifter, which they grasp and pull close to the body, propping it on the 90-90 knee. The person can then return to standing while still holding the item close to the body. This lift is beneficial for someone with poor upper extremity strength, but it would be difficult for someone with poor balance or painful knees. Normal lumbar lordosis and avoidance of spinal rotation should be maintained (Figures 2-25).

Traditional Lift

A traditional lift requires the lifter to place the feet anteriorly-posteriorly on either side of the object being lifted. The lifter goes into a deep squat position, lowering the COG and widening the BOS. The lifter grasps the item, pulls it close to the body, and returns to standing. It is important that the lifter avoids using small back muscles to lift the item to standing; use the lower extremities to return to vertical. Additionally, maintain lower lumbar lordosis (Figure 2-26).

Stoop Lift

A stoop lift is good for items that are below the waist but can be lifted or reached without squatting. It requires less energy to perform and is a bit easier on the knees. The lifter flexes at the hips and knees and maintains lumbar lordosis. The lifter bends and reaches with one of the upper extremities and then returns to standing, avoiding lateral bending of the spine or twisting. Sometimes the lifter can

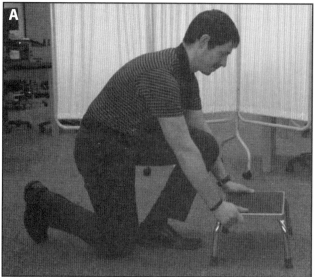

Figure 2-25. Half-kneeling lift.

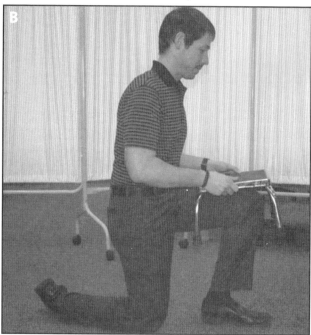

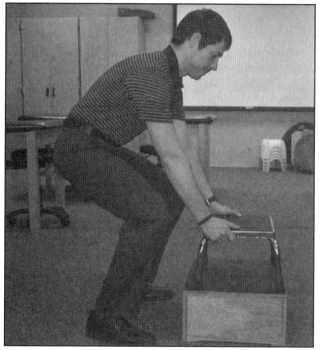

Figure 2-26. Traditional lift.

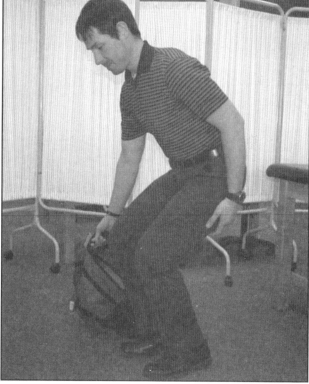

Figure 2-27. Stoop lift.

use only one upper extremity to lift the item, such as suitcases, briefcases, book bags, or shopping bags with handles. In this case the other upper extremity provides counterbalance (Figure 2-27).

Pushing/Pulling

Pushing and pulling utilize the same principles as lifting: get close, get low, and get a wide BOS. You should consider what you are moving. Is it on wheels? What sur-

face are you moving along? How heavy is the object? Try to move the item parallel to the direction the surface runs on and in the direction you want to move it to reduce friction. Pushing is easy when moving an item with wheels, but it may be easier to pull a heavier object. Either way, it will be difficult to get started, as the initial friction will be difficult to overcome (Figures 2-28 and 2-29).

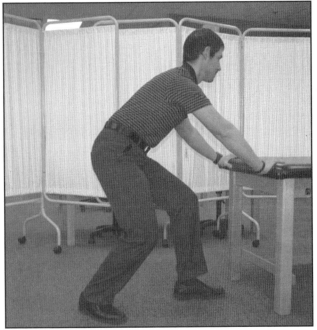

Figure 2-28. Push.

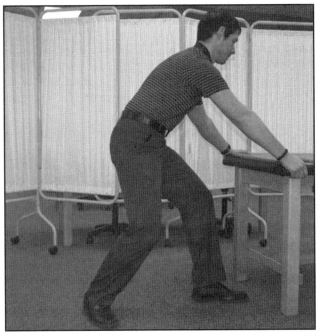

Figure 2-29. Pull.

Reaching Overhead

Think of the last time you had to reach for something on a high shelf. Perhaps you used the tips of your fingers to slide it out to the edge, only to have it tumble off the shelf and on top of you and onto the floor. A clinician once admitted to using a butter knife to slowly edge a box off a high shelf. Perhaps to reach the shelf you stood on a rolling chair or unstable stool. Many people are all guilty of doing something like this in the name of efficiency, but these are all unsafe practices, and the imagined time you are saving is not worth the potential injury.

To safely reach for something overhead, get a steady stool without wheels and stand on it. This will raise your COG and make your COG closer to the object, shortening your lever arm and making it easier to reach and lift the item. If you are reaching for a person to transfer who is on the far side of the bed, move them closer to the edge of bed before transferring. The same applies for transferring a patient out of a chair; scoot the patient forward to the edge of the chair before attempting a lift. Once you lift the item (or patient), pull it close to your body (Figure 2-30). The general guidelines for lifting, pushing, pulling, and reaching can be found in Box 2-3.

SAFETY/RED FLAGS

When performing tasks with your patient, it is important to pay attention to complaints or changes in posture or body mechanics during the treatment session. Be aware of your patient's medical chart and past medical history. If your patient has had bone cancer, for example, lifting items over a certain weight may be contraindicated due to bone brittleness. Additionally, existing fractures, osteoporosis, infection, or preexisting degenerative joint disease may be at least precautions, if not contraindications, for lifting. Likewise, a patient with cardiovascular disease or elevated blood pressure might exacerbate these conditions with certain types of lifts. It would also be worth checking with your patient that he or she has not had any recent falls; a patient with osteoporosis and a recent fall could have a fracture and not know it. This level of caution applies to both practicing how to lift a box, as well as lifting a weight for strengthening exercises. If your patient has any of these diagnoses, it does not mean that he or she is a poor candidate for teaching body mechanics or postural changes, but one must keep in mind what might exacerbate the pain or diagnosis, and avoid or alter these activities.

Additionally, if your patient suddenly complains of pain during your treatment session, it is best to stop the intervention and assess the situation; do not hesitate to alert your supervising physical therapist if the patient's condition changes or worsens, as this may indicate something new or different is happening.

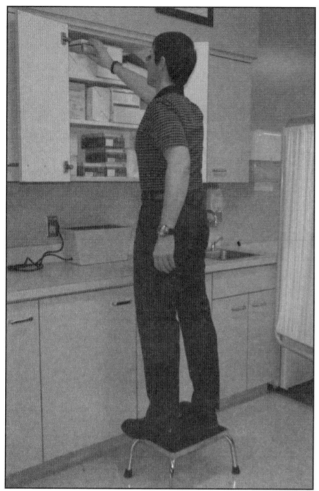

Figure 2-30. Reaching overhead.

Box 2-3

Guidelines for
Reaching, Pulling, and Pushing

- Lower COG.
- Push/pull in straight line.
- Clear objects/obstacles from path.
- Use footstool to reach overhead.
- Pull/move object close to you to shorten lever arm.
- Do not reach and twist simultaneously.

10-second hold for each with 3 verbal cues required to maintain proper positioning. Educated patient on using a footstool while standing in the kitchen to relieve strain on lower back with patient able to teach back and demonstrate posture. Encouraged patient to ensure that prep tables for kitchen are at waist level to avoid excessive flexion or rotation while performing cooking tasks. Patient able to verbalize understanding and teach back exercises and stretches.

A: Patient pain decreased from 6/10 to 3/10 on VAS after MHP treatment. Patient able to teach back HEP and required only 3 verbal cues vs 5 cues last visit.

P: Will see patient for next visit at end of the week. Plan to add bridging and knee-to-chest stretches 5 x 30-second hold next visit. Will have patient review HEP at next visit. PT will reevaluate next week.

Postural Assessment

S: Patient complaining of LBP 8/10 after standing >1 hour. Patient reports that lying down in supine x 30 minutes decreases pain. Patient reports his job requires him to be on his feet much of the day, and he works in construction.

O: Patient posture assessed in standing using plumb line, both in sagittal and frontal planes. Observed rounded shoulders and forward head in sagittal plane and increased lumbar lordosis due to anterior pelvic tilt. Patient performed bridges in hook lying, 3 sets of 10 with a 5-second hold, and performed seated chin tucks 3 sets of 10 with a 5-second hold. Patient required verbal cues x 4 and tactile cueing to perform chin tucks properly. Educated patient about proper body mechanics when performing lifts or daily activities, including lumbar lordosis, using LEs to lift, and avoiding trunk flexion with rotation. Applied TENS unit to lower back to decrease pain while patient performed daily activities: 120pps, 60us, intensity 3, to be worn during the day up to 24 hours. Patient reported pain 2/10 while wearing TENS unit. Educated patient about application, duration of treatment, and safety.

DOCUMENTATION

The following are some documentation examples for body mechanics or postural assessment treatment interventions. These are meant to serve as guidelines for documentation but are not the only way to record your interventions.

Patient Problem: LBP ℝ > 𝕃

S: Patient reports 6/10 pain on VAS. Patient reports he has worse pain when performing his job, which is cook for local restaurant. He reports he is on his feet most of the day, and the only relief comes at home with a hot shower.

O: Patient performed 3 sets of 10 reps of abdominal crunches with a 30-second rest break between each set. Patient then received moist hot pack (MHP) to lower back x 15 minutes with 7 layers of towels and with skin checked every 5 minutes. Patient has no contraindications to this treatment and reported pain 3/10 after MHP. After MHP, patient performed lower back stretches in the form of prone Supermans x 10 with

A: Patient pain decreased from 8/10 to 2/10 with TENS unit. Patient required 4 verbal cues to perform exercises correctly.

P: Will see patient next visit and reassess pain rating and effectiveness of TENS unit.

REVIEW QUESTIONS

1. What happens to your COG when you reach forward? What about when you reach overhead?
2. Provide a brief outline of instructions you would give a patient when educating about proper body mechanics.
3. What are 3 reasons body mechanics and posture are important?
4. Describe 2 types of lifts and when you would use them.
5. When assessing a patient's posture from the frontal plane, what are some deviations you might notice?
6. Describe 1 exercise or treatment you would suggest for a patient with a postural deviation (you select the deviation and the treatment)
7. Write an objective (O) section for the above deviation and treatment described.

REFERENCES

1. Holder NL, Clark HA, DiBlasio J, Hughes C. Cause, prevalence, and response to occupational musculoskeletal injuries reported by physical therapists and physical therapist assistants. *Phys Ther.* 1999;79(7):642-652.
2. Lorenz EP, Lavender SA, Andersson GBJ. Determining what should be taught during lift-training instruction. *An International Journal of Physical Therapy.* 2002;18(4):175-191. Doi: 10.1080/09593980290058580.
3. Darragh A, Campo M, Fros L, Miller M, Pentico M, Margulis H. Safe-patient-handling equipment in therapy practice: implications for rehabilitation. *Am J Occup Ther.* 2013;67(1):45-53. Doi: 10.5014/ajot.2013.005389.
4. Rockefeller K. Using technology to promote safe patient handling and rehabilitation. *Rehabil Nurs.* 2008;33(1):3-9.
5. Guidelines for nursing homes: ergonomics for the prevention of musculoskeletal disorders. *OSHA.* www.osha.gov. Published 2003. Revised March 2009. Accessed August 23, 2018.
6. Gross K, Felson D, Niu J, et al. Flat feet are associated with knee pain and cartilage damage in older adults. *Arthritis Care and Res (Hoboken).* 2011;63(7):937-944. Doi: 10.1002/acr.20431.
7. Franke B. Formative dynamics: the pelvic girdle. *J Man Manip Ther.* 2003;11(1):12-40.
8. Hayhurst C. How PTs are transforming the workplace with ergonomics. *PT in Motion.* 2015;7(5):18-26.
9. Pynt J, Mackey M, Higgs J. Kyphosis seated postures: health beyond the office. *J Occup Rehabil.* 2008;18(1):35-45. Doi: 10.1007/s10926-008-9123-6.
10. Kagen J, Pencek L. Go ahead ... take a stand! Standing on the job offers many favorable benefits. *RDH Magazine.* 2011;31(1):90-101.

Chapter 3

Positioning and Draping

KEY TERMS Contractures | Edema | Friction | Pressure injury | Prone | Shear | Sidelying | Supine

KEY ABBREVIATIONS APTA | AROM | DVT | HOB | PROM | ROM

CHAPTER OBJECTIVES

1. Explain the negative effects that can result from immobility.
2. Describe the various causes and negative effects of pressure injuries.
3. Discuss the necessary procedure to order restraints for a patient, and know the various examples of restraints.
4. Position patients properly for positions of comfort.
5. Describe how to position patients for specific diagnoses.
6. List the reasons for draping a patient.

INTRODUCTION

Positioning is an important and often underestimated part of a physical therapist assistant's job. This chapter briefly discusses the negative effects of immobility, as well as the benefits of range of motion (ROM) and attention to patient sensation. Therapists often play a major role in positioning programs established for immobile patients, and they must always consider what position is best for a patient considering specific treatments and diagnoses.

Draping, too, is a key element of compassionate care. Hospitals and clinics are cold, but temperature is only one reason for properly draping a patient. Therapists must consider, again, what interventions they are doing and why, and then drape their patients appropriately.

OVERVIEW OF MOBILITY AND THE EFFECTS OF IMMOBILITY ON SYSTEMS

Often, mobility is taken for granted, and one only realizes the repercussions of immobility after it has happened. A physical therapist assistant's job is to work with a patient, following a physical therapist's plan of care, to achieve maximum mobility. A physical therapist assistant addresses both the immobility issues that currently exist while attempting to prevent further injuries from occurring. Immobility due to an injury or disease process will inevitably result in problems with other body systems.[1] Some of the complications that can result from prolonged immobility are blood clots, orthostatic hypotension, increased insulin requirements, risk of aspiration, constipation, pressure injuries, decreased muscle mass and strength, loss of joint ROM, difficulty breathing, pneumonia, calcium loss in bones, and a general inability to perform daily activities.[2] It is vitally important that physical therapist assistants work with their patients to promote mobility in whatever form possible so that their patients can avoid comorbidities and have a higher quality of life.

Range of Motion

Range of motion is classified as either passive or active. Passive range of motion (PROM) requires the therapist to

Memolo J.
Procedures and Patient Care for the Physical Therapist Assistant
(pp 31-43). © 2019 SLACK Incorporated.

Box 3-1

Setup and Application of Range of Motion

- Position patient to access the area being treated, to provide patient comfort, and to adhere to proper body mechanics.
- Adhere to the rules of proper draping.
- Explain purpose of activity and acquire consent.
- Complete movements through full or available ROM.
- Move the body slowly and smoothly.
- Evaluate the patient's response after the treatment.
- Position and drape the patient after treatment for proper comfort and safety.

move the patient's joints through the full or available range, either because the patient cannot or should not actively move the joint independently. A patient who has just undergone a shoulder replacement surgery, for example, typically is under postoperative restrictions to not actively move the shoulder for a certain period of time. A physical therapist assistant may then do PROM, so long as the surgeon and supervising physical therapist deem it safe. Active range of motion (AROM) implies that the patient either assists the therapist with the joint movement or performs the movement independently. Range of motion, particularly in its passive form, should not be confused with exercise; it does not increase muscle strength. However, it can be very beneficial for a patient to avoid certain negative effects of immobility, such as contractures, pressure injuries, or difficulty performing daily activities (eg, getting dressed or combing hair). It is important for the physical therapist assistant to be aware of hand placement, the effects of gravity, and patient safety and pain levels during ROM interventions. Box 3-1 includes the setup and application for ROM.

Sensation (Dermatomes) Review

Sensation, or the lack of it, plays a large role in a patient's mobility. The body is equipped with nerves that detect pressure, pain, and touch. These are sensory neurons, and they enter the spinal cord, travel to the brain via sensory tracts, and tell the brain about what is happening to the body. Dermatomes are the striping pattern in which these sensory neurons are arranged, and they help us understand where damage might be located. There are specific sensory tests to check dermatomes, subdivided into superficial, deep, or combined cortical categories.[3] These will be covered in more detail throughout your education, but it is worth noting now that understanding sensation testing and dermatomes will influence how you treat your patient (Table 3-1).

POSITIONING

Consider how long you have been sitting in your chair reading from this textbook. One hour? Two? How many times do you think you have repositioned yourself in that time? You likely have not been aware of your frequent position changes, but that is the beauty of the fully functioning human body. The same thing happens at night when people sleep. Whether people wake up or not, they move in bed and reposition. The body, via pain and sensory receptors, can tell when pressure has built up for too long in one area, and those signals are sent to the brain, which result in a motor response: move. People lean forward, shift from one hip to the other, scoot their bottoms back in the chair, or roll from their right side to their left. This is all the body's effort to reduce pressure on certain bony places.

Physical therapist assistants should be aware of this need to change positions, especially as they encounter patient populations who may not be able to reposition themselves. Positioning is vitally important to maintain proper body function and to avoid secondary complications as a result of immobility. Often, patients who are otherwise unable to reposition themselves are put on a positioning program. The therapist creates and promotes a system of repositioning a patient every so many hours, rotating from prone to supine to left or right sidelying, in order to prevent complications, and the nursing and other caregiving staff are educated on this and encouraged to participate. Recently more studies have been conducted on the benefits (or lack thereof) of repositioning; there is no consensus on how often patients should be repositioned. The Agency for Health Care Policy and Research promotes repositioning the patient every 2 hours, while the European Pressure Ulcer Advisory Panel, the National Pressure Ulcer Advisory Panel, and the National Institute for Clinical Excellence advocate repositioning as needed by the patient.[4] As of a 2015 systemic review, there were no conclusive studies that supported repositioning, yet it is still a foundational aspect of therapeutic prevention and treatment of immobility complications.[4] It is agreed upon that if ischemia, as the result of immobility and pressure, persists for longer than 1 to 2 hours, necrosis takes place and pressure injuries can form.[5] This is an example of applying evidence-based practice to therapy interventions. Although dominant theory supports repositioning, new systematic reviews seem to indicate that repositioning may not prevent immobility complications. This is an area in need of further research so that patient care is maximized.

Pressure injuries, also called *decubitus ulcers*, result from pressure applied to an area of skin over a long period of time. Tissues can be distorted and blood flow can be affected. Friction or shearing forces can also cause or exacerbate these injuries, as well as the patient's comorbidi-

Table 3-1

Sensation Tests

Superficial	Deep	Combined Cortical
Pain Temperature Light touch Pressure	Kinesthesia Proprioception Vibration	Stereognosis Tactile localization Two-point discrimination Barognosis Graphesthesia Texture recognition

ties, such as diabetes, poor sensation, and poor nutrition.[5] Chapter 1 discussed the issue of sensation; a patient who lacks full sensation does not feel pressure build up on his or her bony prominences, and is therefore at higher risk for pressure injuries. In some cases, sensation is intact, but a patient cannot physically reposition. According to the Agency for Healthcare Research and Quality, as of 2014, 2.5 million patients are affected by pressure injuries, and the health care costs surpass $11 billion a year.[6] More than 60,000 patients die as a direct result of pressure injuries, which is why prevention is key.[6]

Pressure injuries are one of the major reasons for positioning (and repositioning) patients, but they are not the only reason. There was once an elderly woman in a skilled nursing facility who lacked mobility on her own. She relied on her caregivers to move her joints through the available ROM. She suffered from severe arthritis, as well, so joint movement was painful. As a result, she had been allowed to lie in her bed in a fetal-like position for many years. Her spine was severely kyphotic. Most notable were her hands—so flexed at the fingers and wrists that her nails dug into the skin of her palms. This woman suffered from severe contractures (bony changes that had occurred in her joints), which prevented normal, full ROM. Unfortunately, there was little therapists could do to address the contractures already present; the only treatment was to attempt preventing further damage to the joints. Box 3-2 includes areas where pressure most commonly builds in the different patient positions.

With proper positioning, therapists aim to avoid the occurrence of contractures. Frequently repositioning not only helps prevent pressure buildup, but it also allows the joints to be moved to a new position, allowing fluid movement and preventing bony changes. It is necessary that therapists put the patient in the most neutral position possible, avoiding excessive flexion or rotation, in order to avoid contractures and to provide support and stability for the body and extremities.[7]

Very often therapists put patients in what is called a position of comfort. It is exactly what it sounds like; it is the

Box 3-2

Soft Tissue Contracture Sites

Supine
- Hip and knee flexors
- Ankle plantar flexors
- Shoulder extensors, adductors, and internal rotators
- Hip external rotators

Prone
- Ankle plantar flexors
- Shoulder extensors, adductors, and internal/external rotators
- Neck rotators (left or right)

Sidelying
- Hip and knee flexors
- Hip adductors and internal rotators
- Shoulder adductors and internal rotators

Sitting
- Hip and knee flexors
- Hip adductors and internal rotators
- Shoulder adductors, extensors, and internal rotators

position that provides the patient the most comfort while you perform your other interventions or when you leave the patient after therapy. Often, the position of comfort is perfectly acceptable for patient positioning. If you are treating a patient for shoulder pain and he or she is more comfortable sitting up rather than being supine, you can accommodate him or her. If a patient has lower back pain, putting a pillow under his or her knees to relieve that pain in supine is also acceptable. Patients who are otherwise healthy or mobile have fewer positioning concerns, and the therapists' concern is making the patient comfortable while providing the necessary treatment.

Box 3-3
Rationale for Proper Positioning

- Prevents injury, pressure, and contractures
- Provides patient comfort
- Provides trunk support and stability
- Provides access to areas to be treated
- Promotes efficient function of body systems

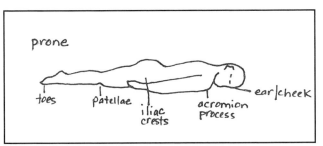

Figure 3-1. Pressure places in prone.

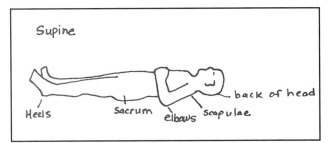

Figure 3-2. Pressure places in supine.

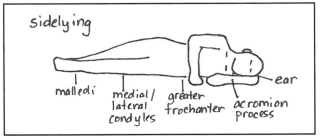

Figure 3-3. Pressure places in sidelying.

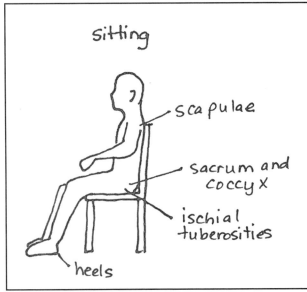

Figure 3-4. Pressure places in sitting.

Often, positioning is about the physical therapist assistant being able to access the body part he or she is treating. Other times, positioning becomes a more involved process. In these cases, when patients are not mobile or lack full sensation, it is the therapists' job to reposition that patient often and to consider the parts of the body that will absorb the most pressure in order to prevent pressure buildup.

In some cases, positioning becomes a factor of maximizing patient function. For example, pediatric patients with cerebral palsy have increased muscle tone, and certain positions can help the patient break out of the typical tonal postures. These patients and others may also have primitive reflexes (those seen normally in developing babies/children but not normal in older children or adults), and positioning can again take the patient out of that nonfunctional position. Previous positioning standards included putting these patients in supine or semirecumbent positions, but newer research indicates that these positions require patients to perform activities against gravity, may promote primitive reflexes, and decrease the patient's ability to perform hand-eye movements or reaching and grasping.[8] Box 3-3 includes the rationale for proper positioning.

Bony Landmarks

Whether a person is sitting or lying down, there are specific bony places on a person's body that experience pressure and its negative effects before other places. When considering each position for a patient, one must also consider what bony prominences should be protected. Bhattacharya and Mishra[5] reported that about 25% of all pressure injuries are found on the sacrum, heel, ischium, and patella.

In supine, the common locations of pressure include the scapulae (including the spines and the inferior angles), the spinous processes, and most commonly the heels or sacrum. In sidelying, the patient is most at risk at the acromion, greater trochanter, and malleoli. A prone patient should be monitored at the clavicles, anterior superior iliac spine, patellae, and tips of the toes. In seated, the ischial tuberosities are most at risk, as well as the heels and sacrum. Figures 3-1 through 3-4 include pictures of areas of pressure in prone, supine, sidelying, and sitting. Table 3-2 includes a list of the most common areas for pressure buildup.

Table 3-2

Most Common Places for Pressure

Area	Supine	Prone	Sidelying	Sitting
Head/Trunk	Occipital tuberosity Spine and inferior angle of scapulae Posterior iliac crests Spinous processes Sacrum Ischium	Forehead Lateral ear Anterior acromion process Anterior superior iliac spine Sternum	Lateral ear Lateral ribs Lateral acromion process	Ischial tuberosities Scapular and vertebral processes Sacrum
Upper Extremity	Elbows: medial epicondyle	Anterior head of humerus	Lateral head of humerus Medial/lateral epicondyles	Medial epicondyle of humerus
Lower Extremity	Posterior calcanei	Tips of toes (dorsum of foot) Patella	Greater trochanter Medial/lateral condyles of femur Medial/lateral malleoli Fifth metatarsal of foot	Calcanei

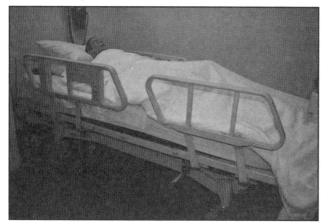

Figure 3-5. A bed rail can be a restraint if the patient is unable to remove it.

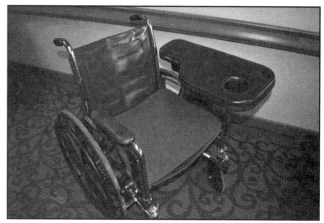

Figure 3-6. A lap tray can also serve as a restraint.

Restraints

When a physical therapist assistant thinks about positioning, he or she should also make sure to avoid creating a restraint. A restraint is anything—physical or chemical—that would prevent a patient from being able to move or change positions on his or her own. Per the Joint Commission, a hospital or facility should only use a restraint when it is clinically justified and when it is relevant to the safety of the patient or staff (Standard PC.03.05.01).[9] Only a doctor or other licensed individual authorized by the hospital or facility can prescribe a restraint in order for one to be used, and a face-to-face evaluation with a physician or licensed caregiver must be conducted at least every 24 hours to renew the order, and at least 1 hour after initiation of the restraint (PC.03.05.05, PC.03.05.11).[9] The least restrictive restraint must be used. One might be surprised what is considered a restraint.

Medicating a person to the point that he or she is unable to move on his or her own is a restraint. Tying a person to their bed with sheets or other devices is likewise a restraint. Some may find it surprising, however, that certain wheelchair cushions, arm troughs, or even raised rails on the side of a hospital bed could also be considered restraints if the patient is unable to remove these on his or her own.

Sometimes what is considered a restraint is implemented for the best of intentions, such as fall prevention or preventing injury to the patient or staff members. A therapist may place a patient in bed with the rails up (Figure 3-5), or the patient may be positioned in his or her wheelchair with a lap tray (Figure 3-6) or a belt buckled across his or her lap. These may be implemented to prevent a fall, although evidence does not support that these are actually preventative, but if the patient cannot lower the rails or remove the belt independently, these are both considered restraints. Unless a physician has ordered such a restraint, one must problem solve in another way.

As they apply to positioning, restraints can also take the form of pillows, towel rolls, bolsters, or other positioning devices, so these must be placed so that the patient can remove them or change positions. Therapists cannot and should not position a patient in a way that he or she cannot move out of. The American Physical Therapy Association's (APTA) position from 2012 states that the use of physical or chemical restraints must be appropriate and not indiscriminate, and that although sometimes restraints may be called for in specific situations, it is unethical to place restraints on a patient without proper evaluation, consideration of alternatives, and communication with the patient and the patient's caregivers.[10]

Supine Position

When a patient is in the supine position, one should first consider those bony landmarks most at risk for pressure buildup. Additionally, physical therapist assistants should be mindful of positioning the body in as neutral a way as possible. Unless there is a specific diagnosis that contraindicates it, a position of comfort is appropriate for your patient. A small pillow under the head is acceptable, although it should not be too fluffy and should avoid excessive neck flexion. A thin pillow under the knees is also appropriate except in certain circumstances (discussed later) to decrease lower back discomfort, but again, excessive flexion of the knees should be avoided. Some kind of towel roll or other positioning boot or device should be used to float the heels off the bed; towel rolls could be placed just proximal to the calcaneus. Towel rolls in the hands could help prevent finger flexion contractures, especially if the patient is prone to finger flexion (Figure 3-7).

Prone Position

The therapist should again aim for as neutral a position as possible when putting a patient in prone. Many patients, especially older ones, have not been in prone for a long time;

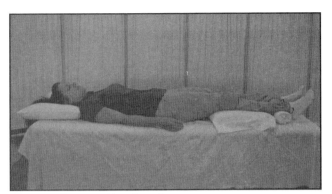

Figure 3-7. Supine position of comfort.

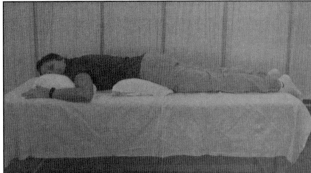

Figure 3-8. Prone position of comfort.

however, it is an excellent position for those with kyphotic postures or for those who sit for prolonged periods, such as in a wheelchair. A small pillow or towel roll can be placed under the patient's forehead, although the patient may opt for no pillow or to turn their head to the side. Some treatment tables and beds have face cutouts, and the therapist can place a thin towel or pillow case around the opening for support and cleanliness. One can put either a pillow under the abdomen or under the anterior lower legs, but not in both locations, to relieve pressure off the back. The patient's upper extremities can either be in a *T* position or down by his or her sides, whichever he or she prefers. If pressure buildup seems likely on the anterior shoulders, additional towel rolls can be added (Figure 3-8).

Sidelying Position

In sidelying, the patient should have proper alignment of the head, trunk, and hips, avoiding excessive rotation of the spine. A thin pillow under the head is appropriate. The patient should not be positioned directly on the shoulders; rather, the shoulder should be rotated slightly forward or back so that the patient is not resting directly on the acromion. Often the bottom lower extremity is slightly flexed and the upper is more flexed, with a pillow placed between the knees to decrease pressure on the medial and lateral knees. Another pillow can be placed across the patient's chest and the arms wrapped around it; again, this is at the patient's discretion. A key for sidelying is that the patient should be able to maintain this position without the use of bolsters or any other restraining device, and you should feel that the patient is safe in this position (Figure 3-9). If you do not feel the patient is safe in this position unsupervised, then this position may not be appropriate for the patient.

Sitting Position

The chair should fit well, with the patient's feet able to touch the floor and the back supportive and allowing for midline positioning of the spine. Pressure on the popliteal space should be avoided, and upper extremity support is appropriate so long as it is not a restraint. If a patient is

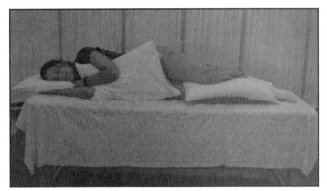

Figure 3-9. Sidelying position of comfort.

sitting while receiving a treatment to the back, requiring the patient to lean forward, the use of pillows for support is necessary. There are positioning devices in chairs, especially wheelchairs, to help promote midline of the trunk, as well as head/neck support and pressure relief and support of the pelvis. These will be discussed in more detail in Chapter 8 (Figures 3-10 [sitting] and 3-11 [sitting and leaning forward]).

Special Positioning

Amputation

Special considerations for positioning should be made for patients who have had amputations of their lower extremities. The following sections discuss 2 specific types of positioning concerns.

Transtibial

A transtibial amputation is one that is below the knee, and the incision is made across the tibia and fibula in the lower extremity. A specific concern for these patients is the possibility that the knee and/or hip could acquire a flexion contracture. It is sometimes painful for postoperative patients with transtibial amputations to fully extend their knees on the affected limb. Either they, an unaware health care staff member, or a family member may slide a pillow under the patient's knee on the amputated side in an effort to relieve pain. This may feel better, but it could cause

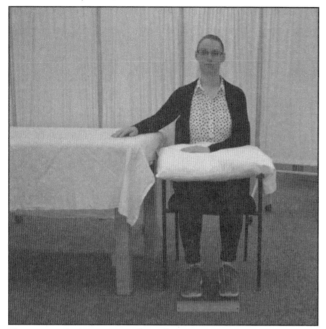

Figure 3-10. Sitting position of comfort.

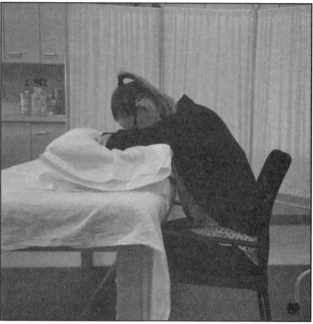

Figure 3-11. Sitting leaning forward position of comfort.

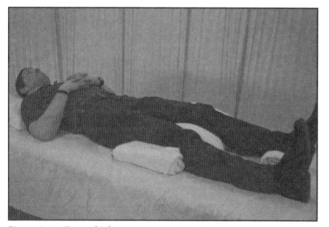

Figure 3-12. Transtibial amputation positioning.

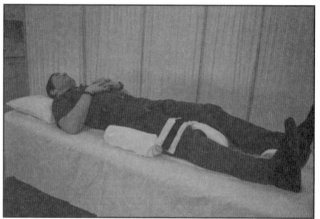

Figure 3-13. Transfemoral amputation positioning.

a knee flexion contracture if this position is prolonged. Likewise, if a pillow is placed under the affected limb, the hip may go into flexion. Prolonged hip flexion is also contraindicated. This patient should avoid prolonged sitting as well for the same reasoning. If the patient has any hope or desire to eventually use a prosthetic, he or she will need that knee and hip to fully extend. Otherwise the limb will not fit into a prosthetic, and the patient's mobility and independence will be negatively affected (Figure 3-12). In this case, then, the knee should be in a fully extended position. The patient could have a pillow or towel roll placed under the unaffected knee for support, but the affected limb should avoid prolonged knee and hip flexion. Prone is an excellent position to place this patient in periodically to counteract the effects of knee and hip flexion. Education is also important so that other caregivers follow this protocol.

Transfemoral

A transfemoral amputation is one that bisects the lower extremity above the knee, cutting the femur. This patient is at risk for hip flexion contractures, as well as external rotation and abduction of the hip. If the patient is allowed to maintain hip flexion, external rotation, and/or hip abduction, he or she will be unable to be fitted for a prosthetic, affecting his or her mobility. As a result, therapists and other caregivers often place a towel roll on the lateral side of the thigh to prevent it from rolling or abducting out, and if the hip is prone to flexion, a light weight (eg, a cuff weight) could be placed across the distal or mid-thigh region to keep it in neutral (Figure 3-13). Prolonged sitting is also contraindicated due to the hip flexion concern. Again, prone is an excellent position for this patient, and other caregivers should be educated so this protocol is followed.

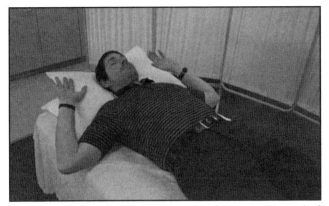

Figure 3-14. Patient with anterior chest and neck burns positioning (end position).

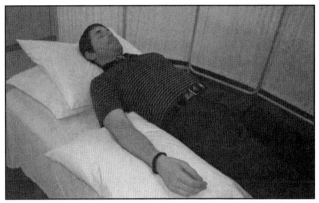

Figure 3-15. Positioning for patient with stroke with a flaccid upper extremity.

Burns

A patient who has suffered from burns must be positioned with consideration of how those burns heal. Healing burns generally result in scar tissue, which is far less flexible than regular, healthy skin. Prolonged positioning for burns over joints should be avoided because contractures are likely to form. For example, a patient with burns across his or her neck and chest should not be positioned with neck flexion or flexion of the shoulders, elbows, and hands, or adduction of the shoulders. The healing tissue will scar down, making it difficult for the patient to move his or her neck into extension or his or her shoulders into abduction. This is another example of how a position of comfort may not be appropriate for the patient. What is comfortable (joint adduction and flexion especially) is not functional. The patient must understand that he or she will undergo some pain or discomfort while preventing contractures. Instead, the patient should be positioned serially to promote more and more extension/abduction, in tandem with gentle ROM, either passive or active. Otherwise, the patient may adopt contractured positions that will require much time, effort, and discomfort to treat; prevention is always easiest and best (Figure 3-14).

Stroke/Hemiplegia

A patient who had a cerebrovascular accident (stroke) will often have one side of the body weaker than the other side—the side opposite the injured side of the brain. Especially in the acute setting, a patient with a stroke often has flaccidity and potential lack of sensation in the affected side, creating concerns with limb safety. A flaccid arm can easily slide off a table; a leg with decreased sensation can be bumped or injured without the patient knowing it. Even when the patient is in a subacute therapeutic setting, his or her affected side is sometimes forgotten or neglected due to decreased function and sensation. In these cases, the limb should be positioned and supported to avoid injury. Towel rolls and bolsters can be great tools to keep a flaccid limb in place. An arm trough or lap tray can also help with upper

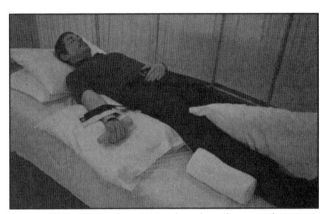

Figure 3-16. Positioning for patient with stroke with increased tone.

extremity positioning in a wheelchair, so long as these do not act as restraints for the patient. The APTA clinical summary on stroke recommends positioning devices such as slings, taping, or wheelchair arm supports as effective methods to initially decrease the risk of shoulder subluxation.[11]

After the acute stage, a patient with a stroke often develops increased tone in the affected limbs. The typical positioning is shoulder adduction and external rotation; supination; and elbow, wrist, and finger flexion. For the lower extremity, the hip typically adducts and internally rotates with knee extension and foot plantar flexion. The therapist should consider these challenges with positioning; the general goal is to position the patient in the opposite of the position of tone.[12] For patients who suffer from increased tone, moving the limb out of the tone positions and supporting it in its new, more neutral positions, is best. For example, a patient with upper extremity flexion tone should be positioned with the shoulder in neutral, with no adduction or rotation, and the elbow, wrist, and fingers should be placed in extension. Again, the use of towel rolls to support the limbs is helpful, and either a towel roll or cone placed in the hand can promote prolonged finger extension (Figure 3-15 with flaccid upper extremity and Figure 3-16 with tone).[12] Some facilities have specialized hand and arm splints to promote elbow, wrist, and

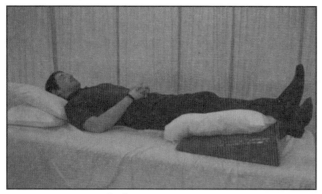

Figure 3-17. Patient with edema positioning.

finger flexion. The same protocol is applied for the lower extremity, using towel rolls to reduce rotation and adduction, and specialized boots are available to reduce plantar flexion. In sitting, the patient is encouraged to sit upright with the affected upper extremity supported on a table or tray with palm down, fingers extended, and elbow straight. The upper extremity can be supported additionally with a pillow or folded towel. The lower extremity may need a pillow under the buttocks on the affected side to keep the foot flat on the floor.

Arthritis

Because arthritis, whether rheumatoid or osteoarthritis, already affects the joints, therapists must be aware of joint positioning and pressure. Prolonged immobility of the joints is not recommended, and it is better to promote gentle ROM, either active or passive, to decrease the risk of contractures. Patients with arthritis may wish to stay immobile for comfort; however, as a therapist, your job is to encourage the patient to be as active as possible within physician recommendations, and your positioning will reflect those recommendations. Again, education is key to encourage the patient's caregivers in supporting these positioning goals.

Orthopedic Conditions

Patients who have had joint replacement surgeries suffer varying amounts of pain with joint movement on the surgical limb. A patient who has undergone a knee replacement, for example, will initially find knee flexion and extension quite difficult. Perhaps you have met someone who had a knee replacement. If so, you know that person was subjected to physical therapy shortly after surgery, possibly the same day. That is because prolonged positioning, the kind that might feel most comfortable to the patient, is problematic for functional activities. If the patient wants to negotiate stairs or get up and down from a low chair or toilet, he or she will need to get as close to normal ROM for that joint as possible. Patients with knee replacements are discouraged from having pillows or bolsters placed beneath the affected knee, and early active assistive and AROM and exercises are encouraged.

Similarly, patients who have had shoulder or hip replacements are equally encouraged to mobilize early. Positioning for total hip arthroplasty avoids hip adduction, rotation, and flexion. Depending on the type of surgery (posterior or anterior approach), the patient will have restrictions on certain movements, so positioning may include the use of bolsters and towel rolls to discourage the patient from performing those taboo positions. A posterior approach contraindicates hip flexion past 90 degrees, internal rotation, and hip adduction.[13] An anterior approach contraindicates hip hyperextension and hip external rotation.[13] Some surgeons apply global precautions, which include both the anterior and posterior approach precautions. Patients, as well as family members or caregivers, should be educated on these precautions, and these precautions should be practiced regularly in therapy interventions even beyond positioning (eg, getting into or out of bed). Recent research has indicated that reduced restrictions or precautions might yield a faster recovery and higher patient satisfaction, but the jury is still out as to whether official precautions will ever be lifted or decreased.[14] In the meantime, physical therapists and physical therapist assistants should follow the surgeon's postoperative protocol and also educate their patients to do the same. Additionally, evidence-based practice per the APTA indicates that these precautions are still to be followed.[13]

Edema

Edema is the accumulation of fluid in the interstitial spaces of the tissue. Patients who suffer from edema require special positioning considerations. Edema can be caused by a number of things, including acute injury such as sprains and strains, lymphatic dysfunction, surgery, cardiac or pulmonary disease, pregnancy, deep vein thrombosis (DVT), and renal or hepatic disease. Depending on the cause of the edema, the general rule of thumb is to position the patient's limb(s) in elevation. Higher than the level of the heart is recommended, and other techniques, which will be discussed later, can be introduced in addition to positioning to reduce edema. There are some contraindications to positioning for edema, however. For example, a patient with a DVT will not be the recipient of any treatment until he or she is cleared for therapy, which would be after the DVT has been treated (Figure 3-17).

Pulmonary Conditions

Patients suffering from pulmonary issues, such as chronic obstructive pulmonary disorder, emphysema, bronchitis, or pneumonia, have increased difficulty breathing when supine or recumbent. That is because in supine, gravity is working against the muscles in the chest that assist with breathing, making the work of breathing harder. Instead, patients with these diagnoses often require the head of the bed (HOB) to be raised to ease the burden of breathing. If your patient has one of these diagnoses, it is likely your patient already positions him- or herself with the HOB

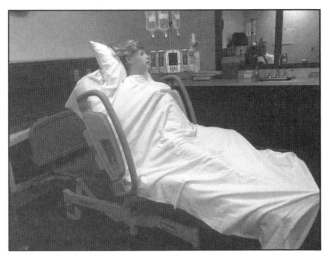

Figure 3-18. Fowler's position for breathing.

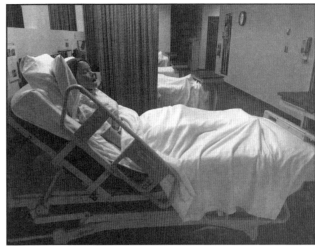

Figure 3-19. Semi-Fowler's position for breathing.

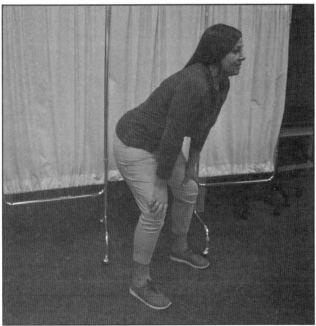

Figure 3-20. Tripod position for breathing.

Box 3-4

Rationale for Proper Draping

- Provides modesty for patient
- Provides warmth for patient
- Allows access to areas being treated
- Protects clothing from being soiled

ventilation distribution; and increases lung volume while decreasing lung secretions.[15] It is important that you read your patient's chart to know if he or she has a pulmonary disease, and to speak with your patient about the best position to facilitate breathing and comfort.

DRAPING

There are several reasons why draping is an important part of patient care. Box 3-4 includes rationale for proper draping. Think of the last time you were in a doctor's office. The nurse gave you a gown to put on, and perhaps you had a sheet to cover your derriere. Consider how exposed you felt, and cold. Modesty and temperature are 2 main reasons for draping your patient appropriately.

In most cases, you will not need your patient to completely disrobe in order for you to perform your treatment or intervention; however, you will need to expose the part of the body you need to treat, which may require some adjustment in clothing. Often, the therapist can tell the patient before the appointment to bring a change of clothes, such as shorts if the therapist needs to access the knee, or a tank top if the shoulder is being treated. However, there are occasions during which the patient is in a hospital gown, namely when they are a patient in the hospital and the therapist works with the patient in the hospital room.

raised without your intervention. This position, with the HOB raised, is called the *Fowler's position*, and anything between the 90 degree upright and supine is called a *semi-Fowler's position* (Figures 3-18 and 3-19).

There are other positions for patients suffering from respiratory distress. The tripod position, in which the patient flexes at the hips and places his or her hands on his or her knees or a table, allows the accessory muscles of the neck and chest to get more air in the lungs (Figure 3-20). This can be done in standing, sitting and leaning forward on the knees, or sitting while leaning forward on pillows on a table surface. For acute respiratory distress syndrome, a 2002 study showed that prone positioning is beneficial because it improves the respiratory mechanics; homogenizes the pleural pressure, alveolar inflation, and

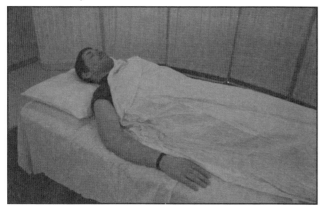

Figure 3-21. Draping to access upper extremity.

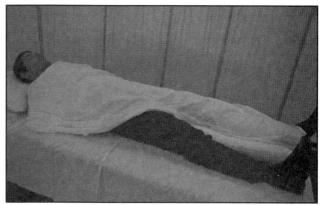

Figure 3-22. Draping to access lower extremity.

In this case, the patient is obviously exposed, and draping should accommodate not only the temperature issue (hospitals are cold) but should also address modesty. If you are performing PROM to the patient's lower leg, you will need to drape across the groin area to protect modesty. Be especially aware of these sensitive areas (gluteals, perineum, and breasts for female patients).

It is also important to consider your patient's cultural or religious preferences for modesty. A Muslim woman may need to be treated only by a woman, while a Muslim man may require a man to treat him. This may also be the case for nuns, or any other person whose garb may not be removed either at all or only with those of the same sex. You will need to be able to adapt to your patient's needs.

Sometimes you will need to transport your patient from one area to another, and this may involve the use of draping to cover the patient during transport. This is again an issue of comfort and modesty.

Access to the part of the body being treated is another reason for draping, but draping also involves protecting the patient's skin or clothing from soiling. For example, you may need to perform an ultrasound treatment to the patient's lower back. Draping the patient to cover his or her upper trunk and lower extremities while leaving the lower back exposed, allows you to perform your intervention; it also allows you to protect the patient's clothing from getting ultrasound gel on their shirt, pants, or skin other than the area being treated. Best practice is to tuck the draping sheet or towel into and over the clothing to protect it.

If the patient is uncomfortable with the exposure required for treatment, education and providing plenty of materials for draping often helps (Figures 3-21 and 3-22).

SAFETY/RED FLAGS

As mentioned before, positioning is a preventative measure that aims to avoid complications such as contractures and pressure injuries. You may enter a patient's room with the intention of performing a specific task, such as bed mobility or sitting on the edge of the bed, only to find that the patient has signs of a pressure injury. You should always check a patient's skin, especially for those patients who are immobile. What should you look for?

Skin that is red and does not blanch is a sign that pressure has already built up. There may already be tissue damage under the epidermis. Repositioning the patient off the area of pressure and alerting the nursing staff, as well as the supervising physical therapist, is the best option. At that point, the staff and your supervising physical therapist can determine the best method of treatment.

If your skin check reveals an open wound, the same procedure would be followed: alert staff and the physical therapist, and in the meantime, reposition the patient off the wound.

A patient who has been in the same position for too long is at risk for contractures. Your treatment session likely will involve moving the patient's joints; if you recognize stiffness, you can communicate this to the supervising physical therapist. Recognition of joint stiffness, or the onset of contractures, can be better addressed before it becomes a problem. Remember that a true contracture is a "fibrosis of connective tissue in skin, fascia, muscle, or a joint capsule that prevents normal mobility of the related tissue or joint"[16(p477)]; joint stiffness that still allows movement through the range is not a contracture, but it can become one if prolonged immobility continues.

DOCUMENTATION

The following documentation examples highlight how one might include positioning and draping in their note.

O: Patient received continuous ultrasound to the Ⓛ patella for pain, 3.3 mHz, 1.2 W/cm², x 8 minutes. Patient positioned supine with towel roll under Ⓑ knees, pillow under head, and heels elevated with towel rolls to prevent pressure and maximize comfort. Patient draped with upper body and lower Ⓡ LE covered with sheet, Ⓛ patella exposed.

O: Patient receiving therapy for Ⓡ transtibial amputation. Performed hip extension, hip internal rotation, and knee extension in supine and sidelying x 3 sets of 10 reps against gravity. After therapy session patient positioned in supine with Ⓡ knee in extension and bolster on lateral thigh to prevent external rotation; Ⓛ knee supported with pillow to relieve strain on the back. Pillow under the head and patient draped with sheet covering Ⓑ LEs.

REVIEW QUESTIONS

1. What are 3 negative effects of prolonged immobility.
2. Why is proper draping necessary for your patient?
3. How would you position and drape a patient with left hemiplegia and a treatment on the right upper extremity?
4. What are some concerns you should have when it comes to using bolsters, towel rolls, bed rails, and arm troughs for positioning? How can you resolve these concerns?
5. Your patient had a total hip arthroplasty on the left lower extremity (posterior approach). What are the rules of positioning? What types of positioning should be avoided?
6. How would you position and drape a patient for an ultrasound treatment to the left scapula?
7. How would you position a patient with burns along his or her left lateral neck, chest, and entire left arm?
8. How would you position and drape a patient for comfort in sidelying?

REFERENCES

1. Mobility. *English Oxford Living Dictionaries*. https://en.oxforddictionaries.com/definition/mobility. Updated 2018. Accessed August 22, 2018.
2. Complications from immobility by body system. *LTC Clinical Pearls: Powered by HCPro's Long-Term Care Nursing Library*. http://www.hcpro.com/LTC-286850-10704/Complications-from-immobility-by-body-system.html. Published November 27, 2012. Accessed August 22, 2018.
3. Bombard T. Neurotrauma review series part 3: what's in a dermatome? Nerves can tell us much about spinal cord injuries. *EMS World*. 2014;43(3):46-49.
4. Moore ZE, Cowman S. Repositioning for treating pressure ulcers (review). *Cochrane Database Syst Rev*. 2015;1:1-17. Doi: 10.1002/14651858.CD006898.pub4.
5. Bhattacharya S, Mishra R. Pressure ulcers: current understanding and newer modalities of treatment. *Indian J Plast Surg*. 2015;48(1):4-16. Doi: 10.4103/0970-0358.155260.
6. Are we ready for this change? *Agency for Healthcare Research and Quality*. http://www.ahrq.gov/professionals/systems/hospital/pressureulcertoolkit/putool1.html. Published April 2011. Updated October 2014. Accessed August 27, 2018.
7. Johnson KL, Meyenburg T. Physiological rationale and current evidence for therapeutic positioning of critically ill patients. *AACN Adv Crit Care*. 2009;20(3):228-240.
8. Stavness C. The effect of positioning for children with cerebral palsy on upper-extremity function: a review of the evidence. *Phys Occup Ther Pediatr*. 2006;26(3):39-53.
9. Joint Commission Standards on Restraint and Seclusion/Nonviolent Crisis Intervention Training Program. *Crisis Prevention Institute*. https://www.crisisprevention.com/CPI/media/Media/Resources/alignments/Joint-Commission-Restraint-Seclusion-Alignment-2011.pdf. Published 2009. Reprinted 2010. Accessed August 27, 2018.
10. Physical and chemical restraints: role of the physical therapist HOD P06-03-17-05. *APTA*. https://www.apta.org/uploadedFiles/APTAorg/About_Us/Policies/Practice/PhysicalChemicalRestraints.pdf. Updated August 7, 2012. Accessed August 27, 2018.
11. Zablotny C, Hershbert J, Parlman K. Stroke. *PT Now*. http://ptnow.org/clinical-summaries-detail/stroke-2#Intervention. Published August 11, 2017. Accessed August 27, 2018.
12. De D, Wynn E. Preventing muscular contractures through routine stroke patient care. *Br J Nurs*. 2014;23(14):781-786.
13. Heislein D. Total Hip Arthroplasty (THA). *PT Now*. http://ptnow.org/clinical-summaries-detail/total-hip-arthroplasty-tha. Published June 14, 2016. Accessed August 27, 2018.
14. Peters A, Tijink M, Veldhuijzen A, Huis in 't Veld R. Reduced patient restrictions following total hip arthroplasty: study protocol for a randomized controlled trial. *Trials*. 2015;16(1):1-6. Doi: 10.1186/s13063-015-0901-0.
15. Pelosi P, Brazzi L, Gattinoni L. Prone position in acute respiratory distress syndrome. *Eur Respir J*. 2002;20(4):1017-1028. Doi: 10.1183/09031936.02.00401702.
16. "Contracture." *Taber's Cyclopedia Medical Dictionary*. 20th ed. Philadelphia, PA: FA Davis Company; 2005.

Chapter 4

Vital Signs

KEY TERMS Apnea | Bradycardia | Diaphoresis | Diastolic | Dyspnea | Febrile/pyrexic | Hypertension | Hyperthermia/hyperpyrexia | Hypotension | Hypothermia | Irregular | Korotkoff sounds | Orthopnea | Orthostatic hypotension | Sphygmomanometer | Syncope | Systolic | Tachycardia | Tachypnea | Thready | Valsalva maneuver

KEY ABBREVIATIONS AHA | CHF | COPD | CVA | ECG | MI | mmHg | SOB

CHAPTER OBJECTIVES

1. Be able to accurately measure each vital sign and use the proper unit of measurement.
2. Describe normal and abnormal ranges/measurements for each vital sign.
3. Understand what causes changes in each vital sign and what is normal or abnormal.
4. Describe why it is important to measure pain and how to assess pain.

INTRODUCTION

A patient was in the therapy gym looking rather weak and pale. The therapist checked her oxygen saturation (SpO_2) and discovered it was at 75% (normal is 90% or higher). The therapist immediately contacted the patient's physician, who ordered the patient to immediately be sent to the hospital. In this case, the therapist knew that performing therapy with this patient was not a good idea. The key to making this important decision was her knowledge of the normal parameters for SpO_2 and the ability to competently check that vital sign in the first place.

Therapists interact with a variety of patients who have a variety of diagnoses and comorbidities. Even if you are seeing a patient for a knee replacement, you should also be aware that he or she has a history of a myocardial infarction (MI) and may need his or her heart rate monitored. A patient you are treating for a cerebrovascular accident (CVA) is at risk of having another stroke and will need his or her blood pressure checked regularly. A patient you are treating for acute lower back pain may also be on oxygen and will need his or her SpO_2 or respiratory rate watched closely. In all of these cases, the physical therapy diagnosis may not require vital sign examination; however, the patient is not just a knee replacement, CVA, or lower back pain. The patient is a whole person with a full medical history. Additionally, vital signs often play a role in setting or reaching goals in the plan of care; therefore, they will need to be documented to show progress or lack of it.

HEART RATE

Heart rate, also known as a person's *pulse*, is the measurement of the number of left ventricle contractions per minute. It is recorded as beats per minute (beats/min or bpm) in documentation. According to the American Heart Association (AHA), the at rest heart rate for normal chil-

Memolo J.
Procedures and Patient Care for the Physical Therapist Assistant
(pp 45-61). © 2019 SLACK Incorporated.

Table 4-1
Normal Resting Heart Rate

Adults (over 10 years old and seniors)	60 to 100 beats/min
Infants	100 to 190 beats/min
Children (under 10 years old)	85 to 205 beats/min
Athletes	40 to 60 beats/min

dren (aged 10 years and older) and adults ranges from 60 to 100 beats/min.[1] This includes seniors, as well. Well-trained athletes may range from 40 to 60 beats/min.[1] Infants and small children register higher pulses, 100 to 190 beats/min for the latter and 85 to 205 beats/min for the former (Table 4-1).[2]

Tachycardia means a fast heart rate, with a resting heart rate of 100 beats/min or greater. Bradycardia is a slow heart rate, denoted by a heart rate of 60 beats/min or less (unless the person is a trained athlete). A heartbeat can be described as weak (poor force), strong (good force), regular (even beats), irregular (both strong and weak beats or uneven beats), or thready (a weak and irregular heart rate).

When performing therapy with a patient, it is sometimes necessary to calculate the age-predicted maximum heart rate, which is the patient's age subtracted from 220 (ie, if the patient is 38 years old, it would be $220-38 = 182$). This is the maximum a person's heart rate should get when performing exercise or activities; a heart rate above this number is dangerous. When having your patient perform an activity, you take a percentage of this maximum number and use that as a goal during therapy. For moderate activity, 50% to 69% of that maximum heart rate number is appropriate; for strenuous activity, up to but not exceeding 90% of that maximum heart rate is acceptable.

Common Diagnoses

Common heart diagnoses include MI, heart failure, and aneurysm. Venous or arterial insufficiency can also be common to therapy patients. An MI results when the flow of blood to the heart is blocked, often from an embolus or plaque that develops from a buildup of fat or cholesterol.[3] Oxygen is deprived from the heart muscle and part of the heart muscle dies. Heart muscle cannot regenerate, so the part that dies is forever affected. If the oxygen is deprived for too long or if too much of the muscle is affected, the patient can die. If the patient survives, the heart will be weaker and less efficient.

If your patient complains of tightness or pain in his or her chest, arm, jaw, or back, or if he or she complains of nausea, shortness of breath (SOB), or sudden dizziness or fatigue, he or she may be having a heart attack, and you should call 911 or push a staff emergency button immediately. Be advised that women often manifest the symptoms of MI differently than men, with more complaints of heartburn or nausea.

Heart failure, also known as *congestive heart failure* (CHF), occurs when the heart muscle is not as efficient as it should be.[4] This can be further complicated by narrowed blood vessels (as a result of plaque buildup) or high blood pressure, and the heart becomes weaker and weaker. Compression (wraps or mechanical) is contraindicated for patients with CHF due to the excessive pressure it places on the heart. Coronary artery disease, hypertension, diabetes and obesity can all cause heart failure. Patients can make lifestyle changes, such as increasing exercise and decreasing salt and body weight, to help control symptoms.

An aneurysm is a bulge in an artery, which can result from high blood pressure, genetic conditions, and trauma that damages arterial walls.[5] An aneurysm can grow and eventually burst if not treated, and a rupture can cause bleeding inside the body and possibly death. The aorta, which is the main artery that carries blood from the heart to the body, is the most common place for aneurysms. An aneurysm here can either occur in the thoracic area or the abdominal area. Early diagnosis and treatment can help prevent death, but aneurysms often grow without symptoms. A therapist once treated a patient in supine and noted excessive pulsing in the patient's abdomen. The therapist brought this to the attention of the physician, and subsequent imaging revealed that the patient had a small aneurysm. The patient had no idea prior to this that she had an aneurysm; she was put on medications and a monitoring routine. Patients with known aneurysms may need surgery, as well as medications that lower blood pressure and relax vessels.

Peripheral vascular disease can present as arterial, venous, or lymphatic. Arterial examples include arteriosclerosis obliterans (also known as *arteriosclerotic vascular disease*), Raynaud's phenomenon, and diabetes mellitus. Venous disorders include acute thrombophlebitis, varicose veins, and chronic venous insufficiency. There are several circulation tests that can be conducted including the Buerger-Allen exercises, the Homan's sign (deep vein thrombosis [DVT] test), claudication, and percussion tests (Box 4-1).[6]

Box 4-1

Homan's, Buerger-Allen, and
Venous Circulation Tests

- Homan's sign (DVT test): grasp the patient's lower extremity and lightly squeeze the calf muscle while simultaneously dorsiflexing the foot (passively). If the patient reports pain with this activity, the patient may have a DVT.

- Percussion test (assesses function of valves in saphenous vein): the patient stands and the caregiver palpates proximal saphenous vein with the fingers of one hand while tapping the distal segment of the vein. If the valves are not functioning, movement of fluid is detected by the proximal fingers. Test bilaterally.

- Buerger-Allen exercises (arterial insufficiency test): (1) lower extremities are elevated 45 to 60 degrees and supported in this position until the skin becomes pale (about 1 minute). A rapid loss of color is abnormal. (2) Patients sit in a relaxed position with feet and legs dangling off edge of chair/bed while performing ankle dorsiflexion/plantar flexion and supination/pronation until color appears. If it takes more than 30 seconds and if the color is red vs pink, this is abnormal. (3) Patients lie quietly for 5 minutes with both legs supported on the bed and with a warm blanket over the legs for 2 minutes.

- Claudication (arterial insufficiency test): patient walks on treadmill at 1 mile/hour until claudication occurs (calf pain with ambulation). Record the time elapsed before pain in the calf is reported and requires ambulation to stop.

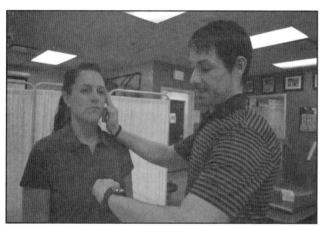

Figure 4-1. Temporal site.

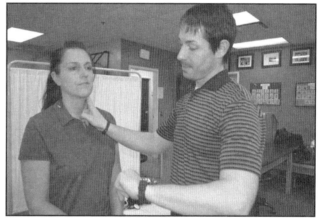

Figure 4-2. Carotid site.

Assessment

You should be aware of the various locations for heart rate assessment. The 2 most common are the radial artery or the carotid artery. Figures 4-1 through 4-8 show the various locations for taking a heart rate, and Box 4-2 describes of the various locations for taking a heart rate with descriptions of locations. These include brachial, dorsal pedal, femoral, popliteal and temporal. Sometimes you will need to locate the pulse in the distal extremities to assess distal circulation. In most cases, however, you will use the radial or carotid arteries to assess pulse. To locate the radial artery, palpate the radial styloid at the base of the thumb and then move your fingers just medial. You will feel a dip after rolling your fingers over the bone. Here you should be able to locate the pulse easily. To locate the carotid artery, slide your fingers down the length of the jaw about 2 inches, starting at the base of the ear. Then slide the fingers just inferior to the jaw bone, anterior to the sternocleidomastoid muscle, and you should feel the carotid pulse.

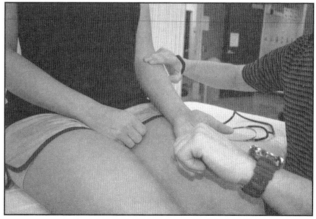

Figure 4-3. Brachial site.

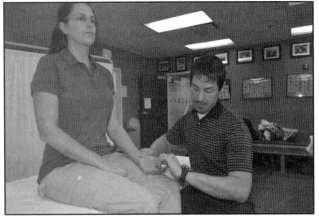

Figure 4-4. Radial site.

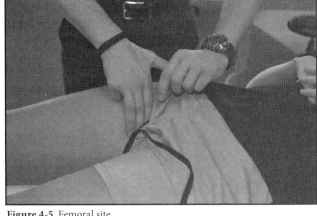

Figure 4-5. Femoral site.

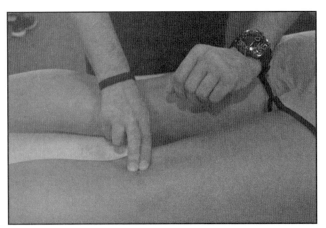

Figure 4-6. Popliteal site.

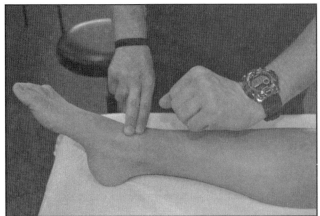

Figure 4-7. Dorsal pedal site.

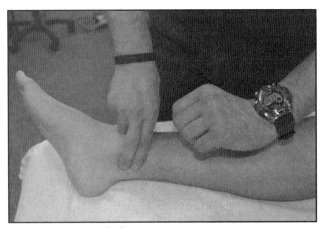

Figure 4-8. Posterior tibial site.

Box 4-2

Descriptions of Pulse Measurement Sites

- Temporal: anterior and adjacent to ear
- Carotid: inferior to angle of jaw and anterior to sternocleidomastoid
- Brachial: medial to biceps in antecubital fossa/medial aspect of midshaft of humerus
- Radial: at wrist on volar forearm and medial to stylus process of radius
- Femoral: at femoral triangle lateral and anterior to inguinal crease
- Popliteal: midline of posterior knee between tendons of hamstrings
- Dorsal pedal: along midline or medial to dorsum of foot
- Posterior tibial: on medial aspect of foot inferior to medial malleolus

Box 4-3

Steps to Measure a Patient's Pulse

1. Wash hands, gather the equipment, and explain the procedure to the patient.

2. Select palpation site, and palpate with the first 2 fingers. Avoid excessive pressure on the artery, and do not use your thumb.

3. Count the beats silently. Measuring for 1 full minute will eliminate error; if you measure for 30 seconds, multiply by 2; if you measure for 10 seconds, multiply by 6. Be aware that the smaller increment of time you measure, the more room for error there is.

4. Record in beats/min, and also note rhythm and volume.

Table 4-2
Factors That Affect Heart Rate

Age	Increased age = decreased heart rate
Sex	Women more than Men
Anxiety/stress	Increased stress = increased heart rate
Environmental temperature	Increased temperature = increased heart rate
Exercise	Increased activity = increased heart rate
Infection	Increased temperature (fever) = increased heart rate
Medications/ disease processes	Varies with medication or disease processes

Box 4-4

Abnormal Heart Rate Responses to Exercise

- Heart rate slowly increasing with exercise
- Heart rate not increasing with exercise
- Heart rate not decreasing after exercise has stopped
- Heart rate declining with exercise
- Heart rate increasing more than expected with exercise
- Heart rhythm or volume changing with exercise

When taking the heart rate, you should first gather your equipment, which is a watch with a second hand or some other time-taking device that allows you to count in seconds. You need to also wash your hands before and after taking the patient's heart rate to follow infection-control protocol. Select the site you plan to check the pulse and palpate over the artery with the first 2 fingers of your hand (pointer and middle fingers). Do not use your thumb, as you will only feel your own pulse rather than your patient's. Do not press too hard, or you will occlude the blood flow and feel nothing. Count the beats in your head silently, the goal being to ascertain how many beats occurred in a minute (60 seconds).[7] You can count beats for 10 seconds and multiply by 6, or you can count for 15 seconds and multiply by 4, or you can count for 30 seconds and multiply by 2.[7] The less seconds you count for, the larger the margin of error in your calculations (ie, counting by 10 and multiplying by 6 is a 6 beats/min margin of error, whereas counting for 30 seconds and multiplying by 2 is only a 2 beats/min margin of error). Make sure to note the rhythm and volume of the heart beat as well as the number of beats in the minute. Box 4-3 includes step-by-step instructions on measuring a patient's pulse.

What Affects Heart Rate?

There are various conditions and factors that can affect a person's heart rate. There are also abnormal heart rate responses to exercise that clinicians should be aware of in order to avoid patient injury or emergency.

Age will affect heart rate; typically the older the patient, the lower the heart rate. This is evident when you look at the normal resting heart rate ranges for different age groups; infants and small children have higher heart rates and the number decreases as age increases. A person's sex also affects heart rate, as women tend to have a higher heart rate than men. Factors such as increased anxiety or stress can make heart rate increase, and exercise will also increase heart rate. Environmental temperature has a direct effect on heart rate; the higher the temperature, the higher the heart rate. If a person has an infection, which often results in a fever, heart rate increases. Finally, certain medications and disease processes will affect heart rate. For example, a patient who has a pacemaker will have his or her heart rate set at a certain range, and it should stay within that range. Table 4-2 includes a list of factors that affect a person's heart rate.

While it is normal for a person's heart rate to increase with exercise, there are some abnormal heart rate responses to exercise. These include the heart rate slowly increasing or not increasing with exercise, the heart rate not decreasing after exercise has stopped, a decline in heart rate with exercise, the heart rate increasing more than expected with exercise, or the heart rhythm or volume changing with exercise. Box 4-4 includes a list of abnormal heart rate responses to exercise.

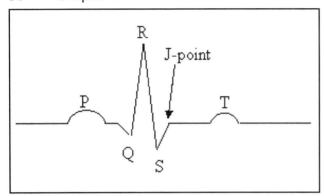

Figure 4-9. An electrical event in an ECG.

S - shortness
O - of
B - Breath

Electrocardiogram Changes

While it is not necessary for a physical therapist assistant to know all the ins and outs of an electrocardiogram (ECG), it is helpful to know what is normal and abnormal. An ECG evaluates the electrical activity of the heart, and an electrocardiograph is the printable representation of that activity.[8] A patient may receive an ECG to find the cause of chest pain, to evaluate potential heart-related problems such as SOB, to identify irregular heartbeats, to determine the overall health of the heart, to see how a pacemaker is performing, or to get a baseline of heart function.

There are certain parts of the ECG that are worth noting. The P wave is the depolarization of the myocardial cells in the atria, initiated by the SA (sinoatrial) node, and it is the first signal on the ECG. The QRS complex is the depolarization of the myocardial cells in the ventricles, and coincides with the repolarization of the cells in the atria. The J point is the end of the QRS complex and the beginning of the ST segment. The T wave is the repolarization of the myocardial cells in the ventricles. The amplitude of the electrical signal is measured on the vertical in millivolts (mV) and the time is measured on the horizontal in milliseconds.[9]

One can measure a person's heart rate on the ECG, as well as measure the time it takes for certain intervals to occur, such as the PR interval and the QT interval. A clinician also looks for changes in rhythm, frequency, and conduction time. Any variation from the normal picture of an ECG indicates something could be wrong.[9] Figure 4-9 includes a picture of an electrical event in an ECG.

RESPIRATORY RATE

Respiratory rate is the measurement of either a person's inspiration (taking in a breath) or expiration (exhaling a breath), but not both. Per the AHA, the normal respiratory rate for an adult is 12 to 16 breaths per minute (breaths/min). The rate increases as age decreases; infants are 30 to 60 breaths/min, and school-aged children are 18 to 30 breaths/min (Table 4-3).

Table 4-3 Normal Resting Respiratory Rate	
Infants	30 to 60 breaths/min
Children	18 to 30 breaths/min
Adults	12 to 16 breaths/min

Just as with heart rate, there are several terms associated with respiratory rate. Dyspnea is difficulty with breathing or SOB. Apnea is the absence of breathing; you may have heard of sleep apnea, when patients temporarily stop breathing during the night and wake up as a result. Orthopnea is difficulty breathing when recumbent; these patients require their head of bed to be raised, and often at home they will tell you they sleep in the recliner. Tachypnea is rapid breathing, typically greater than 20 breaths/min.

Common Diagnoses

There are several common diagnoses associated with the respiratory system, and as a clinician you should be aware of what these are and how they present. Typically, diseases can be categorized into being either obstructive or restrictive. Obstructive diseases are characterized by having a decreased amount of air that can be exhaled from the lungs due to a narrowing or blockage. This, in turn, decreases how much air can be inhaled. Chronic obstructive pulmonary disease (COPD) is an example of an obstructive disease. Chronic obstructive pulmonary disease is a combination of bronchitis and emphysema, and symptoms include a chronic, productive cough, dyspnea, abnormal breath sounds, and apical breathing patterns. Asthma is another obstructive disease, characterized by bronchospasms that result in wheezing, dyspnea, and apical breathing patterns. Cystic Fibrosis is also obstructive, in that the exocrine gland increases the amount and viscosity of lung secretions. These secretions will obstruct the airways unless removed, often via positioning and percussion techniques, and if not removed, the patient will essentially drown.

Restrictive diseases are characterized by having a decreased amount of air being taken in due to poor lung expansion or volume. Diseases include pneumonia, tuberculosis, postural deviations such as kyphosis or scoliosis, or tumors/cancer. Patients with restrictive illnesses present with dyspnea, nonproductive coughs, fatigue, tachypnea, crackles, digital clubbing or cyanosis, and decreased chest wall expansion.

Assessment

When preparing to assess respiratory rate, one should attempt to keep the patient uninformed about what you are measuring. If you tell a patient that you are measuring his or her breathing, the patient may likely change the rate

Box 4-5

Steps for Measuring Respiratory Rate

1. Wash hands, and gather equipment.

2. Do not explain the procedure to the patient to avoid inaccurate results; observe the patient for overt signs of breathing difficulty.

3. Simulate the measurement of the radial pulse while resting the arm on the thorax or abdomen; alternately, rest on patient's shoulder.

4. Count either inspirations or expirations, ideally for 1 full minute to eliminate error; otherwise, count for 30 seconds and multiply by 2.

5. Document as breaths/min, and note also rhythm, depth, and character of respirations.

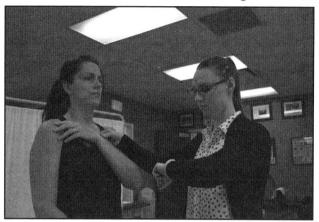

Figure 4-10. Taking a patient's respiratory rate.

Table 4-4 Factors That Affect Respiratory Rate	
Age	Increased age = decreased respiratory rate
Body size/ stature	Obese or kyphotic postures = increased respiratory rate
Exercise	Increased exercise = increased respiratory rate
Positioning	Supine = increased respiratory rate
Disease processes	COPD, asthma, pneumonia (varies with disease processes)

or rhythm of breathing. Instead, it is easiest to tell patients that you are checking their heart rate and then check their respiratory rate instead.

As with heart rate, wash your hands and have access to a watch with a second hand. Simulate taking a patient's heart rate at the radial location and hold the patient's arm against his or her chest. Measure either the inspirations or the expirations, and to be most accurate, measure for at least 30 seconds and multiply by 2. Alternatively, you can place a hand on the patient's shoulder or chest. As with heart rate, the fewer seconds you measure respiratory rate, the less accurate the measurement will be. Respiratory rate is documented as breaths/min, and it is important to also note the depth, rhythm, and character of the respirations. Rhythm is the regularity of the breaths, depth is the amount of air exchanged with each breath, and the character includes deviations from the normal. Abnormal or adventitious breath sounds can be categorized by several terms. Rales, or crackles, are sharp bursts of sound heard on inspiration. These are common in patients with asthma, bronchitis, interstitial lung disease, and early CHF. Pleural rubs sound like brushing or creaking and are heard both during inspiration and expiration. These can be heard in patients with pneumothorax or pleural effusion. Wheezes are described as musical and are most often heard during expiration; rhonchi sound like snorting or gurgling and can be heard during inspiration and expiration. Patients with asthma, chronic bronchitis, CHF, and pulmonary edema often have wheezes or rhonchi. Stridor is also musical in nature and is an inspiratory wheeze, suggesting a blockage in the trachea or larynx; this is a medical emergency. Box 4-5 gives the step-by-step instructions for measuring respiratory rate. Figure 4-10 includes a picture of assessing respiratory rate.

What Affects Respiratory Rate?

There are several factors that affect respiratory rate (Table 4-4). As with heart rate, an increase in age is correlated to a decrease in respiratory rate. Body size and stature also affect respiration; people who are obese often have higher respiratory rates, as do people with kyphotic postures, especially in the thoracic spine (while sitting adopt a kyphotic posture and attempt a deep breath. It is hard to do!). Exercise increases respiratory rate, and positioning, such as supine position, increases respiratory rate due to the effects of gravity. As already discussed, certain diseases such as COPD, asthma, and pneumonia can affect respiratory rate.

If your patient's respiratory rate does not increase with exercise, is slow to decrease after exercise concludes, or is irregular in rate or rhythm during or after exercise, these are points of concern and should be noted in both your documentation as well as your communication with your supervising physical therapist and the nursing or other medical staff.

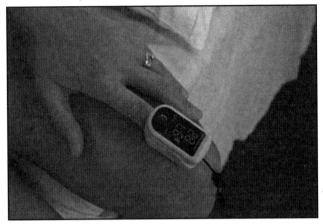

Figure 4-11. A pulse oximeter.

OXYGEN SATURATION

Oxygen saturation is a method by which clinicians can measure how much oxygen is in the blood (Figure 4-11). Normally, red blood cells carry oxygen to all of the internal organs and throughout the rest of the body. People obviously need oxygen to stay alive, so this is an important measurement. For this measurement, clinicians typically use a pulse oximeter. These come in all sizes and they also often measure heart rate as well. For more accurate readings, a patient may have blood drawn to assess his or her arterial blood gas, but this is a test physical therapist assistants do not do.

Normal SpO_2 should range from 95% to 100%. Oxygen saturation is not affected by age, as heart rate, blood pressure, and respiratory rate may be. Measurements are documented in percentages, but are often referred to as SpO_2 (eg, a physical therapist's goal may read: "maintain $SpO_2 >$ 98%").[10]

Assessment

Wash your hands and make sure the pulse oximeter has been cleaned with an alcohol wipe. Place the oximeter over the patient's fingertip, often the forefinger or the ring finger. There are versions that clip on the earlobe. If a patient has finger nail polish, you may need to remove this, as the polish could interfere with the oximeter's ability to read the SpO_2.[10] Other factors such as lighting or temperature can affect the reading as well.[10] If the patient has poor circulation or cold hands, the reading may not be accurate.[10] The patient will wear the oximeter for a few seconds to let it measure the SpO_2 and heart rate. Patients can wear these throughout treatment sessions to monitor saturation, and these are often used to not only assess for safety concerns but also for goal achievement. Box 4-6 includes the step-by-step instructions for measuring SpO_2.

What Affects Oxygen Saturation?

Certain factors can affect SpO_2. As mentioned earlier, simple things like nail polish, bright lighting, or temperature can cause the readings to be inaccurate. Also, many disease processes can affect the readings; since oximeters measure the amount of oxygen in the blood, any pulmonary or cardiovascular disease can cause the saturation to be low. Exercise can make a patient's SpO_2 drop, especially at initiation of activity, unless or until they become acclimated to that activity. Patients who live higher elevation areas may have a lower SpO_2. If the patient has poor circulation to the measurement site, the readings could be inaccurate; these patients include those with hypotension, hypothermia, or vasoconstriction. Patients with cardiac arrhythmias may not have accurate readings, as well as those with jaundice or deeply pigmented skin.

BLOOD PRESSURE

Blood pressure is noted by 2 numbers, known as the *systolic number* (the top number) and the *diastolic number* (the bottom number). The systolic number measures the pressure in your blood vessels when your heart beats. The diastolic number indicates the pressure in your vessels between beats, or when your heart rests. Blood pressure is measured using a stethoscope and a sphygmomanometer (blood pressure cuff), and the unit of measurement is millimeters of mercury (mmHg).

The Centers for Disease Control and Prevention and the AHA define normal adult resting blood pressure as less than 120/80 mmHg.[11] Unlike heart rate and respiratory rate, blood pressure tends to get higher with age. Infants range between 72 to 104 for systolic and 37 to 56 for diastolic, while children tend to range from 97 to 120 for systolic and 57 to 80 for diastolic. The AHA recently updated its blood pressure guidelines.[12]

If a patient has hypertension, his or her blood pressure is high. Per the AHA, elevated blood pressure begins at 120 to 129 for systolic and less than 80 for diastolic. Stage 1 hypertension is 130 to 139 for systolic and 80 to 89 for diastolic, stage 2 is greater than 140 for systolic and 90 for diastolic, and hypertensive crisis is defined as anything greater than 180 for systolic and 120 for diastolic. There are various causes for hypertension, but the most common include a decrease of elasticity in the blood vessels and/or a buildup of plaque in the arteries that narrow the vessels. Table 4-5 includes the updated numbers for blood pressure categories.

Hypotension is low blood pressure and is generally represented by a blood pressure reading of less than 90/60 mmHg.[13] There are various causes for hypotension, including dehydration, pregnancy, heart valve problems, endocrine problems, medications, infection, and malnutrition.

Orthostatic hypotension is a sudden drop in blood pressure as a result of position change. The Mayo Clinic[14] defines orthostatic hypotension as a drop of 20 mmHg in the systolic blood pressure or a drop of 10 mmHg in the diastolic blood pressure within 2 to 5 minutes of standing up, or if standing causes signs and symptoms of orthostatic hypotension. A patient who has been in bed for several days, for example, and then decides to get up (possibly due to therapy asking him or her to sit up), may suffer a drop in blood pressure. This can result in a minor symptom of dizziness, or it could result in a more significant problem of losing consciousness. It is normal for anyone's blood pressure to temporarily drop with a positional change, but for patients who suffer from orthostatic hypotension, the heart is unable to pump the blood fast enough to recover, blood (and oxygen) does not get to the brain, and dizziness or loss of consciousness results. Again, patients who are pregnant, dehydrated, on beta blockers, or who have been on prolonged bed rest can suffer from this problem.

Think of the last time you had to pick up something heavy, perhaps a box of books or a large piece of furniture. When you went to lift this heavy item, did you hold your breath? Likewise, think about a time you needed to pop your ears. You probably held your nose and blew out, as if trying to blow up a balloon, to make your ears pop. The Valsalva maneuver is when a person forcefully expires against a closed glottis, which in turn temporarily increases intrathoracic and intra-abdominal pressure and affects venous return, cardiac output, and heart rate.[15] This pressure increases until the breath is released, which causes a sudden drop in the intrathoracic pressure. A sudden increase in cardiac output and aortic pressure results from this, and these changes in cardiac output can affect blood pressure. Blood pressure will initially rise and then drop. A sudden drop in blood pressure can cause syncope (fainting).

The Valsalva maneuver can be done on purpose, such as the example of popping one's ears, or it can be done unintentionally, as in the example of moving something heavy. In therapy, therapists note this most often when patients are performing a task that is difficult or requires strain. Patients will hold their breath while performing a leg lift

Table 4-5
Normal Resting Blood Pressure

Infants	72 to 104/37 to 56 mmHg
Children	97 to 120/57 to 80 mmHg
Adults	Less than 120/80 mmHg
Elevated	120 to 129/less than 80 mmHg
Hypertension stage 1	130 to 139/80 to 89 mmHg
Hypertension stage 2	Greater than 140/greater than 90 mmHg
Hypertensive crisis	Greater than 180/120 mmHg

or when doing core exercises. The therapist should cue the patient to breathe during his or her activity in order to avoid this change in intrathoracic pressure.

Common Diagnoses

There are several diagnoses that can cause high or low blood pressure. As mentioned previously, high blood pressure is often caused by a hardening or narrowing of the arteries. Atherosclerotic cardiovascular disease is the hardening and thickening of the arteries due to the buildup of fat and cholesterol in the vessels, which makes the vessels lose elasticity and become narrow. The less elastic and the narrower the vessels, the higher the blood pressure. Aneurysm, which was mentioned earlier in the Heart Rate section, can often be the result of hypertension, and a rupture could lead to death if untreated. Arteriosclerosis obliterans is the occlusion of arteries, especially those supplying blood to the extremities, again due to the buildup of plaque.

Assessment

Figure 4-12 illustrates how to take a person's blood pressure. Box 4-7 includes the step-by-step instructions. First, you must wash your hands and gather your equipment. You will need a stethoscope and a sphygmomanometer (blood pressure cuff), as well as alcohol wipes to clean the equipment before and after use. You should position your patient so that the upper extremity you are using to measure is resting and relaxed; ideally, the patient is seated and the upper extremity is supported. Typically, blood pressure is taken in the left upper extremity, unless there is cause to do otherwise. Reasons to not take blood pressure in an extremity would include the patient having an intravenous drip; a shunt, such as for dialysis; if the patient has had surgery on that extremity or lymph nodes removed on that side, such as with a mastectomy; or if the patient has had a CVA or stroke and the left upper extremity is affected.[16] In those cases you would use the right upper extremity, and it is also possible to take blood pressure in the lower extremity.

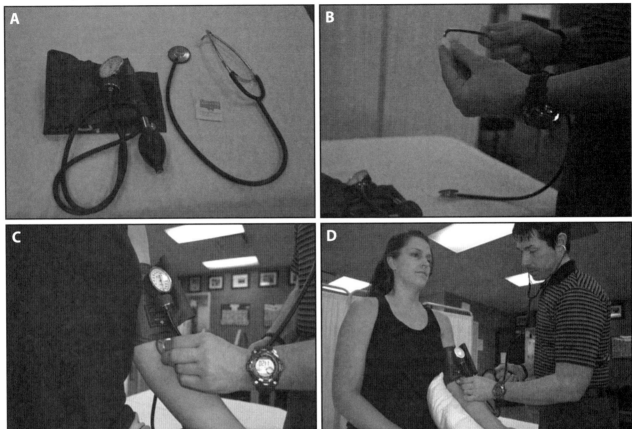

Figure 4-12. The steps for taking a patient's blood pressure.

Box 4-7

Steps to Measure a Patient's Blood Pressure

1. Wash your hands, and collect the equipment. This includes a stethoscope, a sphygmomanometer, and alcohol wipes if assessing blood pressure manually.

2. Clean the equipment.

3. Have the patient sit quietly for at least 5 minutes prior to assessing blood pressure; the patient should be seated with the (left) upper extremity supported on the table or other surface, approximately at the heart level.

4. Remove clothing in the area prior to applying the cuff; the cuff should be placed approximately 1 inch superior to the antecubital space and such that the gauge can be easily seen and read.

5. Determine the inflation number via palpation of the radial pulse while inflating the cuff to 70 to 80 mmHg, and then continue to inflate until the radial pulse is not palpable. Continue to inflate to 30 mmHg above the number at which you can no longer palpate the radial pulse.

6. Deflate the cuff, and have the patient wait 30 to 60 seconds.

7. Place the stethoscope bell over the brachial artery, and listen for the pulse; then reinflate the cuff to the number that was 30 mmHg over the number at which the radial pulse was not palpable.

8. Listen for the Korotkoff sounds, and note the readings for the systolic and diastolic number.

9. Record as mmHg, as well as the patient position and extremity used. Clean the supplies after the assessment.

	Table 4-6 Korotkoff Sounds	
K1	First tapping sound heard (systolic)	
K2	Sounds softer and longer and swishing sound	
K3	Sounds crisper and louder	
K4	Sounds muffled and softer	
K5	Sounds disappear (last sound is diastolic)	

Table 4-7 Factors That Affect Blood Pressure	
Artery diameter/ elasticity	The less elastic, the higher the blood pressure. The narrower the artery, the higher the blood pressure.
Exercise	Increased exercise = increased blood pressure
Age	Increased age = increased blood pressure
Positioning	Prolonged recumbent positions = orthostatic blood pressure If patient is supine, blood pressure may be higher than if seated.
Emotion/ stress	Increased anxiety or stress = increased blood pressure

The blood pressure cuff should be the correct size for the patient; there are different sizes for infants, children, adults, and those who are obese. Clean the cuff, ear tips, and diaphragm of the stethoscope. The cuff should be positioned on the upper extremity at heart level, just superior to (about 1 inch above) the antecubital space. This will occlude the brachial artery. The cuff should be tight enough to stay in place, but know that inflating it will make it tighter. If you have not taken the patient's blood pressure before, there is a method to determine the amount of pressure needed to occlude the brachial artery and aids in avoiding over inflation of the cuff. Palpate the radial pulse. While monitoring the pulse, inflate the cuff rapidly to 70 to 80 mmHg. Inflate the cuff in increments of 10 mmHg until the radial pulse is no longer palpable. Continue to inflate the cuff to a measurement that is 30 mmHg above the pressure where the pulse was last palpated; this will be the highest level the cuff should be inflated when taking the actual blood pressure.[17]

Now deflate the cuff, and wait 30 to 60 seconds. Place the stethoscope bell over the brachial artery, and listen for the pulse. Then slowly inflate the cuff while listening for the pulse to disappear. This is when you will stop inflating the cuff.[18]

Slowly deflate the cuff; watch the gauge on the sphygmomanometer to ensure you get an accurate reading. Your readings will be based on Korotkoff sounds. As you inflate the cuff, you occlude the artery. Then, as you slowly release the pressure, the blood flow resumes. The Korotkoff sounds are the tapping or thumping sounds one hears as the cuff is deflated.[18] There are 5 phases, as indicated in Table 4-6; for your purposes, you will need to pay attention to the first tapping sound and the last sound. The first sound is the first clear tap heard as the cuff is deflated. This is often the time when you hear the pulse again in the stethoscope and is defined as the systolic number. The diastolic number is noted when the last audible sound is heard, or just before the pulse completely disappears because blood flow has fully resumed.

Do not round your numbers up or down; record the exact numbers you note when you hear the first and last sounds.

After taking your reading, fully deflate the cuff and remove it. Follow up by cleaning your equipment again.

What Affects Blood Pressure?

There are several factors that can affect blood pressure (Table 4-7). As mentioned earlier in regards to artery diameter and elasticity, there is an indirect relationship between elasticity and diameter and blood pressure readings. The more narrow the vessel, the higher the pressure. Likewise, the less elastic the vessel, the higher the pressure. As with heart rate and respiratory rate, exercise can cause blood pressure to rise, and changes are most often seen in the systolic number. Blood pressure tends to increase with age, often due to a correlated decrease in exercise/activity and poor dietary habits. Prolonged recumbent positions can cause orthostatic hypotension when patients begin to change positions. If the patient is supine, the blood pressure reading may be higher than in seated, and if the extremity being tested is dependent, the blood pressure reading will be higher. Fear, anxiety, stress, and pain can increase blood pressure readings as well.

There are abnormal responses that a person should be attentive to. A slow or no increase of the systolic number with exercise is not normal. Neither the systolic nor diastolic numbers should decrease with exercise. Likewise, the systolic number should not decrease with exercise in normal situations. During exercise, if the diastolic number increases by more than 10 mmHg, this should be of concern.

Table 4-8
Normal Body Temperature

Normal	97.8°F to 99°F
Febrile	Greater than 99°F

Table 4-10
Factors That Affect Temperature

Time of day	Circadian rhythm = decreased temperature in the morning and increased in the evening
Illnesses	Infections or illness = increased body temperature
Food/fluid consumption	Warm foods and smoking = increased oral temperature readings
Exercise	Increased exercise = increased body temperature
Environment	Increased temperature outside = increased body temperature
Pregnancy/ menstruation	Both = increased body temperature

Table 4-9
Locations to Take Temperature

Ear	More accurate
Rectal	Considered most accurate
Axillary	Least accurate (0.5°F to 1.0°F below rectal, ear, and temporal)
Temporal	More accurate
Oral	Most common but not always as accurate (0.5°F to 1.0°F below rectal, ear, and temporal)

TEMPERATURE

Temperature can be read in degrees of Fahrenheit or Celsius. Normal body temperature ranges from 97.8°F to 99°F for a healthy adult. Hypothermia is a low body temperature, noted by being less than 94°F. Hyperthermia (also known as *hyperpyrexia*) is too high a body temperature, noted as greater than 106°F. If a patient is febrile, that means they have a fever (or temperature greater than 99°F). A patient with a fever could also be described as pyrexic. Normal body temperature ratings are listed in Table 4-8.

Assessment

Wash your hands, and gather your equipment. There are a variety of tools to assess body temperature, such as mercury glass thermometers, ear or oral electronic thermometers, or a temporal lobe thermometer. Glass thermometers are not commonly used anymore due to the hazards of mercury if the glass breaks. Most clinics use one of the electronic forms of assessment. These have probes on the tips that either measure the temperature inside the mouth or ear canal or on the temporal lobe of the patient.

There is a variety of locations to take temperature, and some are considered more accurate than others (Table 4-9).

The 2 most common locations are the mouth and ear. Ear thermometers are popular for use with pediatric patients, as young children have difficulty holding a thermometer in their mouths long enough to get an accurate reading. Temporal lobe thermometers are also popular with the pediatric community. Other locations to check temperature include the axilla and rectum. The rectum is often used for young children and infants because it is considered the most accurate location for a temperature reading. It is also, however, the most uncomfortable. The axilla is considered the least accurate location, and is often not used. It is important in your documentation that you include the site used for temperature measurement as well as the type of thermometer used.

What Affects Temperature?

Various factors can affect temperature (Table 4-10). The time of day the measurement is taken can affect the reading because the circadian rhythm causes a slight decrease in temperature in the mornings and an increase in the evenings. Parents with sick children know this to be true; fevers are always worse at night. Food or fluid consumption can affect the reading, as warm foods, drinks, or smoking can make an oral temperature reading high. One should wait at least 15 minutes after smoking, eating, or drinking before taking a temperature if one is doing so orally. Exercise can increase internal temperature due to the increased metabolic rate. The environment, too, can affect temperature readings; readings may be higher on hot days. Pregnancy or menstruation can increase body temperature, as can various infections and disease processes. A higher body temperature is one of the first indicators that an infection is present.

It is normal for temperature to increase with exercise, but it should decrease as activity decreases. Body temperature that does not increase or decreases during activity is abnormal.

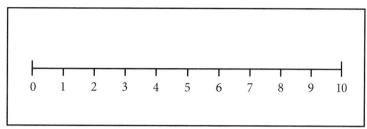

Figure 4-13. Numeric pain rating scale.

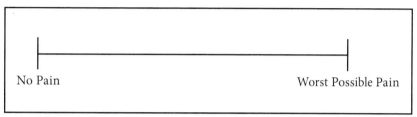

Figure 4-14. Visual analog scale.

PAIN ASSESSMENT

Pain is often called the fifth vital sign, although health care providers have begun to debate the validity of this title. A patient's pain is a major factor in how well they perform tasks in a therapy setting, and so, whether or not you classify pain as another vital sign, it is important to assess. There are various methods for assessing pain. Of course, the goal is for the patient to have no pain, or at least less pain, but measurement of pain can give an indication of what the patient can tolerate and can also be a means to show progress (or lack of it) if it is a part of the goals set by your supervising physical therapist. For example, the physical therapist might set a goal that the patient will be able to perform his or her seated lower extremity exercises x 15 reps each, with a pain rating no greater than a 4/10.

Recently, the opioid epidemic has been an issue of major concern. As doctors, therapists, and other health care workers began asking more about pain, the number of prescriptions for opioids also increased. According to the Centers for Disease Control and Prevention, prescriptions for opioids increased dramatically from 2006 to 2010 and then tapered off; however, the supply of prescription opioids is still high in the United States, and 1 in 5 patients with pain-related diagnoses are prescribed opioids in doctors' offices.[19] As a result, opioid addiction (including both prescribed medications as well as illegal drugs such as heroin) has become a widespread problem, and the American Physical Therapy Association launched a campaign in June of 2016 to endorse the use of physical therapy as an alternative to opioid medications.[20] While it is important to acknowledge a patient's pain and record ratings in documentation, physical therapist assistants can encourage patients to look beyond prescriptions to control or manage pain.

Assessment

The most common way to assess pain is via the numeric pain rating scale, which is measured on a 0 to 10 scale (Figure 4-13). A rating of 0 indicates no pain, and a 10 indicates the worst pain the patient has ever felt. Some patients have a difficult time assigning numbers to their pain, however, and a more simple visual analog scale can be used (Figure 4-14). This is simply a line that goes from "no distress" to "unbearable distress," and a person makes a mark along the line that indicates how bad his or her pain is at the time. There are various forms of graphic or faces pain rating scales, which show a series of faces or images ranging from smiling (no hurt), to slightly frowning (hurts even more), to a crying face (hurts worst). There are also more complex and detailed scales that do more than assign a number or rating to the pain. These scales attempt to get at what the pain actually feels like, how often it occurs, what prompts the pain, and what makes the pain feel better. The McGill Pain Questionnaire is an example of this type of assessment, which provides descriptive words for the pain (such as pounding, cutting, scalding, or aching) and also asks what exacerbates the pain. A numerical rating is calculated based on the patient's responses, but it does provide more detail than a simple 0 to 10 pain rating. Even if you do not use a complex scale such as the McGill Pain Questionnaire, it is worthwhile to assess more than the severity of the pain. Discussing onset, location, severity, as well as what alleviates the pain will help you better educate the patient on pain management and avoid exacerbations if possible. If, for example, you know that the patient's pain increases with his or her wound care treatment, you may suggest the patient premedicate (take pain medication prior to the treatment session) so he or she can better tolerate the intervention.

Box 4-8
Assessment of Pain

- Pain onset
- Duration of pain
- What makes it worse or better (movement, time of day, medications, exercises/activities)
- Exact location of pain
- Whether pain radiates or spreads
- What activities of daily living or social activities are affected by pain
- Results of pain questionnaire or pain scale rating

Table 4-11
Factors That Affect Pain

Medications	Pain medications = decreased pain temporarily
Emotions	Increased stress or anxiety = increased perception of pain
Activity/exercise	Increased activity or exercise = exacerbated pain

---

The important issue to consider when asking patients about their pain is clear communication. You need to be able to clearly verbalize or demonstrate what the scale is and how the pain is rated. Simply asking the patient, "what is your pain?" is too general, and asking, "on a scale of 0 to 10, what is your pain?" is only slightly less vague. You need to explain what the numbers mean in order for your patients to give you the most accurate rating. Additionally, you should consider the cognitive status of your patients and select a pain rating scale that is appropriate for their level of understanding, taking into consideration whether they are visual, verbal, or literate (English or otherwise).

Also know that pain is a subjective issue. You may ask one patient, who has just had abdominal surgery, about her pain, and she tells you it is a 3 or 4 out of 10. Maybe her pain medications are effective, or maybe she just has a high threshold for pain. On the other hand, you may see a patient who is sitting comfortably watching television. When you ask what his pain is, he tells you it is a 10 out of 10. Perhaps he does not understand the scale and you need to reeducate him, or perhaps he has a low threshold for pain. Box 4-8 includes how one conducts a general assessment of pain.

What Affects Pain?

There are several factors that can affect a patient's pain level and his or her perception of pain (Table 4-11). As previously mentioned, a patient's pain rating is highly subjective. No 2 people will report their pain as the same, even if they both have the same diagnosis or procedure and the same physician. The medications your patient is taking will also affect his or her pain. If a patient just took a pain pill 30 minutes prior to coming to physical therapy, his or her pain rating might be less than if he or she had not taken anything for pain. A patient's emotions or stress level can also affect perception or rating of pain; the more stressed or worried a patient is, the higher the pain rating might be. Bear in mind that activity may exacerbate pain. A patient may rate his or her pain at a 2/10 at rest, but that rating

climbs to 8/10 with activity. This does not mean that you should not have the patient perform his or her exercises; however, it does mean that the patient may need to take rest breaks, may need to premedicate in preparation for therapy, or may need a pain-controlling intervention as a part of his or her therapy (such as a transcutaneous electrical nerve stimulation unit or an ice pack).

SAFETY/RED FLAGS

Vital signs are a therapist's way to determine that a patient is appropriate for therapeutic interventions and a means to assess that patient's response to the interventions. As it is unlikely that you will encounter many patients without comorbidities, monitoring vital signs allows the physical therapist to determine if the patient is achieving goals while also avoiding exacerbation of those comorbidities.

A patient with a history of heart disease or MI should be carefully monitored during therapy sessions. As mentioned earlier in the Heart Rate section, patients who demonstrate or complain of nausea, dizziness, chest pain, or arm or jaw pain, should cease therapy immediately and be placed in a safe and comfortable position while vitals are monitored. It may be necessary to call a staff emergency or call 911, especially if the pain worsens or the patient loses consciousness. Refer to Chapter 12 for additional information on how to handle emergencies, including the use of an automated external defibrillator or basic life support/cardiopulmonary resuscitation.

Often, clinicians can note a patient's breath sounds. Typically, auscultation (listening via a stethoscope) of the lungs happens in a respiratory evaluation, although sometimes a clinician can hear these sounds without the use of a stethoscope. If you note any new or changing breath sounds, you should document these, as well as alert your supervising physical therapist and the nursing staff. Figure 4-15 includes common posterior locations for auscultation of breath sounds, and Table 4-12 incudes descriptions of breath sounds.

As with the patient example provided at the beginning of the chapter, it is significant if the patient's SpO_2 is

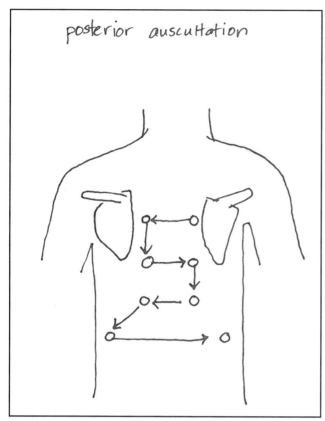
posterior auscultation

Figure 4-15. Typical locations for posterior auscultation.

Table 4-12 Common Breath Sounds	
Rales/crackles	Popping or crackling sounds at the end of inspiration; associated with pneumonia or bronchitis
Wheezes	Musical and continuous in nature; associated with COPD or asthma
Rhonchi	Low-pitched, rattling sounds like snoring; associated with pneumonia or cystic fibrosis

below the normal range. Typically, patients whose SpO_2 is below 90% to 88% should stop therapy and should be cued to work on breathing exercises, positioned to help with breathing, or, if needed, should have their oxygen increased or have nursing staff intervene. Per the American Physical Therapy Association, there are no known regulations that prohibit physical therapist assistants from using oxygen for patients, so long as oxygen has been prescribed and the parameters set by the physicians are being followed.[21] For example, a patient may be wearing oxygen at 2 liters but demonstrates SOB and the SpO_2 is measured at 85%. First, a clinician should check that the patient's nasal cannula is in the nose; this happens a lot more than you would think! Once that has been assured, the therapist can often cue the patient to take deep breaths: in through the nose and out through the mouth. This maximizes the oxygen intake and the carbon dioxide elimination. If necessary, the therapist can often adjust the oxygen (either from the wall or oxygen canister), as long as it does not exceed the parameters set by the physician. Often a doctor will document that a patient can receive oxygen at 2 to 5 liters, or 2 liters at rest and up to 5 liters with activity. If continued monitoring of oxygen shows no improvement when following the doctor's parameters, notify nursing staff immediately, or, in emergency situations, call 911 or pull the staff emergency button/cord at your facility.

Safety concerns for blood pressure include taking the blood pressure in an extremity not affected by stroke, surgery, shunts, or intravenous lines. Doing so would be contraindicated and the therapist should select the other upper extremity or a lower extremity, if necessary, to assess blood pressure.

Patients who are prone to orthostatic hypotension should be monitored carefully during position changes. A patient with this condition could easily lose consciousness and fall. Likewise, patients who demonstrate hypotension (not as a result of position change) or those who show hypertension should be monitored by medical staff prior to therapy interventions, especially if these readings are different from the patient's norm. Some patients do run low blood pressure and are asymptomatic; uncontrolled high blood pressure is still considered a safety concern.

Physical therapists often withhold therapy when a patient is febrile, or the patient performs less strenuous activities. Consider how you felt the last time you had a fever; did you want to walk around or perform exercises? Depending on how high the temperature is will affect what, if anything, a therapist can do with patients. A change in temperature from the patient's norm should be documented, and it would be worthwhile to communicate with nursing staff that the patient's status has changed.

A patient's pain can affect his or her ability to perform in therapy interventions. While therapists should be understanding of a patient's pain and adjust their interventions accordingly, the fact that the patient has pain does not necessarily mean that therapists do not do any therapy with that patient. There are some interventions therapists could perform that may decrease pain, and therapists also will need to remind the patient that mobility will ultimately help the patient be healthier and stronger and will mitigate other complications down the road.

If you suspect a patient has a DVT, you should not do therapy with that patient. Signs/symptoms of a DVT include redness (erythema) in the area, warmth, swelling, and pain or tenderness in the area. The most common area for a DVT is in the calf. You may see a therapist perform a Homan's test to determine if a blood clot is present. Be aware that this test is not consistently accurate, and any suspected DVT should be brought to the attention of the nursing staff, supervising physical therapist, and/or physician for further investigation via ultrasonography or venography.[22]

To perform the Homan's test, the patient is supine, with the suspected affected limb at 90 degrees of hip and knee flexion. Simultaneously dorsiflex the patient's ankle while giving a light squeeze to the calf muscle (gastrocnemius). If the patient reports pain or jerks the leg away, and the patient displays other signs and symptoms of a blood clot, there is a chance a blood clot is present. A positive Homan's sign/test should be documented and nursing staff should be alerted immediately. All therapy interventions are stopped until the patient has been cleared for activity.

DOCUMENTATION

Two examples are provided to represent common vital sign documentation.

Diagnosis: Ⓡ TKA S/P One Week

O: Patient performed quad sets 3 x 10, SLR 3 x 10, heel slides 3 x 10, with < 2 cues required to maintain form. Performed seated LAQ 2 x 10. Measured ROM at -10 degrees extension and 94 degrees flexion. Patient reported pain at 3/10 at rest but increased to 8/10 with exercises. Vitals monitored during session; HR 78 bpm and BP 129/68 mmHg. No c/o dizziness during session. Applied ice pack to Ⓡ knee after therapy session to control pain. After 5 minutes, patient reported pain decreased to 4/10.

Diagnosis: Deconditioning After Pneumonia

O: Patient RR prior to treatment 18 breaths/min. Patient wearing O_2 via nasal cannula at 1 L. Checked SpO_2 prior to treatment and at 94%. Patient performed seated exercises 2 x 10: LAQ, knee extensions, hip abd, hip add, and toe taps, all with yellow theraband for resistance. Patient performed 3 sit to stands with CGA required and use of arms on armrests. Patient reported feeling SOB after; RR 22 breaths/min and SpO_2 89%. Cued patient to perform breathing exercises x 5 minutes. Remeasured and RR 19 breaths/min and SpO_2 93%.

REVIEW QUESTIONS

1. What do the systolic and diastolic numbers in blood pressure represent?

2. What is the normal at rest heart rate range for an adult?

3. What is an abnormal response of blood pressure to exercise?

4. Describe the proper procedure for taking a patient's heart rate.

5. How does one measure pain?

6. What is a normal range for respiratory rate for a resting adult?

7. Describe why it is important to assess a patient's SpO_2.

8. You take your patient's blood pressure prior to exercise (while at rest). The patient then rides the stationary bike for 20 minutes. What would you expect the patient's blood pressure to read immediately after exercise (in relation to her resting blood pressure)?

9. Before you take a patient's blood pressure, what are some safety concerns to consider or avoid?

10. Describe the functioning of patients with COPD using the *International Classification of Functioning, Disability and Health.*

11. Your friend comes to you complaining of lower back pain, exacerbated by a weekend of moving. Your friend consulted his doctor who recommends surgical intervention immediately; however, you have read that surgical intervention may not adequately resolve lower back pain. Write a PICO (Patient, Intervention, Comparison, and Outcome) statement that addresses this problem, and then find a scholarly article that addresses your PICO statement.

REFERENCES

1. All about heart rate (pulse). *American Heart Association.* https://www.heart.org/en/health-topics/high-blood-pressure/the-facts-about-high-blood-pressure/all-about-heart-rate-pulse. Updated July 31, 2015. Accessed November 7, 2017.

2. Normal values in children. *ACLS Medical Training.* https://www.aclsmedicaltraining.com/normal-values-in-children/. Updated 2018. Published August 28, 2018.

3. Heart attack. *Mayo Clinic.* https://www.mayoclinic.org/diseases-conditions/heart-attack/symptoms-causes/syc-20373106. Printed May 30, 2018. Accessed August 28, 2018.

4. Heart failure. *Mayo Clinic.* https://www.mayoclinic.org/diseases-conditions/heart-failure/symptoms-causes/syc-20373142. Published December 23, 2018. Accessed August 28, 2018.

5. What is an aneurysm? *National Heart, Lung, and Blood Institute.* https://www.nhlbi.nih.gov/health-topics/aneurysm. Accessed August 28, 2018.

6. Chang CC, Chen MY, Shen JH, Lin YB, Hsu WW, Lin BS. A quantitative real-time assessment of Buerger exercise on dorsal foot peripheral skin circulation in patients with diabetes foot. *Medicine (Baltimore).* 2016;95(46):e5334. Doi: 10.1097/MD.0000000000005334.

7. Measuring heart rate. *PT Direct.* http://www.ptdirect.com/training-delivery/client-assessment/taking-heart-rate-measurements. Accessed August 28, 2018.

8. Health library: electrocardiogram. *Johns Hopkins Medicine.* https://www.hopkinsmedicine.org/healthlibrary/test_procedures/cardiovascular/electrocardiogram_92,P07970. Accessed August 28, 2018.

9. Price D. How to read an electrocardiogram (ECG). Part one: basic principles of the ECG. The normal ECG. *South Sudan Medical Journal.* 2010;3(2):26-28.

10. Howell M. The correct use of pulse oximetry in measuring oxygen status. *Nursing Times.* www.nursingtimes.net/clinical-archive/assessment-skills/the-correct-use-of-pulse-oximetry-in-measuring-osygen-status/199984.article. Published March 1, 2002. Accessed August 28, 2018.

11. Measuring blood pressure. *Centers for Disease Control and Prevention.* https://www.cdc.gov/bloodpressure/measure.htm. Published 2014. Updated July 30, 2018. Accessed November 7, 2018.

12. Understanding blood pressure readings. *American Heart Association.* https://www.heart.org/HEARTORG/Conditions/HighBloodPressure/KnowYourNumbers/Understanding-Blood-Pressure-Readings_UCM_301764_Article.jsp. Updated November 30, 2017. Accessed August 28, 2018.

13. Low blood pressure (hypotension). *Mayo Clinic.* https://www.mayoclinic.org/diseases-conditions/low-blood-pressure/symptoms-causes/syc-20355465. Published March 10, 2018. Accessed November 7, 2018.

14. Orthostatic hypotension (postural hypotension). *Mayo Clinic.* https://www.mayoclinic.org/diseases-conditions/orthostatic-hypotension/diagnosis-treatment/drc-20352553. Published July 11, 2017. Accessed August 28, 2018.

15. Mistovich J. Why the Valsalva Maneuver breaks SVT and causes syncope. *EMS1.com.* https://www.ems1.com/ems-products/cpr-resuscitation/articles/397955-Why-the-Valsalva-Maneuver-breaks-SVT-and-causes-syncope/. Published April 22, 2008. Updated February 28, 2016. Accessed August 28, 2018.

16. Centers for Disease Control and Prevention. National Health and Nutrition Examination Survey (NHANES). Health Tech/Blood Pressure Procedures Manual. *Centers for Disease Control and Prevention.* https://www.cdc.gov/nchs/data/nhanes/nhanes_09_10/BP.pdf. Published May 2009. Accessed August 28, 2018.

17. Pickering D, Stevens S. How to measure and record blood pressure. *Community Eye Health.* 2013;26(84):76.

18. Maley C. Intro to blood pressure. *American Diagnostic Corporation.* www.adctoday.com/blog/intro-blood-pressure. Published July 16, 2013. Accessed August 28, 2018.

19. Opioid overdose: prescription opioid data. *Centers for Disease Control and Prevention.* https://www.cdc.gov/drugoverdose/data/prescribing.html. Updated August 30, 2017. Accessed August 28, 2018.

20. APTA Launches #ChoosePT Campaign to Battle Opioid Epidemic. *PT in Motion News.* http://www.apta.org/PTinMotion/News/2016/6/7/ChoosePTCampaignLaunch/. Published June 7, 2016. Accessed August 28, 2018.

21. Oxygen administration during physical therapy. *APTA.* www.apta.org/OxygenAdministration. Updated August 12, 2014. Accessed August 28, 2018.

22. Ambesh P, Obiagwu C, Shetty V. Homan's sign for deep vein thrombosis: a grain of salt? *Indian Heart J.* 2017;69(3):418-419.

Chapter 5

Infection Control

KEY TERMS Acute | Airborne | Chronic | Contact | Droplet | Isolation | Local | Medical asepsis | Nosocomial | Pyogenic | Septic | Surgical asepsis | Systematic

KEY ABBREVIATIONS CDC | *C difficile* | HAI | MRSA | OSHA | PPE | SDS | VRE

CHAPTER OBJECTIVES

1. Describe the importance of and proper method for handwashing.
2. List and explain the various types of isolation and the proper precautions to avoid each.
3. Describe and be able to perform the proper order of donning and doffing personal protective equipment (PPE).
4. Set up a sterile field, and understand the considerations of keeping it sterile.
5. Identify safety data sheets (SDS) and other policies/procedures for clinic/facility safety.

INTRODUCTION

A patient enters the hospital to have a knee replacement after enduring years of pain and cortisone shots. The surgery goes well, and after the surgery, physical therapy is ordered. The physical therapist assistant comes in the next day following the physical therapist's evaluation to get the patient up and to work on range of motion prior to the patient's discharge; however, the physical therapist assistant notices that the incision looks inflamed, and there is an indication of pus along the incision. The patient reports an increase in pain, and girth measurements indicate an

increase in swelling in the area. The physical therapist assistant reports this to the supervising physical therapist as well as the nursing staff, and it is determined that the patient has acquired an infection, which will require the new knee hardware to be removed and a round of antibiotics to be started immediately. Physical therapy is put on hold, and the patient cannot leave the hospital as planned.

Nosocomial infections, sometimes called *health care-associated infections* (HAIs), have been a problem for patients and clinicians for some time. Per the Centers for Disease Control and Prevention (CDC), over 700,000 people acquired infections while in US hospitals as of 2014, and infections were the cause of over 75,000 deaths per year.[1] In response to this, in 2008, payer sources, such as Medicare, began requiring hospitals and other facilities to bear the burden of cost for infections or complications acquired by patients while in that facility. For example, if a patient enters the hospital to have his or her appendix removed, but the patient contracts pneumonia while recovering in the hospital, that facility must pay for the patient's care without reimbursement from Medicare. The 2009 estimated cost of HAIs was $28 billion to $45 billion, depending on the health care venue.[2]

Medicare and Medicaid include a list of HAIs and complications for which they will not pay, including pneumonia, pressure injuries, falls, urinary tract infections, deep vein thrombosis, surgical site infections, and foreign objects left in surgical sites.[3] Some private insurers have also adopt-

Memolo J.
Procedures and Patient Care for the Physical Therapist Assistant
(pp 63-74). © 2019 SLACK Incorporated.

Table 5-1 Vectors for Disease Transmission	
Animal	Rabies, plague
Human	Methicillin-resistant *Staphylococcus aureus* (MRSA), influenza
Food	Food poisoning (*Escherichia coli*, *Salmonella*)
Insect	Malaria (mosquito), Lyme disease (tick)
Prenatal/in utero	Sexually transmitted diseases
Soil	Tetanus, hookworm
Water	Typhoid, hepatitis A
Blood	HIV, hepatitis C

ed this policy. These financial penalties have put the focus on the facilities and the health care providers to take measures to avoid spreading infections. The CDC estimated that preventative measures for HAIs could save facilities anywhere from $5.7 billion to $31.5 billion, not an insignificant number.[2] Preventative measures include adopting aseptic handwashing techniques, donning the appropriate personal PPE, and following the correct procedures of isolation for different types of illnesses and infections.

ASEPTIC TECHNIQUES

Infection control is an attempt to prevent the spread of microorganisms that transmit illness. It can be broadly aimed to support asepsis, which is the absence of microorganisms that cause disease.[4] In physical therapy, physical therapists most often use medical asepsis, which is the attempt to contain microorganisms to a specific area, object, or person (such as with the use of PPE or patient isolation). The most common aseptic technique that therapists use to prevent the contraction or dissemination of infection is PPE. This equipment includes gowns, gloves, head coverings, glasses, face shields, masks, and shoe coverings. One of the other most commonly effective methods of maintaining medical asepsis is via handwashing.

Surgical asepsis is what people think of when a patient has a surgery; there is an attempt to make all objects, persons, and areas clean. Physical therapists do not often engage in surgical asepsis; however, common applications include the set up and use of sterile fields and gloves.

A microorganism or pathogenic agent can present as a variety of vectors. Table 5-1 includes a list of all the possible vectors or microorganisms.[5]

INFECTION CONTROL

Infection control can include a variety of preventative methods such as handwashing, isolation procedures, and the use and set up of sterile fields. Table 5-2 lists the CDC's recommended standard precautions for infection control.

Handwashing

Do you ever go into a public bathroom and observe people's handwashing habits? Some people just run their hands under the water, and others may forgo washing hands at all. As a health care provider, you will never be able to watch someone wash his or her hands incorrectly again without shuddering.

There was a time when it was not understood that handwashing was an essential part of hygiene and safety. These days people are surrounded by antibacterial soaps, alcohol rubs, and germ-eliminating wipes. Until 1847, however, when Dr. Ignaz Semmelweis determined that handwashing decreased the mortality rate of new mothers shortly after childbirth, handwashing was not the norm.[6] In the mid-19th century, 5 in 1000 women died in labor when delivering at home; the number increased by 10 to 20 times that in hospitals.[6] The causes were fevers, abscesses, and sepsis within 24 hours of the babies' births. The simple source of the infections was the doctors themselves. They went from performing an autopsy on a newly deceased mother to examining a mother in labor. Semmelweis realized that the doctors were the harbingers of infection, and he required all doctors and students to wash their hands. The mortality numbers dropped precipitously. Unfortunately, not all of Semmelweis' colleagues bought into his hypothesis, especially since it implied that the doctors were complicit in spreading infection. Not until later in the century were Semmelweis' ideas proven to be true.[6]

Thankfully, handwashing is enforced in health care practice now, and there is a correct procedure for washing hands. The CDC details the process, as well as occasions when someone should wash his or her hands. These include before and after preparing food; before eating; before and after caring for someone with an infection; before and after performing wound care; after using the toilet; after chang-

Table 5-2 **Standard Precautions**	
Perform hand hygiene	Follow guidelines for handwashing.
Use personal protective equipment	Wear gloves, gowns, masks, respirators, shoe coverings, head coverings, face shields.
Follow respiratory hygiene/cough etiquette	Cover coughs/sneezes with tissues and dispose of properly; wash hands or use an alcohol-based hand rub; provide masks for sick patients.
Ensure proper patient placement	Follow isolation precautions (contact, droplet, airborne, airborne plus contact).
Properly handle and clean/disinfect patient care equipment/instruments/devices and environment	Follow environmental infection control guidelines and disinfection/sterilization guidelines.
Handle textiles/laundry carefully	Follow environmental infection control guidelines to avoid infection spread.
Follow safe injection practices	Follow isolation precautions and safe injection protocol.
Ensure health care worker safety, including handling of sharps	Follow sharps safety protocol: no bending, recapping, or breaking of needles; dispose of in sharps container; report incidents or contact with infectious materials immediately.

ing diapers or assisting patients with post-toileting hygiene; after blowing your nose, coughing, or sneezing; after touching animals or their waste; after handling pet food; and after touching garbage.[7]

Recently, the Food and Drug Administration revealed that the soap people use at home does not need to be antibacterial. The Food and Drug Administration has not been convinced that the soap is safe, and they found no evidence that it is more beneficial than regular soap and water in eliminating germs. This rule excluded alcohol wipes or hand sanitizer, and it also did not include the soaps used in health care settings.

The appropriate procedure for washing one's hands (for medical asepsis; surgical asepsis handwashing is more laborious) begins with turning on the water. It can be warm or cold. Apply soap to your hands, and lather by rubbing your hands together vigorously. Be sure to scrub the backs of your hands, as well as between the fingers and under your nails. It is not recommended that health care workers have long or false nails, and it is difficult to adequately clean under these for infection control.

Perform this scrubbing for 20 to 30 seconds. It is about the time it takes to sing "Happy Birthday" twice. Scrubbing creates friction, which aids in removing microbes from your skin. Rinse your hands under the water, being sure to not shake your hands off in the sink. It is best to rinse from proximal to distal. Use a clean paper towel to dry your hands, and then use the same paper towel to turn off the water. Current CDC recommendations note that letting the water run and turning if off after rinsing wastes water and

paper towels, and they also indicate there is no evidence that it improves health or decreases the risk of infection.[8] In that case, you could turn off the water after soaping your hands, then turn the water on to rinse and off again after rinsing. Figure 5-1 shows pictures of the step-by-step procedure for washing hands,[8] and Box 5-1 has the written instructions.

The alternative to washing with soap and water is to use an alcohol rub or wipe. These dispensers are ubiquitous in health care settings, easily found on patient room walls and in hallways. You will observe that instead of handwashing, many clinicians pump sanitizer into their hands when entering and again when exiting a patient's room. This is generally an appropriate practice. However, in certain patient care situations, such as wound care procedures or when treating patients with highly communicable diseases, or any time your hands are visibly soiled, it is best practice to wash your hands rather than apply an alcohol rub. Even if you wore gloves, handwashing is important and necessary to maintain infection control. Box 5-2 includes a list of occasions when it is best practice to wash one's hands. Recall that no one, not even physicians, are exempt from these standards.

There was once a very well-respected doctor working at a hospital; he was also well-liked by his patients. A clinician noted, however, that this doctor did not wash his hands, nor did he apply alcohol rub, prior to entering a patient's room. He might shake the patient's hand, or those of the patient's family members.

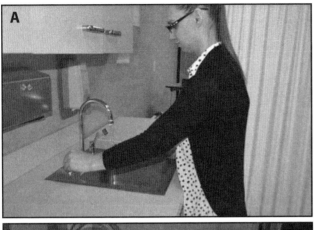
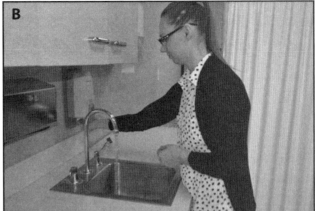
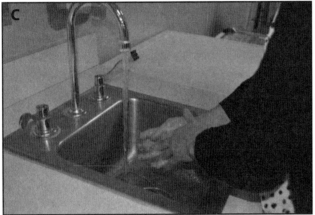
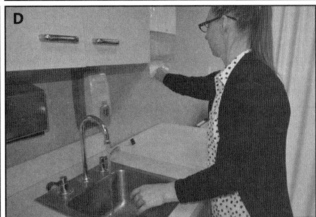

Figure 5-1. Steps of handwashing.

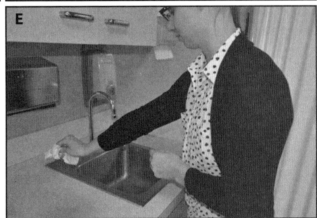

Box 5-1
Handwashing Procedure

1. Remove jewelry from hands/wrists.
2. Turn on the water to preferred temperature; wet hands.
3. Apply soap to hands, and wash with hands pointed down.
4. Scrub for 40 to 60 seconds, including palms, between fingers, fingernails, and dorsum of hand.
5. Rinse hands, again with hands pointed down.
6. Dry hands with paper towel; use the paper towel to turn off the water, and then discard the paper towel.

Box 5-2
When to Wash Hands[7]

- Before, during, and after preparing food
- Before eating food
- Before and after patient care
- Before and after treating a wound
- After using the toilet
- After blowing nose, coughing, or sneezing
- After touching an animal, animal food, or animal waste
- After touching garbage

Table 5-3
A Breakdown of Isolation Precautions

Type	Examples	Room	Equipment	Patient Transport
Contact	MRSA, vancomycin-resistant *Enterococcus* (VRE), *Clostridium difficile*, lice, Zika	Private or share room with patient with same infection	Dedicated equipment in room; wear mask with Zika; gown and gloves	Minimize transport
Droplet	Mumps, group A *Streptococcus*, influenza	Private room	Mask if within 3 feet; no gown or gloves required unless skin lesions present	Minimize transport; mask patient when transporting
Airborne	Measles, tuberculosis	Private room with negative airflow	N95 mask; no gown or gloves required	Minimize transport; mask patient when transporting
Airborne Plus Contact	Chickenpox, herpes zoster, smallpox	Private room with negative airflow	N95 mask; gown and gloves required	Minimize transport; mask patient when transporting

No one, not even the most respected physician, is exempt from infection control procedures. Patients should be educated that they have the right to request a health care worker, even a doctor, to wash his or her hands prior to patient care. The patient will be the one to suffer if the health care worker does not comply.

Types of Isolation

Another way health care workers maintain infection control is to observe isolation procedures. Most hospitals and health care facilities have procedures and plans in place for patients with certain communicable diseases and infections. Many times, a brightly colored sign will be placed on the door of the patient's room, alerting anyone entering of the isolation status and what the policy for that isolation dictates. Table 5-3 includes a breakdown of isolation precautions.

You will observe that health care providers generally do comply with these policies. If the isolation status requires those entering the room to wear gowns and gloves, most nurses, therapists, and physicians will follow the policy. The family members of the patients are the ones who do not follow the policies, and they frequently become the ones to transmit infection. A clinician noticed that a husband often left his wife's hospital room to get coffee or snacks from the family area. He never wore a gown or gloves, as was required, since his wife suffered from *C difficile*, a highly infectious illness that causes severe diarrhea, especially in older adults or those with compromised immune systems.[9] He came and went from her room with no handwashing and no PPE. The clinician stopped him prior to entering his wife's room and asked him, "Do you not see the sign on your wife's door that you need to wear a gown and gloves every time you enter and remove them every time you leave?" The man replied, "I thought that was only for the nurses."

It is vitally important, then, that not only health care workers are educated on the importance of infection control. This man was unknowingly transmitting the bacteria from his wife all over the hospital floor, including the family area where other patients' families congregated or acquired snacks and beverages. Infection control is for everyone.

Contact

Contact isolation is for patients with illnesses such as MRSA, VRE, *C difficile*, Zika, or respiratory syncytial virus.[10] Patients with lice or impetigo are also under contact isolation. These are all examples of infections that can be spread by touching the patient or items in the patient's room. Health care workers who interact with these patients should be sure to wear a gown and gloves while in the patient's room, and then remove these just before exiting the room. They should also wash or sanitize hands when entering and leaving the room. Ideally, visitors should check in with the nursing staff prior to entering the room. The patient is typically in a private room, and the equipment in the room is dedicated to that patient (such as the gait belt, stethoscope, and sphygmomanometer).[11] If the patient must leave the hospital room, he or she should wear a mask and gloves.

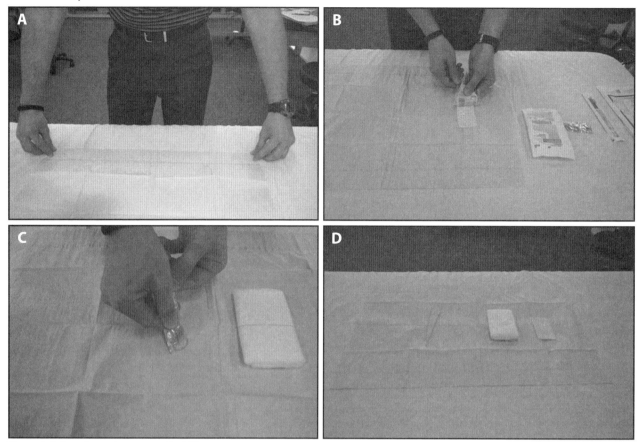

Figure 5-2. Steps for setting up a sterile field.

Droplet

Droplet isolation is required for patients with pneumonia, influenza, whooping cough, or bacterial meningitis.[10] These are all examples of infections that are spread in droplets caused by sneezing or coughing. Health care workers are required to wear a mask while in the room, which should be discarded after leaving the room.[11] Hands should be washed or sanitized before entering and after leaving the room.

Airborne

Patients with tuberculosis and measles are put in airborne isolation rooms.[10] These are examples of infections that are spread through the air from one person to another. The patients will be placed in a negative air pressure room (where the air is sucked outside the building rather than redistributed in the air ducts) and the door should remain shut. Health care workers will need to be fitted for a National Institute for Occupational Safety and Health–approved N95 or higher level respirator to wear while in the patient's room.[11] The mask, as well as other PPE worn in the room, must be removed when leaving the room. Health care workers should also wash or sanitize hands before entering and after leaving the patient's room. The patient should wear a mask if he or she must leave the room, and visitors will also need to wear a mask.

Airborne Plus Contact

Patients with chickenpox, smallpox, or disseminated herpes zoster (in immunocompromised patients) fall in this combination category. Patients must be in a private room with negative airflow and the door closed, and an N95 mask is also required. Gown and gloves are required and the patient should have minimal transportation. If the patient must be transported, he or she must wear a mask.

Sterile Field

Physical therapists, and often physical therapist assistants, play a role in wound care. When physical therapists do play a role, they are often required to set up a sterile field. A sterile field is a site for placing all the equipment and supplies needed for wound care and dressings. By definition, the field and the objects on it should remain sterile, meaning that several rules and procedures must be followed. Figure 5-2 depicts setting up a sterile field, and Box 5-3 includes setup guidelines for a sterile field.

First, consider the room in which you will be doing the wound care. If the room has many people—patients and clinicians—passing through, the field may not remain sterile. It may be best to select a private treatment room, or a place where a curtain can be drawn, to decrease the likelihood of cross-contamination.

Second, you must set up the sterile towel or drape. These are usually in sterile packaging, and once open, you are allowed to touch the outer 1 inch of the drape without considering it contaminated. Once there was a student who, during a practical examination, had to set up a sterile field. She opened and placed the drape appropriately, but, in her nervous state, she then swept her hands over the towel to smooth it out. She had just contaminated the sterile field!

When setting up the equipment or supplies, you should consider in what order you will need to use them.[12] It is best practice to set up the supplies with the items you will use first toward the front, and the items you will use last in the back. This will prevent you from reaching over the sterile field, which causes it to become contaminated.

Other actions that can contaminate a sterile field include turning your back on it, sneezing or coughing, putting non-sterile items on the field, moving the sterile field, leaving the sterile field unattended, or preparing the sterile field too far in advance of the treatment time.

You should not place unopened packages of supplies (eg, Kerlix [Cardinal Health], Vaseline, or saline) on the field; these packages are nonsterile and will contaminate the field.[12] When opening the items to put on the sterile field, you should open them away from you and drop them onto the field. This includes tweezers, scalpels, scissors, or any other supplies that are packaged. Saline should be poured into a sterile receptacle, and whatever is not used will be discarded after the treatment. Ointments, medicines, and lotions should be dispensed directly onto the field, again with any leftovers discarded afterwards.

Some clinicians wear nonsterile gloves to set up the sterile field; however, if this is the case, these should be discarded prior to treatment and sterile gloves should be donned (put on). The application of sterile and nonsterile gloves will be covered in the next section. Hands should be washed prior to the application of the sterile gloves. Gloves that have been contaminated should be doffed (take off) and new ones donned. Additionally, the clinician should wear a sterile gown. The front of the gown is considered sterile from the chest level to the level of the sterile field.[12]

PERSONAL PROTECTIVE EQUIPMENT

Personal protective equipment is a required safety accessory for treating patients with various infections and diseases. This protects you as well as the other patients you will be treating that day, so it is especially important that you know how to don and doff your equipment. Gloves, gowns, masks, shoe covers, head covers, and face shields are all examples of PPE.

Gloves

In your health care practice you will encounter sterile and nonsterile gloves. Nonsterile gloves are those not used for sterile purposes, but are necessary for isolation precautions.

Box 5-3
Guidelines for Setting Up a Sterile Field

- Do not sneeze, cough, or reach over the field.
- The 1-inch border around the field is considered nonsterile (and so can touch to open/place the field); avoid any sterile items touching this border.
- Do not turn your back on the field or leave the field unattended.
- If a nonsterile item touches the sterile field, you must redo the field setup.
- PPE considered sterile are front and sleeves of gown and gloves.
- Place the items to use on the field in order of use.
- Maintain hand hygiene and general cleanliness of area used for sterile field setup.

Sterile gloves are used for sterile treatment procedures, such as setting up a sterile field as described in the previous section. Gloves come in a variety of sizes and can be either latex or nonlatex, powdered or nonpowdered. The intention of wearing gloves is to protect your hands from whatever infectious materials you may come in contact with, and also to protect the patient from your germs.

Gowns

A gown is usually a bright blue or yellow garment to be worn over your clothes to protect yourself from infectious materials. They generally tie in the back; some have holes to slip over your head and some must be tied behind the head. They are made to be easily removed, and the tie straps can be torn to make removal easier. Bear in mind that these gowns do not breathe, and they, along with all of the other PPE, become very hot.

Masks

A mask can be firm or soft, and either has elastic straps or ties for the back of the head. Masks protect your mouth and nose from the transmission of infectious materials. They act as a filter and barrier. N95 masks are specialized masks for patients with airborne diseases such as tuberculosis, and these must be specially fitted to the health care worker prior to use.

Eyewear

Some masks come with face shields attached. Otherwise, it may be necessary to wear goggles or some other kind of eye protection. Again, these are to protect you from infectious materials that may splatter or be ejected from the patient via coughing or sneezing.

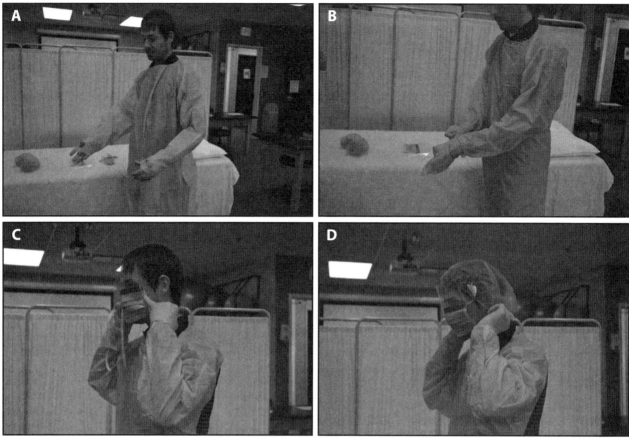

Figure 5-3. Step-by-step pictures of the application of PPE.

Donning/Doffing

There are special procedures for donning and doffing PPE. Figure 5-3 shows how to apply PPE, and Figure 5-4 demonstrates the process of applying sterile gloves; Boxes 5-4 and 5-5 cover the step-by-step procedures for donning and doffing gloves and PPE. Donning equipment can be less significant, unless you are performing sterile treatments; doffing is very important in order to prevent contamination when you have treated patients in isolation. Figure 5-5 demonstrates how to correctly doff PPE. Also keep in mind that your specific facility may have its own policies or procedures for donning and doffing PPE, and these should be followed. This text provides the basic procedure.

To don your PPE, consider whether you are performing a sterile treatment or not. If you are, you will apply your sterile gown first and your gloves last, following sterile procedure. If you are also wearing sterile face coverings (goggles or mask), these are donned first, and then the gown, and finally the gloves. For gown application, it is common to have a second person assist with application to prevent contamination.

If you are not performing a sterile treatment, the order in which you apply your PPE is less significant. It is important to ensure that your body is covered appropriately; isolation gowns, for example, typically come in one size. If you are a particularly tall or large individual, the gown may not fit you correctly. Also, the gown cuffs sometimes ride up a person's arm, exposing skin during treatment. A trick to avoid this is to stick your thumb through a hole in the gown sleeve. Some gowns come with this hole pre-made; others do not and you can punch a small hole using your thumb to accommodate.

Doffing PPE is of significance after treating a patient with chicken pox, tuberculosis, or VRE. First, you should remove your gown. Ties can often be broken rather than untied. Cross your hands over your shoulders and grab the gown, pulling it away from your body and turning it inside out as you do so. Remove it from your arms, keeping the gown turned inside out, and roll it up into a ball. Once you discard the gown, you can remove the gloves. With one gloved hand, grasp the other glove on the outside, then pull it off, turning it inside out as you go. Using your ungloved hand, grasp the other glove on the inside, pulling it off and turning it inside out. Once you discard your gloves, you can then remove your mask and head covering, if you wore them.

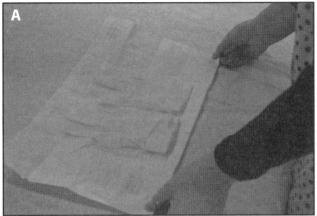

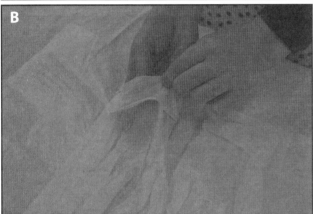

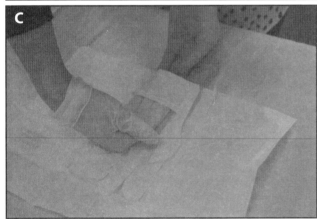

Figure 5-4. Step-by-step pictures of the application of sterile gloves.

Box 5-4

Application and Removal of Sterile Gloves

1. Wash your hands.
2. Open sterile glove packet, and arrange gloves so cuffs are facing you without touching the outer surface of the gloves.
3. Apply the first glove: grasp the cuff that is folded inside out. Do not touch the outer surface of the glove. Slide the glove onto the hand.
4. Apply the second glove: using the now gloved hand, you can touch the outer (sterile) surface of the glove but not with your ungloved hand. Slide fingers inside the cuff (so you are touching the outer surface of the glove but not the inside out portion of the cuff), and pull the glove onto your hand.
5. Once both gloves are on, you can adjust the fingers/fit because the outside of the gloves are both sterile.
6. To remove gloves: using gloved hand, pull one glove inside out; using the ungloved hand, reach inside the glove and pull it off inside out. Discard properly.
7. Wash your hands

Box 5-5

Application and Removal of Personal Protective Equipment

1. Wash your hands.
2. Know what PPE to apply according to the patient's isolation status.
3. To apply the gown, pull the sleeves to the wrist and tie the gown behind the neck and around the waist.
4. Apply the mask or fitted respirator, if applicable.
5. Apply the goggles/face shield, if applicable.
6. Apply clean gloves; make sure the cuffs go over the sleeve of the gown. Sometimes therapists will poke a hole through the end of the sleeve with their thumbs to ensure the gown sleeves will not slide up the arm.
7. Remove gloves: pull the gloves inside out, and be sure to refrain from touching the outside of the gloves with ungloved hands. Discard properly.
8. Remove eye protection, if applicable.
9. Remove gown: untie or break the ties on the gown, and then remove by touching the inside of the gown and wrapping up inside out. Alternatively, you can remove the gown at the same time you remove the gloves, pulling the gown off while the gloves are still on, and then turning everything inside out. Discard properly.
10. Remove mask/respirator, if applicable.
11. Wash your hands.

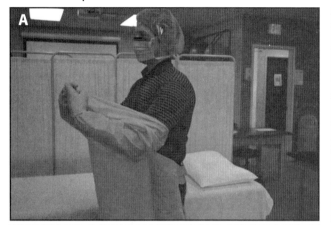

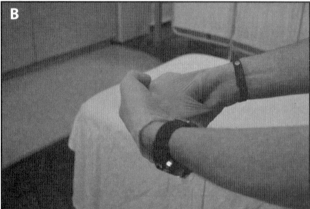

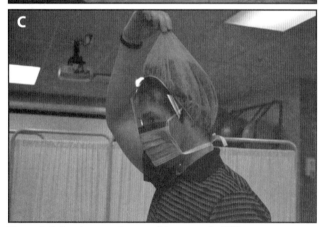

Figure 5-5. Step-by-step pictures of the removal of PPE.

Disposal of Contaminated Items

Once you have doffed your PPE, you will need to discard of it correctly. Typically, a biohazard container (Figure 5-6), which should be nonporous and leak-proof, is present in the patient's room so you can easily doff and discard your PPE as you exit the patient's room. Sometimes these biohazard containers are located just outside the patient's room. There should also be biohazard containers for discarded bandaging or wraps if wound care or edema dressing was performed.

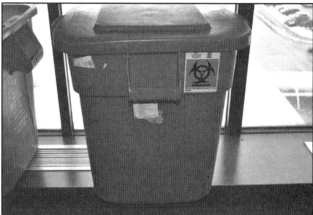

Figure 5-6. A biohazard container.

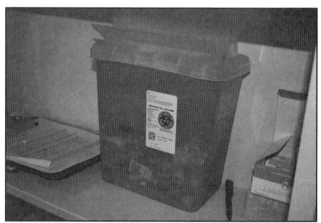

Figure 5-7. A sharps container.

Infection control also includes the proper disposal of sharps, especially needles of any type. Although therapy staff do not typically administer or use needles during therapy practice, with the exception of dry needling, therapists should know how to dispose of these items properly. Sometimes needles are inadvertently left in a patient's room or bed by a member of the nursing staff. These go in a designated sharps container, which is often found on the wall in the patient's room. Otherwise, a stand-along sharps container should be utilized to properly dispose of these items (Figure 5-7).

As mentioned earlier, some patients have dedicated equipment in their rooms, such as stethoscopes and gait belts. Other equipment may need to be sterilized, and this would be placed in the appropriate containers labeled for sterilization. Sharps, such as scalpels, should be placed in the sharps container, typically on the wall in the patient's room. Equipment that is not dedicated to the patient should be cleaned with alcohol wipes (including the ear tips and diaphragm of stethoscopes, plastic reusable gait belts, pulse oximeters, and other reusable equipment). And always remember to wash your hands after leaving a patient's room!

SAFETY/RED FLAGS

There are always things to worry about or be aware of when treating patients with infections or diseases. Safety is the most important aspect, which is why it is vitally important that you wear the appropriate PPE, follow isolation precautions, wash your hands often, and discard of materials appropriately.

As mentioned earlier, family members may not follow the isolation precautions as they should. Education is necessary to ensure infections are not spread throughout a facility. Additionally, health care workers, including physicians, sometimes need friendly reminders to wash their hands and follow procedures; we can all become slack in our adherence, but we need to stay vigilant.

Sometimes during patient care or transport, spills or accidents can happen. If you are in a patient's room or with a patient (whether he or she is in isolation or not) and he or she vomits, is incontinent of bowel or bladder, or bleeds, it is necessary to call the hospital or facility cleaning department to have someone specially trained come to clean up and disinfect the area. These employees should also wear gloves and possibly gowns when cleaning up spills.

Safety Data Sheets, Policies, and Procedures

Safety Data Sheets, formerly known as *Material Safety Data Sheets,* are required at any place of work that houses hazardous chemicals (Figure 5-8). The Occupational Safety and Health Administration (OSHA), a part of the US Department of Labor, states that every chemical manufacturer, distributor, or importer provide SDS for every chemical made to users of those chemicals.[13] The SDS were revised in 2012 to be more user-friendly.[13] The SDS are now broken down into sections; sections 1 through 9 contain information about the properties of each chemical, including identification, hazards, composition, safe handling practices, and emergency control measures.[13] Sections 9 through 11 and 16 contain information such as physical and chemical properties, stability and reactivity, toxicological information, exposure control information, and information about the date of preparation or revision.[13] Sections 12 through 15 are consistent with the UN Globally Harmonized System of Classification and Labeling of Chemicals, but this portion is not enforced by the OSHA.[13]

The goal of the SDS is to allow chemical users quick and easy access to information about the chemicals they use, especially those related to safety concerns. Hospitals, skilled nursing facilities, and outpatient clinics, as well as any other health care related facility, use chemicals; these are most often the chemicals used for cleansing. Per the OSHA, employers must have the SDS readily accessible, either by binders or computers, with easy access even in

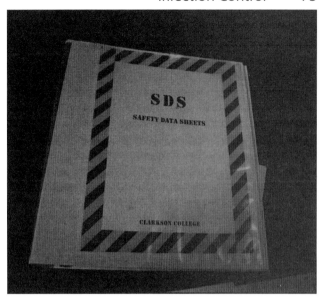

Figure 5-8. An SDS.

case of power outages.[13] Often, employers designate a specific staff member to be responsible for obtaining and/or maintaining the SDS. Most health care facilities include information about the SDS in orientation, and all employees should be aware of where to access and how to read or interpret the information in the SDS.

Additionally, each facility may have its own specific policy regarding either hazardous materials or infection control procedures. The information provided in this chapter is based on recommendations by the CDC and other health care organizations, but your specific facility may have its own additions or policies. Again, these are often reviewed during orientation.

DOCUMENTATION

When documenting treatment of patients in isolation, you should include what material you donned and doffed, as well as any other infection control procedures you followed. If you are documenting the setup of a sterile field, you should include what materials were used and in what order. As with all documentation, your goal is to represent what you did and how, so you can replicate that the next treatment session (if need be), as well as for both a demonstration of compliance and a means for reimbursement.

O: Patient in contact isolation for MRSA. Donned gloves and gown prior to entering patient's room to perform exercise and gait training. Patient able to ambulate 60 feet with FWW SBA x 2 and 3 verbal cues required to increase step length. Patient performed seated LAQs, ankle pumps, and marches, 10 x 3 repetitions each to improve strength in LEs. Prior to leaving patient's room, doffed gown and gloves and disposed in biohazard container.

REVIEW QUESTIONS

1. List the steps necessary to properly wash hands.
2. Describe the rationale for handwashing.
3. What is a vector? Provide 2 examples of vectors.
4. Your patient is in droplet isolation; describe the proper PPE you should wear and other isolation procedures you should follow.
5. List 2 diseases that fall under airborne isolation.
6. In what order should you doff your PPE?
7. What are 3 things to avoid when setting up a sterile field?
8. What are 4 components of SDS?

REFERENCES

1. Healthcare-associated infections: HAI Data and Statistics. *Center for Disease Control and Prevention*. https://www.cdc.gov/hai/surveillance/index.html. Updated January 9, 2018. Accessed August 30, 2018.
2. Scott R. The direct medical costs of healthcare-associated infections in U.S. hospitals and the benefits of prevention. *Center for Disease Control and Prevention*. https://www.cdc.gov/HAI/pdfs/hai/Scott_CostPaper.pdf. Published March 2009. Accessed August 30, 2018.
3. Hospital-Acquired Conditions. *Center for Medicare and Medicaid Services*. https://www.cms.gov/Medicare/Medicare-Fee-for-Service-Payment/HospitalAcqCond/Hospital-Acquired_Conditions.html. Updated August 30, 2018. Accessed August 30, 2018.
4. Asepsis. *The Free Dictionary*. http://medical-dictionary.thefreedictionary.com/medical+asepsis. Accessed August 30, 2018.
5. Soil-transmitted helminth infections. *WHO*. http://www.who.int/mediacentre/factsheets/fs366/en/. Published February 20, 2018. Accessed August 30, 2018.
6. Markel H. In 1850, Ignaz Semmelweis saved lives with three words: wash your hands. *PBS NewsHour: Health*. May 15, 2015. http://www.pbs.org/newshour/updates/ignaz-semmelweis-doctor-prescribed-hand-washing/. Accessed August 30, 2018.
7. When & how to wash your hands. *Centers for Disease Control and Prevention*. https://www.cdc.gov/handwashing/when-how-handwashing.html. Updated March 7, 2016. Accessed August 30, 2018.
8. Show me the science—how to wash your hands. *Centers for Disease Control and Prevention*. https://www.cdc.gov/handwashing/show-me-the-science-handwashing.html. Updated July 22, 2015. Accessed August 30, 2018.
9. C. difficile infection. *Mayo Clinic*. http://www.mayoclinic.org/diseases-conditions/c-difficile/home/ovc-20202264. Published June 18, 2016. Accessed August 30, 2018.
10. What are transmission-based precautions? *Association for Professionals in Infection Control and Epidemiology*. http://professionals.site.apic.org/what-are-transmission-precautions/. Accessed August 30, 2018.
11. Infection control: standard precautions for all patient care. *Center for Disease Control and Prevention*. https://www.cdc.gov/infectioncontrol/basics/standard-precautions.html. Updated January 16, 2017. Accessed August 30, 2018.
12. AORN Recommended Practices Committee. Recommended practices for maintaining a sterile field. *AORN J*. 2006;83(2):402-410.
13. OSHA Brief: hazard communication standard: safety data sheets. *United States Department of Labor, Occupational Safety and Health Administration*. www.osha.gov/Publications/OSHA3514.html. Published 2012. Accessed August 30, 2018.

Chapter 6

Wounds

KEY TERMS Blanch | Erythema | Exudate | Granulation | Inflammatory phase | Primary intention | Proliferative phase | Remodeling phase | Secondary intention | Slough | Staging

KEY ABBREVIATIONS DTPI | NPUAP

Chapter Objectives

1. Describe each phase of healing, including length of time as well as what happens during each phase.
2. Understand the various underlying causes of wounds.
3. Classify wounds according to type or size.
4. Describe the process of treating or healing wounds, including bandages, dressings, and other healing methodologies.
5. Identify safety concerns or red flags when performing wound care or identifying patients at risk for wounds.
6. Document a wound care intervention in the appropriate section of a SOAP (Subjective, Objective, Assessment, Plan) note.

Introduction

You have been asked by your supervising physical therapist to see a patient recently admitted to the hospital. The patient was in a skilled nursing facility prior to admission and has been immobile for several days due to having pneumonia, which has worsened (thus, her hospitalization). The physical therapist performed an evaluation on the patient yesterday, and the physical therapist wants you to get the patient sitting on the edge of the bed. In the patient's room, you help her log roll to her left side in preparation for sit-

ting up. It is then you notice an area of significant redness on the patient's sacrum. Upon palpation, the area does not blanch, and the patient reports some tenderness in the area. You alert the nursing staff immediately, and you also notify your supervising physical therapist.

This often happens to physical therapist assistants, even when they are not intending to perform wound care. Physical therapist assistants sit someone up or roll them in bed only to discover the beginnings or exacerbation of a wound. In this case, the physical therapist assistant still may not perform wound care to this patient; however, it is the physical therapist assistant's job to notify nursing staff and the supervising physical therapist. The physical therapist assistant should also be able to educate the nursing staff, the patient, and the patient's family members, if necessary, on how to avoid making the wound worse and how to prevent future wounds.

Phases of Healing

That paper cut you got on your finger when you opened this book is a wound. It is an acute wound, you could call it traumatic even, but because you are likely relatively young and healthy, that wound will heal quickly and without intervention.

Wounds heal via primary or secondary intention. Primary intention means that a wound has clean edges

Memolo J.
Procedures and Patient Care for the Physical Therapist Assistant
(pp 75-86). © 2019 SLACK Incorporated.

Phase	Duration	Actions
Inflammatory	First 24 to 48 hours	Vessels contract and blood clot or scab form to stop blood loss. Vessels dilate to allow fluid carrying nutrients, white blood cells, antibodies, and enzymes necessary for healing enter the injured area.
Proliferative	3 to 24 days	New tissue generated by fibroblasts. New blood supply created and granulation tissue hopefully evident.
Remodeling/ Maturation	21 days to 2 or 3 years	Epithelial cells reduce the size of the wound, and the edges contract. Scar forms, and scar tissue reorganizes to be smaller and stronger.

Table 6-1

Phases of Healing

that can easily be approximated, and these are healed by applying sutures, staples, or steri-strips. Secondary intention is where physical therapy gets involved. In these cases, the wound edges are jagged and not easily approximated. The wound is large and/or deep, with possible tunneling or undermining. The wounds may need to be packed with material to encourage the wound to heal from the inside out. Otherwise, the body may form a scab over the top of the wound, considering the healing more or less complete but leaving unhealed tissue beneath.

Whenever someone acquires a wound, whether it results from pressure, a paper cut, or a car accident, his or her body responds immediately. Healing is generally subdivided into 3 phases: the inflammatory, the proliferative, and the remodeling or maturation phases.[1] Table 6-1 includes the phases of healing and details about each phase. Sometimes there is a fourth phase added between inflammatory and proliferative, called the *destruction phase.*

It might be best to refresh one's memory on the anatomy of the skin. Recall that the outermost layer is the epidermis, which is avascular and regenerated every 2 to 4 weeks. The next layer is the dermis, a vascular layer rich with nerves, connective tissue, elastin, collagen, and fibroblasts. It also contains receptors for heat, cold, pain, pressure, itches, and tickles. The next layer is sometimes called the *hypodermis* or the *subcutaneous layer.* This contains adipose tissue, blood vessels, and connective tissue, and it protects the organs below while providing insulation. Below the subcutaneous layer you will find fascia, muscle, bone, and organs.

The first phase of healing is the inflammatory phase. This begins immediately after injury and lasts up to 3 days.[1] Some view inflammation as a negative thing; when someone sprains his or her ankle, therapists rush to decrease the swelling with elevation and ice. However, inflammation is the emergency response of the body, and to some degree, it is necessary for the rest of healing to continue.

During the inflammatory phase, the body attempts to stop blood loss via vasoconstriction, which creates a scab or blood clot. Once this has occurred, the vessels dilate again

and fluid carrying cells necessary for healing enter the injured area. This yields the classic signs of inflammation: redness, swelling, heat, and pain. Histamine and prostaglandins in the wound area are the culprits for this response.[1]

Some clinicians state there is a destructive phase; others lump these events into the inflammatory phase. If you are the type to subdivide, then the Destructive phase is the time when the body sends in specialized cells to clean up the wound in hopes to prevent infection. White blood cells release chemicals that digest bacteria. This phase lasts 1 to 6 days, so it overlaps with the inflammatory phase.

The proliferative phase begins after the inflammatory phase and lasts 3 to 24 days, and this is when new tissue is generated by fibroblasts.[1] The new tissue is made up of extracellular matrix and collagen. New capillaries form to provide blood supply to the wound (called *angiogenesis*), and this appears as granulation tissue, a beefy red tissue that indicates good blood flow. The wound should grow stronger as the fibroblasts reorganize the tissue.

Finally, the remodeling or maturation phase occurs. This lasts anywhere from 21 days up to 2 or 3 years.[1] During this phase, the epithelial cells begin to reduce the size of the wound by making the edges contract and pull together. Macrophages reorganize the collagen to make it neater and more flexible. A new scar is red or pink, but in time it will fade to white, meaning that the scar is done reorganizing. However, scar tissue is not as strong as uninjured skin.

TYPES OF WOUNDS AND CAUSES

Amputations, Traumatic Wounds, and Surgical Wounds

Amputations can occur because of traumatic events, such as car accidents, or they can result from progressive or circulatory illnesses, such as diabetes. Whatever the cause, however, an amputation leaves a large incision. In an oth-

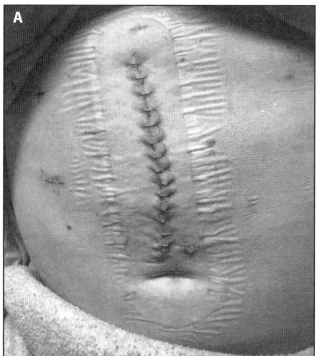

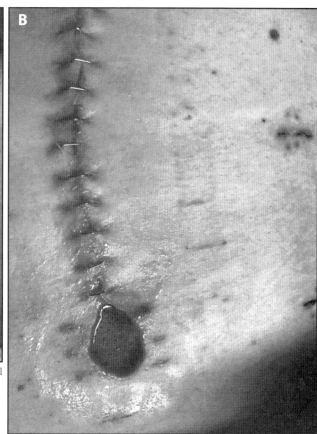

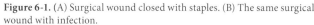

Figure 6-1. (A) Surgical wound closed with staples. (B) The same surgical wound with infection.

erwise healthy individual, such as a person who lost a limb due to a car accident, the incision should heal without any additional intervention. The wound is sutured and should heal by primary intention. However, patients with circulatory issues will have difficulty healing, and they may need wound care to assist in that endeavor.

The same applies to general traumatic wounds. Someone can slice his or her finger open with a knife, be shot by a gun, or be impaled by a metal rod. Again, many of these wounds are healed by primary intention, and otherwise healthy individuals will heal with little complication. Wounds with jagged edges or significant depth may need additional wound care and may need to be healed via secondary intention.

Surgical wounds may fall under this category; sometimes surgery is the result of a traumatic event. Other times, the surgery is not caused by trauma, but a wound still exists and must heal. Typically, these are healed via primary intention; however, some surgical wounds become infected and do not heal properly, requiring additional wound care intervention. Figure 6-1A shows a surgical incision closed with staples; Figure 6-1B depicts the same wound with an infection.

Pressure Injuries

It was mentioned in a previous chapter that pressure or friction can cause or exacerbate pressure injuries. Per the National Pressure Ulcer Advisory Panel (NPUAP), pres-

sure ulcers, also known as *bedsores* or *decubitus ulcers*, are now officially called *pressure injuries*.[2] Pressure injuries are wounds acquired due to pressure in certain bony locations over a long period of time.[2] A 2011 study indicated that around 33% of patients in hospitals and community care populations acquire pressure injuries.[3] Recall from an earlier chapter how it was discussed that positioning (and repositioning) is an important aspect of patient care. That is because a patient staying in one position over a period of time will have pressure build up, especially over bony prominences, and if that patient also has other comorbidities, such as poor circulation, poor sensation, or paresis/paralysis, a pressure injury is likely in that patient's future. Other risk factors include advanced age, incontinence, and poor nutrition/hydration. The same 2011 study found that elderly or intensive care unit patients with pressure injuries are 2 to 4 times more likely to die, possibly due to complications from the injuries and possibly due to those patients' other comorbidities.[3] Again, prevention is best, but if a pressure injury has already formed, wound care must be performed. Depending on the size and shape of the wound, healing by primary intention could be possible. However, it is more likely that healing by secondary intention will occur, as pressure injuries are generally deep and have edges that are difficult to approximate. Figure 6-2 includes pictures of pressure injuries in various stages. Box 6-1 lists risk factors associated with pressure injuries.

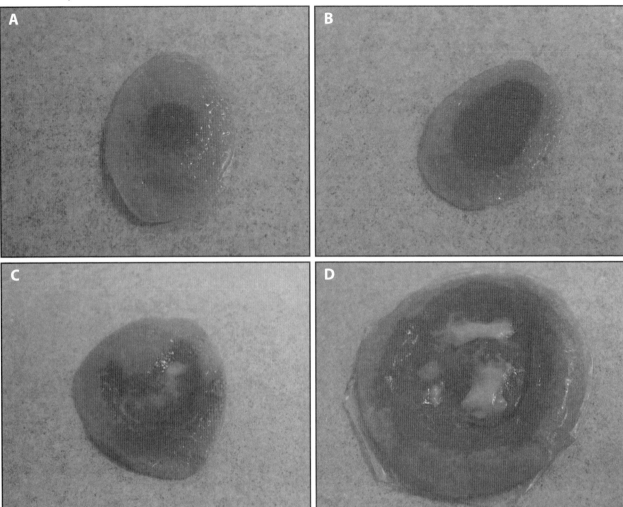

Figure 6-2. The 4 stages of pressure injuries.

Box 6-1

Risk Factors Associated With Pressure Injuries

- Pressure over bony prominences
- Shear/friction forces on skin
- Poor nutrition/hydration
- Areas of tissue lacking or with decreased sensation
- Incontinence
- Metabolic or systemic disorders (eg, diabetes)
- Reduced mobility or contractures
- Use of tobacco products

Wounds can be classified depending on the type they are. It is important to classify wounds as a part of your wound documentation. Pressure injuries are classified via staging. The NPUAP provided updated staging at a 2016 conference.[2] Rules of staging include numerically classifying the stages based on the deepest type of tissue exposed, classifying the wound as either a deep tissue pressure injury (DTPI) or unstageable if the wound base cannot be otherwise classified, and documenting but not staging a mucosal membrane.

Stage 1 pressure injuries are identified as nonblanchable areas of erythema on intact skin. The epidermis is not broken, and if erythema is not yet noted, there may be a change in sensation, temperature, or firmness of the tissue that indicates pressure. Purple or deep maroon colors indicate a DTPI vs a stage 1 injury.

A stage 2 injury is described as the partial thickness loss of skin with an exposed dermis. The wound bed is red or pink, possibly moist, or it could be a fluid-filled blister. Deeper tissues are not yet visible, nor is granulation tissue, slough, or eschar.

Stage 3 injuries demonstrate a full thickness loss of skin with adipose tissue visible. Slough and/or eschar could be noted, and undermining or tunneling may also be present. Fascia, muscle, and bone are not yet visible.

Table 6-2

Pressure Injury Stages

Stage 1	Nonblanchable area of redness on intact skin; change in sensation, temperature, or firmness of tissue
Stage 2	Exposed dermis with red/pink, moist wound bed, or blister
Stage 3	Adipose tissue visible, as is slough/eschar, if present, and undermining or tunneling
Stage 4	Full loss of epidermis and dermis, with fascia, muscle, bone, tendon, or cartilage visible
Unstageable	Skin or tissue loss present, but unable to determine extent due to wound bed being obscured

A stage 4 injury is a full thickness loss of skin plus exposed fascia, muscle, tendon, ligament, cartilage, or bone. Slough, eschar, tunneling, and/or undermining are possible.

Some wounds are classified as unstageable, which indicates that there is skin or tissue loss, but the extent of loss is undeterminable due to something obscuring the wound. Eschar or slough are the common culprits, and if these are removed (via debridement and other wound care methods), the wound can then become available for staging.

The NPUAP also include a classification of a DTPI, which is defined as a persistent nonblanchable deep red, maroon, or purple discoloration.[2] The skin may be intact or not intact, and the injury occurs as the result of prolonged pressure and shear where muscle and bone meet. This definition might also be changed if the therapist can observe underlying tissue, such as granulation, fascia, or muscle, or the wound could be unstageable if obscured by eschar or slough. Table 6-2 includes details on each stage of pressure injury classification.

Venous Stasis Ulcers

Venous stasis ulcers are a result of blood and fluid collecting in the lower extremities, often due to veins being unable to push the fluid back up toward the heart or possibly due to the valves in the veins not working correctly to prevent fluid backflow.[4] Lower extremities staying in a dependent position exacerbate this problem. Edema forms in the lower extremities, and other signs and symptoms include lower extremity heaviness, aching, itching, pigmentation, and ultimately ulceration. The ulcers are common to the medial aspect of the lower leg, especially just superior to the medial malleolus.[4]

Common measures taken to prevent and treat venous stasis ulcers are compression bandaging or wraps, as well as elevation of the limbs. Additionally, educating the patient on increased mobility to facilitate muscle pumping can be helpful. Once an ulcer forms, additional wound care treatment must be applied, including dressings and medications, as needed.

Diabetic Ulcers

Once there was a patient who came to the wound care clinic to have his diabetic ulcer treated. His shoe was removed along with his sock. The physical therapist assistant inspected his foot, only to find a beer bottle cap stuck to the bottom of his foot. He had no idea it was there, nor did he know how long it had been there. The bottle cap had already begun a new wound, so now the physical therapist assistant needed the supervising physical therapist to reevaluate the patient due to a change in status.

It is not uncommon for a patient with diabetes to suffer from a foot ulcer; the American Podiatric Medical Association indicates that about 15% of patients with diabetes will acquire a foot ulcer.[5] The American Podiatric Medical Association also asserts that diabetes is the leading cause of nontraumatic lower extremity amputations in the United States.[5] This is due to a lack of feeling, poor circulation, friction or pressure on the foot, and foot deformities.

A patient with a foot ulcer may eventually need a toe removed if the wound does not heal properly. Then that patient may acquire an infection, and the foot will need to be removed. Then possibly the leg below the knee is removed, and then the leg above the knee. Although prevention is best, once a wound forms, it is the therapist's duty to treat and educate the patient. If wound care is involved and the patient is compliant with instructions, amputations can sometimes be avoided. It is also worth knowing that diabetic ulcers tend to heal slowly due to the underlying complications of diabetes, so these wounds require frequent and long-lasting attention. Therapists can educate their diabetic patients about daily foot inspections, keeping the feet clean, wearing diabetic shoes, off-loading areas of pressure, and maintaining proper diet and activity to minimize the symptoms of diabetes.

Burns

Burns can result from sunlight, chemicals, electricity, or fire, and they mainly occur in the home or workplace.[6] The World Health Organization estimates that there are 180,000

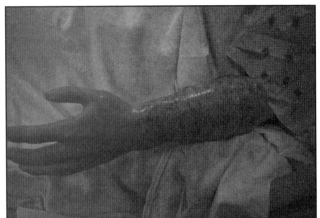

Figure 6-3. First degree burns.

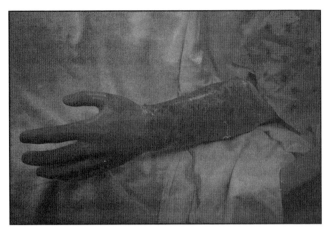

Figure 6-4. Second degree burns.

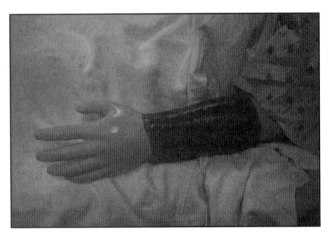

Figure 6-5. Third degree burns.

epidermis and the dermis.[7,8] These burns result from spills or splashes of scalding liquid and can take between 1 and 3 weeks to heal depending on how much tissue is affected.[8] The deeper the injury, the less acute pain is felt. Red, white, or splotchy skin color occurs, as well as pain and swelling. The wound area can look moist, and blisters often develop. These burns can also cause scarring. Scarring can be severe, possibly hypertrophic, and there is an increased risk for contractures.[8]

Third degree burns go beyond the dermis into the subcutaneous layer of the skin.[7] These are also called *full thickness injuries* and are a result of scalding from immersion, flames, chemicals, or high-voltage electricity.[8] The burned area can look white or black and charred, and the skin can also look waxy or leathery. Nerves are typically destroyed, which causes numbness. Healing can take a long time and may not occur at all if the burn affects more than 2% of the total surface area of the body.[8] With full thickness burns, the risk of contractures, as well as significant scarring, is high.[8]

Burns can also be classified in terms of the amount of area affected. This is called the *Rule of 9s* (Figure 6-6).[8] The body is divided into parts, and a percentage number is applied to each area (to total 100%). The areas are either 9% or multiples of 9. The larger the surface area affected, the higher the mortality rate. The rule is slightly adjusted for children to account for larger heads and smaller legs than adults.[9] If patients have greater than 30% to 40% of their total body surface area involved, they are at a significantly higher risk to die from their injuries.[9]

DOCUMENTING WOUNDS

Classification of wounds is just one way to document wounds properly. Box 6-2 includes information you should include when documenting a wound.

burn-related deaths per year.[6] Depending on the severity of the burn, a burn can be as mild as a sunburn or as severe as that which can result from a house fire. More will be discussed in a later section about how burns are classified, and another chapter deals with the emergent care of burns, but the wound care for burns differs a bit from traditional wound care. Figures 6-3, 6-4, and 6-5 are pictures of a first degree, second degree, and third degree burn, respectively.

Only pressure injuries are staged; other wounds are classified in different ways. Burns, for example, are classified in terms of depth and the size of the area affected. One way of classifying burns is in terms of first, second, or third degree injuries.[7] This classification system is being slowly replaced by the labels of *superficial, superficial partial thickness, deep partial thickness*, and *full thickness*.[8]

A first-degree burn is that which affects only the outer layer of the skin (epidermis).[7] Redness, swelling, and pain are hallmarks of a first degree burn, and a sunburn is a classic example. First degree burns will blanch with pressure. These burns will heal in several days with no scarring. This is also known as a *superficial burn*.[8]

A second degree burn, sometimes called a *superficial partial thickness burn* or a *partial thickness burn*, affects the

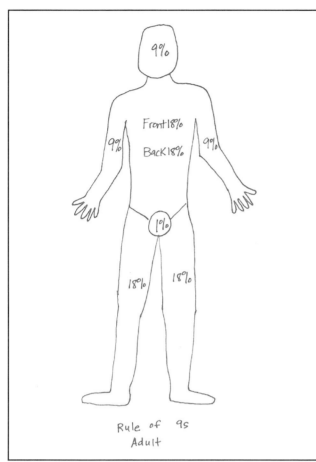

Figure 6-6. The Rule of 9s for an adult.

Box 6-2

Wound Descriptors for Documentation

- Wound stage, if applicable, or classification of wound (eg, laceration, abrasion, puncture, burn)
- Size (length, width, diameter)
- Tunneling/undermining (use o'clock method)
- Smell
- Exudate (amount and color)
- Wound edges (eg, macerated, hair loss, pale/blanched)
- Signs of edema/swelling (amount and location)
- Necrotic tissue (eschar) or slough (amount and location)
- Granulation tissue (amount and location)

Wound Healing

As mentioned earlier, wounds can be healed via primary or secondary intention. Secondary intention healing incorporates physical therapy (or nursing) wound care procedures above and beyond traditional incisional care provided with primary intention healing.

Wounds can have (and hopefully will have) granulation tissue, which is the beefy red tissue present when normal healing occurs. The red color is due to vascularization and circulation. However, a wound can also have necrosis (eschar) present, which is dead (often black) tissue. Slough, which can be yellow or other colors, is tissue that is falling away and sometimes is viscous in nature. This tissue is also dead or dying. A wound can have too much exudate, or fluid, and if the wound is due to or exacerbated by incontinence, maceration may occur; dressings may need to take into account absorption of excess exudate.

Basic wound care incorporates debridement (if necessary), wound cleaning, wound dressing, and other therapies as needed (eg, electrical stimulation or whirlpool). Wound debridement means that the wound requires more than just cleansing. This applies to the aforementioned necrotic tis-

sue or slough. If too much of this tissue is present, it may be necessary to debride the wound, or remove the dying or dead tissue, so healthy granulation tissue can grow.

Sometimes the wound can be debrided using a warm whirlpool to soften and loosen up the dead tissue, although the use of a whirlpool is decreasing due to the risk for cross-contamination. Another hydrotherapy tool is the pulsatile lavage system, which is like a water gun used to loosen dead tissue. Once the dead tissue is loosened up, additional sharp debridement may be necessary. Sharp debridement involves the use of scalpels or scissors to cut away the necrotic tissue or slough; be sure to check with your state practice act, as some states do not allow physical therapist assistants to perform sharp debridement. Another option is chemical debridement, which uses enzymes to soften or dissolve the dead tissue. These can be applied as topical medications directly to the wound or sometimes in the whirlpool, but care must be given as this process can also damage healthy tissue nearby.[10] Once debridement is performed, or if it is not necessary, the wound still must be cleansed. This may simply be a matter of using sterile saline or a gentle antibacterial cleanser to prepare the area for medications, dressings, and bandages.

If a wound is not healing properly, and especially if that wound is large, deep, or has irregular edges, a wound vacuum machine may be indicated. A wound vacuum creates negative pressure in the wound while also suctioning out debris and infectious material. Figure 6-7 depicts a wound vacuum collection canister, and Figure 6-8 shows the wound vacuum connected to a patient.

Dressings and Bandaging

It is impossible to list all the various medications, dressings, and bandaging options available for wound care treatments. New dressings and medications are always being developed and tested; however, all dressings aim for the

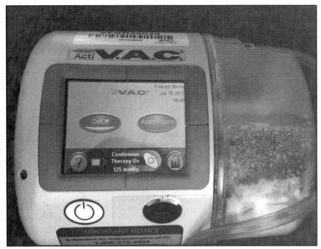

Figure 6-7. A wound vacuum collection canister.

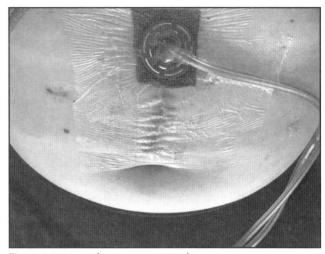

Figure 6-8. A wound vacuum on a wound.

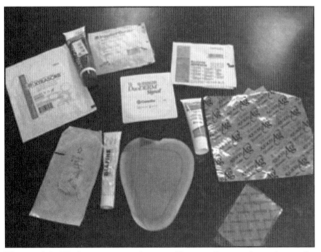

Figure 6-9. Various contact, intermediate, and outer layer items for wound dressings.

same goal: to facilitate wound healing while protecting the wound and preventing infection. Application of dressings generally follows the same procedure. Often, some kind of topical medication is first applied to the wound. Topical medications can be antibacterial or antimicrobial, and some have honey or silver in them, such as Silvadene (silver sulfadiazine). Some medications encourage epithelialization, like hydrogels, and others assist with debridement, such as Travase (proteolytic enzyme), Debridace (papain and urea), and Collagenase.[10] Some dressings are impregnated with silver or other medications to assist with wound healing. This first application is called the contact layer.

An intermediate layer is used for absorption of exudate and offers protection to the wound. It has also been supported that wounds heal best in a slightly moist environment, so this layer assists with providing that. The intermediate layer includes gauze sponges, absorbent ABD pads, or burn dressings.

Finally, an outer layer is applied to hold everything in place and to offer additional protection. Kerlix (Cardinal Health), Ace wraps (Ace), or Tubigrips (Molnlycke) are examples of outer layers. Figure 6-9 includes pictures of various contact, intermediate, and outer layers. Box 6-3 details the steps for applying a wound dressing.

It is important to pay as much attention to the removal of dressings as the application. Gloves should be applied, and it may be necessary to use scissors, with the blunt edge against the skin. As you remove the dressing, it is worth noting the number of layers, the sequence, and the amount of drainage on the dressing. When removing the contact layer, it may be necessary to moisten the dressing, so it can be removed without damaging any new granulation tissue. Best practice indicates that loosening the edges first and then pulling toward the center of the wound allows for the least injury to the wound. Once the old dressing is removed, you should also remove your gloves and apply clean ones to avoid cross-contamination. Once the wound is exposed, you can perform your wound assessment before applying a new dressing.

Modalities for Wound Healing

In addition to traditional forms of wound healing, such as topical medications, dressings, and bandages, there are alternative or supplemental methods of assisting with wound healing. Therapeutic modalities, such as ultrasound, electrical stimulation, and laser, have all been used, with varying degrees of success, to promote wound healing.

A 2014 literature review found that high-frequency ultrasound sped up the healing for stage 1 and 3 pressure injuries, as well as venous stasis ulcers.[11] Ultrasound parameters required a 20% or pulsed duty cycle, although intensity levels varied from 0.5 to 1.0 W/cm^2 between the 2 studies.[11] Frequency also affected healing; 3 times a week or more resulted in faster healing.[11] Electrical stimulation has

Box 6-3

Procedure for
Application of a Wound Dressing

1. Remove previous dressing. Note order in which materials were applied.

2. Cleanse wound as dictated by the physical therapist's plan of care.

3. If allowed by your state practice act, perform debridement. Note that some states do not allow sharps debridement of wounds by physical therapist assistants.

4. Set up a sterile field.

5. Apply the contact layer: could be medications for healing, Vaseline, pain medication, etc. Also includes dressing in direct contact with wound.

6. Apply the intermediate layer: gauze, sponges, ABD pads, etc.

7. Apply the outer layer: Kerlix, Ace wraps, Tubigrips, etc. Ensure tension is not so much to occlude blood flow.

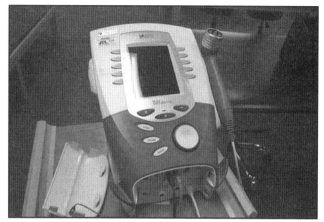

Figure 6-10. Laser for wound care.

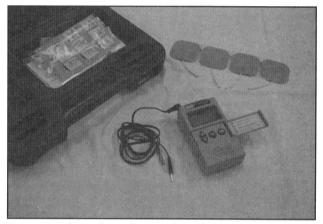

Figure 6-12. Electrical stimulation machines for wound care.

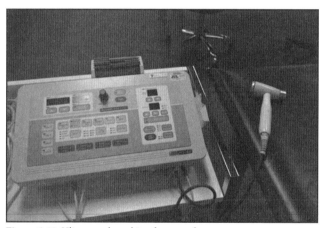

Figure 6-11. Ultrasound machine for wound care.

been used in various forms to assist with wound healing. A 2013 study compared various types of electrical stimulation, including high volt, alternating current, and transcutaneous electrical nerve stimulations. In all but 2 of the studies, wounds clearly healed faster with fewer incidences of infection.[12] Low level laser therapy demonstrated improved wound contraction in superficial or partial-thickness wounds in a 2004 study.[13] Parameters were 8 J/cm^2 and treatment time of 2 minutes 5 seconds.[13] Wound healing was theorized to result from increased fibroblast proliferation as a result of the treatment. Other modalities, such as hydrotherapy (including whirlpools and pulsed lavage systems), wound vacuums, and ultraviolet C light have been used with success in healing wounds, especially those that may otherwise take more time or have more complications. It will depend on your patient care setting and that location's equipment as to what you will have access to and what you can do with your patients. Figures 6-10, 6-11, and 6-12 include pictures of modalities used for wound healing.

Compression

Patients who suffer from lymphedema (or edema of any kind), or those who have venous stasis ulcers, may benefit from compression. Compression assists with moving fluid that has collected in the lower extremities back up toward the heart, where it can be pumped and redistributed throughout the body in a more normal way. In this way, compression can assist with treating or preventing venous stasis ulcers. Compression can also help with formation of a residual limb after amputation, and with scar tissue formation, especially in patients with burns. Compression can come in the form of Ace bandages or compression bandages, as well as custom or prefabricated compression garments and intermittent compression pumps.

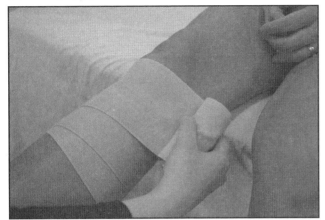

Figure 6-13. A spiral wrap.

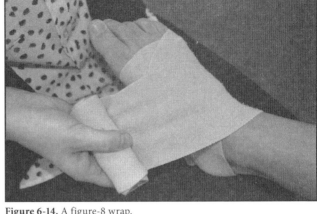

Figure 6-14. A figure-8 wrap.

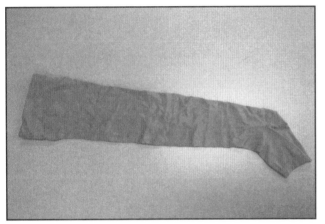

Figure 6-15. A compression garment.

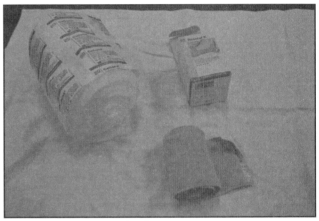

Figure 6-16. A compression bandage.

Compression bandages can vary in the amount of stretch they provide. Long-stretch bandages provide resting pressure, or an inward force on a limb at rest. The long-stretch bandages can stretch to around 140% of their original length, and Ace bandages are an example of long-stretch bandages. Short-stretch bandages do not stretch as much, only up to about 60% of their original length. These provide working pressure, meaning a person walking or moving will have a muscle contract against an inelastic bandage. This accelerates what happens naturally in the body when a person moves and the calf is contracted. In all types of compression, the compression gradient must be considered. Generally speaking, more pressure should be applied distally and less proximally to promote the distal to proximal movement of fluid from the extremities to the heart.

Compression bandages can be applied in one or multiple layers, with each layer adding an increase in compression. These bandages can be applied utilizing a spiral (Figure 6-13) or a figure-8 pattern (Figure 6-14) in order to evenly distribute pressure and avoid cutting off circulation. An alternative to this would be to use an off-the-shelf or custom fitted compression garment, which is like a sleeve or sock that the patient can wear for longer periods of time to reduce edema. Off-the-shelf versions include a pressure gradient according to the patient's needs; custom-fitted garments are the result of detailed measurements on the therapist's part, usually done once the patient has plateaued with his or her edema reduction. These garments assist in maintaining edema reduction. Figure 6-15 includes a picture of a compression garment.

Intermittent compression pumps use a sleeve and a machine to inflate the sleeve (Figures 6-16 and 6-17). The sleeve inflation is intermittent and helps to replicate the normal muscle pump. These can be very simple or complex, with options of making the compression sequential as well as uncorking for lymphedema patients.

It is worth noting that in cases of compression, a clinician should not only measure and document aspects of the wounds being treated, but he or she should also measure girth before and after compression treatment to demonstrate change, if any, in this area.

Scar Management

As mentioned earlier, compression garments are an option for compression and are often used for scar tissue management. Some garments are off the shelf, meaning they are a general size and have a premeasured amount

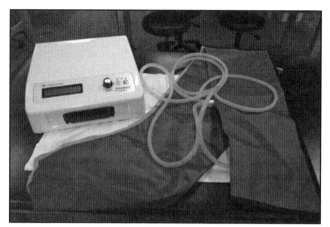

Figure 6-17. A compression pump.

of compression. However, a clinician can measure a patient for a custom garment, as well. In either case, the compression against scar tissue can help decrease the size and height of scars. Patients who have suffered from burns often wear compression garments to help decrease the size and height of their burn scars. Proper fit of the garment is vital, as is comfort, so the patient will be compliant. In postoperative cases, or with patients who develop hypertrophic or keloid scars, the use of a silicone gel sheet or a topical self-drying silicone gel can be used to yield a flatter, softer scar while also protecting the scar tissue.[14] A 2009 study indicated that topical gel was just as effective as the gel sheeting, while also being more convenient and easy to apply.[14]

SAFETY/RED FLAGS

Whenever performing wound care, there are some safety concerns to keep in mind. Any significant changes in the wound that are not for the better should be reported to the supervising physical therapist, as well as the nurse or physician, as is warranted. This may be a change in status and the plan of care may need to be altered.

Additionally, you should keep in mind the underlying cause of the wound and recall the factors that can affect wound formation or healing. Nutrition, hydration, pressure, diabetes, maceration (continence), and the patient's general health all affect wound healing. It is important that you can recognize the risk factors for wounds and be able to educate your patients on how to avoid wounds. Box 6-4 lists various factors that can affect wound healing.

As in the example provided in the beginning of this chapter, you may be the first to come across a wound or the signs that a wound is beginning. Off-loading the area of pressure is the first step, followed by alerting the supervising physical therapist and the nursing staff.

In patients with deep vein thromboses, compression is contraindicated. It is also contraindicated for patients with congestive heart failure, and it is not a good choice for patients with wounds that result from arterial insufficiency.

DOCUMENTATION

Clinicians assess wounds according to various descriptors. Specifically, wounds are documented based on the stage of the wound (if a pressure injury), the size (length, width, diameter), the specific location of the wound, the wound edges, any tunneling or undermining present, exudate (amount and color), necrotic tissue, odor, surrounding skin status, and characteristics of wound healing (eg, granulation tissue, slough, or wound contraction). Clinicians use the clock face to indicate where different qualities are located on the wound. For example, a wound with yellow slough in the upper left side of the wound may be described as being from the 8- to 10-o'clock position. A tunnel measuring 3 mm in length may be present at the 3-o'clock position.

O: Stage 3 pressure injury on Ⓡ buttock just superior to ischium, 5 cm x 3.2 cm x 1.2 cm. Wound edges with some blanching noted at the 4-o'clock position. Tunnel of 3.4 cm measured at the 2-o'clock position. Small amount of serisanguinous exudate present with dressing change. No necrotic tissue noted and no odor, but 10% yellow slough observed between the 8- and 9-o'clock positions. Sixty percent granulation tissue observed at the 3- and 6-o'clock positions. Applied new dressing with contact layer of bacitracin, silver nitrate, with tunnel packed. Intermediate layer of ABD pad and Tegaderm (3M); outer layer of Kerlix. Patient denied pain during treatment.

A: Wound decreased in size from previous measurement of 5.2 cm x 3.4 cm x 1.5 cm. Granulation tissue increased from 50% to 60%. Yellow slough decreased from 15% to 10%.

Review Questions

1. What happens during the inflammatory phase and approximately how long does this phase last?

2. What are 3 common types of wounds?

3. What does it mean if a pressure injury is classified as stage 2? What about stage 4?

4. What is the benefit or purpose of the contact layer of dressings?

5. List 5 risk factors for wounds.

6. Document a wound care intervention in the appropriate section of a SOAP note using the following information. Add information as needed to complete the note.
   ○ Size: 1.2 cm x 2.4 cm x 0.7 cm. Previously measured at 1.3 cm x 2.6 cm x 1.0 cm. Sixty-five percent necrosis from the 3- to 12-o'clock positions. Thirty-five percent red granulation tissue from the 12- to 3-o'clock positions. Moderate sanguinous exudate on dressing. Polysporin (bacitracin/polymyxin B), Kerlix gauze, Tegaderm, and Tubigrip applied.

7. Describe how you would assess a wound once you remove the dressing.

8. You have been tasked with creating a wound prevention plan for an 85-year-old man who is not very mobile. What are some of the recommendations you would make? Who would you implement this plan with (other than the patient)?

9. Locate and read a systematic review or other evidence-based summary for the treatment of diabetic ulcers. What does it recommend?

References

1. Brown A. Wound management 1: phases of the wound healing process. *Nursing Times*. www.nursingtimes.net/clinical-archive/wound-management-1-phases-of-the-wound-healing-process/7000047.article. Published 2015. Accessed August 31, 2018.

2. NPUAP pressure injury stages. *National Pressure Ulcer Advisory Panel*. http://www.npuap.org/resources/educational-and-clinical-resources/npuap-pressure-injury-stages/. Published 2016. Accessed August 31, 2018.

3. Reddy M. Pressure ulcers. *BMJ Clin Evid*. 2011;2011:1901.

4. Simon DA, Dix FP, McCollum CN. Management of venous leg ulcers. *BMJ*. 2004;328(7452):1358-1362. Doi: 10.1136/bmj.328.7452.1358.

5. Diabetic wound care. *American Podiatric Medical Association*. https://www.apma.org/Patients/FootHealth.cfm?ItemNumber=981. Accessed August 31, 2018.

6. Burns. *World Health Organization*. http://www.who.int/mediacentre/factsheets/fs365/en/. Published March 6, 2018. Accessed August 31, 2018.

7. Burns. *Mayo Clinic*. http://www.mayoclinic.org/diseases-conditions/burns/basics/symptoms/CON-20035028. Published July 24, 2018. Accessed August 31, 2018.

8. Morgan ED, Bledsoe SC, Barker J. Ambulatory management of burns. *Am Fam Physician*. 2000;62(9):2015-2026.

9. Chemical hazards emergency medical management. Burn triage and treatment–thermal injuries. *US Department of Health and Human Services*. https://chemm.nlm.nih.gov/burns.htm. Updated November 10, 2017. Accessed August 31, 2018.

10. Sarabahi S. Recent advances in topical wound care. *Indian J Plast Surg*. 2012;45(2):379-387.

11. Bolton L. Evidence corner: high-frequency ultrasound speeds. *Wounds*. 2014;26(10):306-308.

12. Thakral G, Lafontaine J, Najafi B, Tala TK, Kim P, Lavery LA. Electrical stimulation to accelerate wound healing. *Diabet Foot Ankle*. 2013;4. Doi: 10.3402/dfa.v4i0.22081.

13. Hopkins J, McLoda T, Seegmiller J, et al. Low-level laser therapy facilitates superficial wound healing in humans: a triple-blind, sham-controlled study. *J Athl Train*. 2004;39(3):223-229.

14. Puri N, Talwar A. The efficacy of silicone gel for the treatment of hypertrophic scars and keloids. *J Cutan Aesthet Surg*. 2009;2(2):104-106.

Chapter 7

Special Equipment and Environments

KEY TERMS Fowler's position | Micturate | Ostomy | Semi-Fowler's position | Stoma | Trendelenburg position

KEY ABBREVIATIONS ADL | CPR | CVC | DVT | G tube | Hct | Hgb | HOB | ICP | ICU | INR | IV | NG tube | ORIF | PEG tube | RBC | WBC

CHAPTER OBJECTIVES

1. Identify and describe some of the basic equipment encountered in patient care settings.
2. Identify the important lab values for patients noted in charts, and apply these to therapy interventions.
3. List and apply understanding of the various precautions or contraindications for physical therapy interventions as they apply to patient care equipment.
4. Properly document patient care interventions, considering the equipment used.

INTRODUCTION

By the time most people reach adulthood, they have seen or been inside a hospital at least once. Perhaps your grandmother or parent was ill. Perhaps you or your significant other were giving birth. Perhaps you visited the Emergency Department after you accidentally cut your hand with a knife. If you have not yet been inside a hospital or seen a hospital room, you have likely seen one on TV. There are a lot of monitors and tubes. Equipment is plugged in, making the room look cluttered. Seriously ill patients end up in the intensive care unit (ICU), with even more monitors and tubes.

All of this equipment can be overwhelming, especially when you are tasked to perform a physical therapy intervention with a patient connected to all of those monitors and tubes. How exactly do you get the patient up and walking when the patient is connected to multiple pieces of equipment? What if something gets unplugged, dislodged, or pulled out?

The good news is that you often do not have to do interventions with seriously ill patients on your own. Intensive care unit nurses (and hospital nurses in general) are very good about providing assistance, and another option is to co-treat with another therapist (occupational therapist, physical therapist, etc). The other good news is that this equipment is not as daunting as it seems, and with familiarization and practice, you will become an old pro at getting patients up and moving even when they are connected to 12 pieces of equipment.

Whether your patient is only on oxygen or has 4 different tubes or lines, treatment will begin with a review of the patient's medical chart and an assessment of the equipment in the room so you can generate a strategy for treatment. The goal is to not unplug or pull out anything that you should not while still achieving the goals of the therapy intervention. A quick look at what you are dealing with will help you to be safe and efficient. Additionally, monitoring the patient and asking for assistance is key; sometimes you cannot do it alone, and sometimes the patient needs a break.

Memolo J.
Procedures and Patient Care for the Physical Therapist Assistant
(pp 87-101). © 2019 SLACK Incorporated.

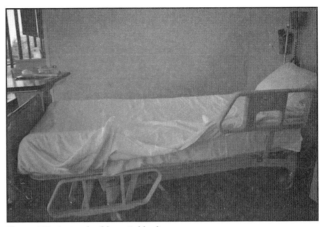

Figure 7-1. A standard hospital bed.

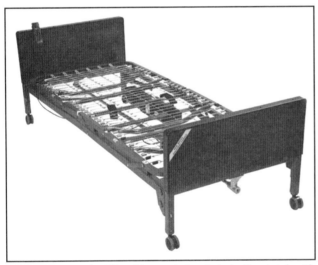

Figure 7-2. A Delta Ultra Lite semi-electric bed. (Reprinted with permission from Drive Medical.)

THE INTENSIVE CARE UNIT

The ICU is a specialized hospital area for patients who are critically ill. These patients are often connected to the usual pieces of equipment, like intravenous lines (IVs) and oxygen. However, these patients are also connected to chest tubes, arterial lines, ventilators, heart monitors, catheters, and more.

As a result of their critical status, these patients are not as active as those in standard hospital rooms. Patients in the ICU need and should have therapy interventions, but these interventions will be less intense and will be shorter in length than those for noncritical patients. It is also necessary that you monitor the patient's response to the interventions and provide rest breaks or stop treatment altogether if the patient is not responding well.

Sometimes patients are placed in critical care units, which are similar to ICUs, or they can be placed in cardiac/coronary care units. Children who need specialized care are placed in pediatric intensive care units, while newborns have their own specialized location in the neonatal intensive care unit. Even though the population might change, the equipment is often the same in each unit. Box 7-1 includes protocol for treating patients in the ICU.

HOSPITAL BEDS

A hospital room, no matter its specialization, always has a hospital bed. However, beds can be specific to a patient's diagnosis or needs, and it is important to be familiar with the different types. Most hospital beds, especially the specialized versions, are electric; however, there are some standard hospital beds that are still adjusted manually.

Standard Beds

A standard hospital bed (Figure 7-1) has the capability of adjusting the head and foot of the bed up and down, as the patient needs for treatment or comfort. Most are electric and have controls on the rail of the bed, as well as on a separate remote or call light control. The entire bed also can be raised or lowered to assist with patient care and transfers. Often the entire bed can tilt, so the feet are lower than the head or vice versa. Rails are typically on both sides of the bed and can also be raised or lowered to provide easier access to the patient or to prevent the patient from rolling out of the bed. Keep in mind that rails can become restraints, and a doctor's order is required to restrain a patient. Nonelectric beds also are adjustable; these have turn cranks on the foot of the bed that can raise or lower the head, the foot, and the entire bed. Figure 7-2 shows a semi-electric bed.

Standard beds have wheels to roll the bed from one room to another and brakes to prevent rolling when it is not needed. These beds also have a cardiopulmonary resuscitation (CPR) button or function that makes the mattress firm in case CPR is needed. Various hooks are on the underside of the bed, from which to hang catheter bags, and the foot of the bed can house intermittent compression pumps. The bed controls include a call button for nursing staff in case the patient or clinician requires assistance, and usually the remote includes television controls as well.

Turning Frame (Stryker Wedge Turning Frame)

This bed is specifically for patients with spinal cord injuries or surgeries that prevent them from turning or moving in bed on their own. This bed allows for a change of position from supine to prone without patients moving themselves; patients can remain in spinal traction throughout the turning process.[1] Think about a pancake being flipped; the movement is not sudden, but a patient is literally rotated from supine to prone and back again. This bed can also place the patient in Trendelenburg or reverse Trendelenburg position as needed.

Advantages of this bed include the fact that a patient can be repositioned to decrease pressure (and therefore decrease the risk of pressure injuries) without negatively affecting the spine or interfering with traction.[1] This bed also allows for easy access to the patient for clinical or therapeutic interventions. One person can easily reposition the patient, and the bed can be easily wheeled to another location. The bed itself does not take up a great deal of space.

However, the bed only allows for patients up to 250 pounds (lbs), and there are risks of friction or shearing forces as the patient is rotated from supine to prone and back.[1] The patient is at an increased risk of contractures due to the positioning in this bed. However, this bed is not commonly seen due to new advances in technology.

Air Fluidized Support Beds

Air fluidized support beds (Clinitron) have silicone-coated beads in a mattress, which are suspended by heated air.[2] The sensation is like being on a waterbed. These beds are indicated for patients with wounds or at risk for wounds, as the air suspension decreases pressure, friction, and shearing forces. This bed is also used with patients who are immobilized for long periods of time or who are healing from recent skin grafts or burns.

An advantage of this type of bed includes the decreased pressure, which could decrease costs of topical wound treatments and help treat or prevent wounds.[2] The warm air is relaxing and comfortable for patients, and the air can be turned off to create a firm surface for other clinical or therapeutic interventions. However, the mattress is punctured easily, and the patient can become dehydrated from the warm air. The bed sometimes cannot be raised or lowered, although newer versions of the Clinitron brand do have a high/low adjustment option.[2] Older versions also allow for potential pooling of fluids in the lungs, but newer versions have head of bed (HOB) articulation to decrease these respiratory risks. The bed is rather large, and because it is a specialized bed, it can be expensive.

Posttrauma Mobility Beds

A posttrauma mobility or RotoRest bed (Arjo) is situated on a rotating platform. Think about a baby cradle that rocks the child gently from left to right; the posttrauma mobility bed does much the same. The patient is strapped into the bed to prevent him or her from falling off, and there are bolsters to keep the patient in position while the bed rocks. The rocking can be moved in increments, and it can also be paused for up to around 30 minutes.[3]

This bed can rock up to 62 degrees in either direction, which helps address and prevent upper respiratory complications related to immobility, such as pneumonia.[3] Additionally, the bed eliminates the need for health care providers to rotate or reposition a patient to prevent pressure injuries, and the oscillation helps maintain proper bowel and bladder function. Patients with thoracic or lumbar fractures, skeletal traction, or cervical traction are good candidates for this bed.

Contraindications to use this bed include patients who are post–cardiac surgery, patients with bronchospasms, patients with intracranial hypertension, and patients with multiple rib fractures.[3] Additionally, patients who normally suffer from motion sickness may not enjoy this bed, and the bolsters in the bed can prevent physical therapy mobilization. This bed is rather large, especially as it oscillates, and so sufficient space is needed in the room.

Low Air Loss Beds

A low air loss bed is a segmented mattress with individually filled air bladders. Each bladder can be controlled or adjusted to the patient's needs.[4] These beds are ideal for patients with pressure injuries or who are at risk for pressure injuries, since the bladders can be adjusted to reduce pressure on certain areas. This bed is often adjustable for the HOB and other positions; however, transferring a patient in and out of this bed requires adjusting the bladders just so.[4] The individual bladders can be replaced, which eliminates the costly problems of puncturing that come with the air fluidized support beds. Low air loss beds, just like the air fluidized beds, have a CPR function to make the bladders deflate quickly for a hard surface, and many have the technology to prevent air loss in the case of power outages.[4]

Negative aspects include that this bed can still be punctured and that patients with cervical, thoracic, or lumbar traction or fractures cannot maintain proper alignment in this bed. Also, the clinician still needs to adjust the pressure or reposition the patient regularly to prevent pressure injuries.

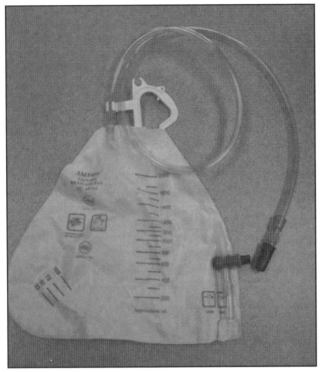

Figure 7-3. A Foley catheter.

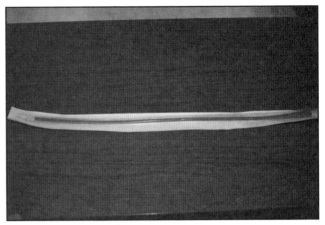

Figure 7-4. A straight catheter.

Bariatric Beds

Bariatric beds are becoming more and more available in the hospital setting due to the rapid rise in obese patients. Bariatric beds are wider, longer, and made of more heavy-duty materials than their nonbariatric counterparts; they often reach 54 inches wide, 88 inches long, and can hold up to 1200 lbs.[5] Like standard beds, bariatric beds generally come with electronic controls, with the capability of raising the head or foot of the bed as well as the entire bed. Many bariatric beds take into consideration the increased difficulty of repositioning or moving these patients, and offer features that assist with these interventions. Medical supply companies are now also making specialty beds with bariatric patients in mind; these can offer air bladders or lateral rotation components to prevent pressure injuries and to prevent nosocomial pneumonia, respectively.[6]

URINARY CATHETERS

Urinary catheters are devices that can be either internal or external (if the patient is male) and drain urine from the bladder to be collected in a bag. Sometimes this is due to a patient having a surgery; it is not uncommon for patients put under general or spinal anesthesia to have a catheter inserted, as the patient temporarily loses the ability to control the emptying of his or her bladder. These catheters are generally removed shortly after surgery or once sensation and movement has returned to the lower half of the body, so the patient can empty his or her bladder voluntarily.

However, some patients permanently lose the ability to empty their bladders voluntarily; patients who have suffered a spinal cord injury, for example, may lose this ability. Some disease processes or even advancing age can affect the ability to micturate voluntarily, either on a temporary or permanent basis.

Whatever the cause, a catheter may be necessary for your patient. It is typical to enter a patient's room and see a catheter bag hanging from the hospital bed. As mentioned before, it is best practice to survey a patient's room quickly to ascertain what equipment you will be working with when treating, transferring, or ambulating with your patient.

There are several types of catheters, and knowing what type you are working with will help you avoid complications or injury. A Foley catheter (Figure 7-3) is an indwelling or internal catheter. A tube is inserted into the urethra and then into the bladder, where it is held in place by a small balloon inflated with air or sterile saline. The tube has holes to drain the urine into the catheter bag and to irrigate the bladder. To remove the Foley catheter, the air or sterile saline must be removed first. Any yanks or tugs on the catheter tubing when the balloon is inflated will yield pain.

A suprapubic catheter is inserted directly into the bladder via an incision in the lower abdomen. The catheter is held in place by a few small stitches and tape, so accidental removal is possible. An external catheter is only appropriate for male patients, and it is essentially like a condom placed over the penis and held in place with adhesive or a strap. For patients who need more long-term use of a catheter but do not want or need the suprapubic option, a straight catheter (Figure 7-4) can be used to empty the bladder, and then can be immediately removed to increase patient independence and function.

In addition to assessing what type and where the catheter and its bag are located, you should take a quick peek at the urine. Light urine is a sign of good hydration; the darker yellow the urine, the less hydrated the patient. If the urine is cloudy, the patient may have an infection; likewise, if blood is present, something may be amiss.

OSTOMIES

Ostomies are surgically created openings in the abdomen that allow fecal material to be eliminated without passing through the rectum.[7] A stoma is the end of the small or large intestine that can be seen protruding from the abdomen. As with patients who have catheters, ostomies can be temporary or permanent, depending on the reason for having them. Ostomies are named for where the opening is created. A colostomy is an opening in the colon; an ileostomy is an opening in the small intestine; and a urostomy is a means of diverting urine away from a malfunctioning bladder via a section of the small or large intestine.[7]

Ostomies have several options for collection bags; generally patients wear these all the time (Figure 7-5). Collection pouches can have an open end, which is clamped and can be emptied while attached, or a closed end, which can be discarded after each use. All collection systems have some kind of skin barrier to which the collection pouch attaches and that protects the skin from the stoma output.

VENTILATORS

Sometimes patients have difficulties breathing on their own. Sometimes patients are fully incapable of breathing without assistance; in other cases, patients need help with breathing at night when they sleep. Whatever the reason, these patients will have or use some kind of ventilator (also sometimes referred to as a *respirator*) to maintain normal oxygen exchange in the body. Otherwise, the patient will suffer from dyspnea, hypoxemia, or some other breathing-related disorder that could result in organ or brain damage.

Ventilators are classified as being invasive or noninvasive. Noninvasive ventilators include volume-cycled ventilators, pressure-cycled ventilators, flow-cycled ventilators, time-cycled ventilators, continuous positive airway pressure ventilators, and bilevel positive airway pressure ventilators.[8]

Volume-cycled ventilators deliver a certain volume of air (typically set by respiratory therapist) and then allow for passive exhalation. Patients with acute respiratory distress or bronchospasms are good candidates for this type of ventilator.

Pressure-cycled ventilators give a preset pressure of air and also allow for passive exhalation. There is a decreased risk of lung damage with this type of ventilator, but the tidal volume delivered can change with lung resistance and poor patient compliance.[8] This is used for patients who have short-term ventilator needs.

Flow-cycled ventilators deliver oxygen until a preset flow rate is achieved during inhalation. A time-cycled ventilator delivers oxygen over a preset time period, but these are not used as often as volume or pressure-cycled ventilators.[8]

Continuous positive airway pressure ventilators require the patient to exhale against resistance and provide a continuous flow of oxygen at the same pressure during inhala-

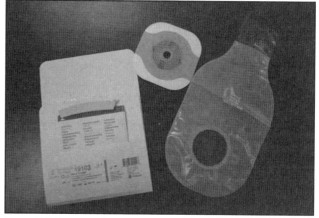
Figure 7-5. An ostomy bag.

tion and exhalation to keep the airway open.[9] This is for patients with obstructive sleep apnea, and is not considered a true ventilator because it does not assist with breathing.

Bilevel positive airway pressure ventilators deliver oxygen at 2 pressures for inhalation and exhalation, and are good for patients with neuromuscular diseases. They have a timed mode and a backup system that helps initiate breaths, especially at night when the patient is sleeping.

Invasive ventilators are those that deliver oxygen through an endotracheal tube inserted either into the patient's nose, mouth, or through a tracheostomy. These deliver oxygen on a time cycle to ensure the patient takes a minimum number of breaths per minute. These can be adjusted to allow patients to take their own breaths if able. Invasive ventilators are often permanent. A drawback is that they can override the body's own initiation of cleaning out mucus from airways, and patients with these types of ventilators will need some kind of humidification to avoid excessive drying out of the respiratory tract.

There are also various modes of ventilator settings. Assist-control ventilation is where each breath is either an assist or control breath, all of the same volume.[9] Synchronized intermittent-mandatory ventilation has a minimum number of breaths per minute, but the patient partially breathes on his or her own.[9] Pressure-controlled ventilation allows the patient to determine the inflation volume and frequency of respiration, but not the pressure; it can be used to augment spontaneous breathing.[9]

There are many more options for ventilator types and modes than listed here; your responsibility is to read the patient's chart, be familiar with the type or set up of the ventilator, and consult nursing staff for assistance when uncertain. Patients with ventilators are not contraindicated for therapeutic interventions; they are, however, less likely to tolerate strenuous activities. Positioning of the patient is important, as is awareness of the ventilator tubing to ensure it is not kinked or pulled out of either the machine or the patient. Alarms will sound if the airway is obstructed, if the tubing is removed, if the respiratory pattern changes, or even if the patient coughs. Figure 7-6 shows a portable ResMed Astral ventilator.

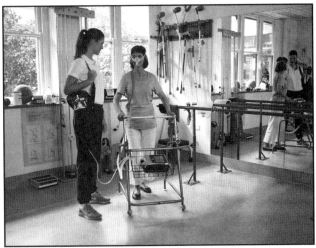

Figure 7-6. A ResMed Astral ventilator. (Reprinted with permission from ResMed.)

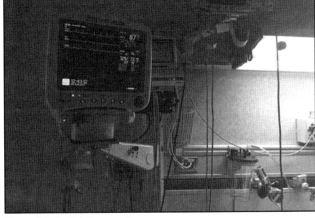

Figure 7-7. A vital sign monitor.

Monitors

When you walk into a patient's room, you may be overwhelmed by all of the monitors in the room. It is important to know what information these monitors provide because that information may influence how much or what type of therapy you provide. Some monitors assess heart rate, blood pressure, and respiratory rate or oxygen levels; others measure pressure in a vein or in the skull.

The most common monitor is the vital signs monitor (Figure 7-7). This monitor measures and displays heart rate, respiratory rate, oxygen saturation (SpO_2), and blood pressure. Sometimes temperature and cardiac patterns are also displayed. These monitors can be limited to the room, but there are portable versions that a patient can take with them while ambulating in the hallway or when transferred to another area, such as the Radiology Department or therapy gym. Sometimes the nursing staff sets alarms for ranges on the monitor, so the alarm will sound if the patient goes below or exceeds the range preset. This is handy for a therapist because you can observe the patient's physiological responses to interventions and make changes if necessary.

A pulmonary artery catheter, also known as a *Swan Ganz catheter*, is inserted through a large vein, to the right atrium of the heart, into the right ventricle, and out through a pulmonary artery.[10] This allows the health care staff to learn about the pressure in the right side of the heart and the arteries of the lungs. This catheter also allows for blood samples to be taken to measure blood oxygen flow. The physician selects which vein to insert the catheter into, but most often it is in the neck, groin, or below the collarbone.[11]

The normal values for the right atrium are 0 to 8 mmHg; normal values for the right ventricle are 15 to 25/0 to 8 mmHg.[10] Normal values for the pulmonary artery are 15 to 25/8 to 12 mmHg, and normal values for the pulmonary capillary wedge pressure are 9 to 23/1 to 12 mmHg.[10]

While a patient is wearing a pulmonary artery catheter, activity is limited by the location of the catheter in order to avoid dislodging or damaging the catheter or the vein in which it is placed.

An intracranial pressure monitor (ICP) is placed in cases of traumatic brain injury, brain tumor, or brain hemorrhage. Normal pressure is between 5 to 15 mmHg, and anything greater than 20 mmHg is considered abnormal.[12]

Intracranial pressure monitors can be classified as either invasive or noninvasive. Invasive types of ICPs include implantable transducer catheter systems, telemetric systems, and fluid-filled systems. Noninvasive ICPs include an impedance mismatch, a tympanic membrane displacement, a transcranial Doppler, a near infrared spectroscopy, an optic nerve sheath diameter, a fontanometry, and a pulsed phase lock loop technique.[13]

Exercise or therapy is not strictly contraindicated for patients with ICPs; however, the Valsalva maneuver or isometric exercises should be avoided, and the HOB should stay above 30 degrees.[14] You should also avoid head to chest neck flexion, Trendelenburg's or prone positions, and excessive hip flexion.[14]

A central venous catheter (CVC), sometimes known as a *central venous access device*, allows medications, blood, nutrients, and fluids to be entered directly into the blood.[15] They are also used for extracting blood samples for testing. Patients who are receiving chemotherapy drugs often have CVCs placed to prevent repetitive sticks for blood draws and medication administration.

An indwelling right atrial catheter, also known as a *Hickman catheter*, is placed in one of the veins under the collarbone and, like the CVC, is used for drawing blood, administering medications (eg, chemotherapy), and providing nutrition and fluids.[16] This catheter also allows for fewer needle sticks.[17]

For the CVC and the indwelling right atrial catheter, the patient should avoid having the site of the catheter insertion submerged under water, and if showering, the patient

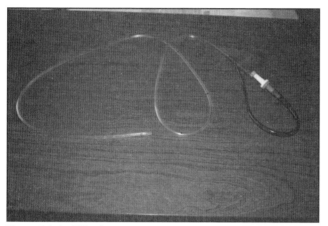

Figure 7-8. An NG tube.

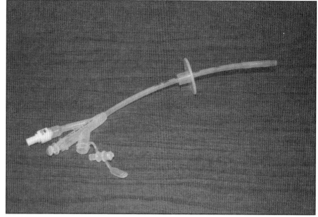

Figure 7-9. A PEG tube.

should protect and cover the site of insertion. As a therapist, you should avoid pulling or tugging on the insertion site to avoid removal or disruption of the catheter. Lifting weights or repetitive movement of the arm on the side of the catheter is contraindicated.

An arterial line monitors blood pressure continuously, which is especially helpful for those with pressure instability and for those who may need medication intervention to treat blood pressure changes.[18] The catheter is typically inserted into the radial artery. Exercise is not contraindicated, but the therapist should again be aware of not disrupting or pulling on the catheter.

FEEDING DEVICES

A nasogastric (NG) tube (Figure 7-8) passes through the nostril and into the stomach. It allows for the emptying of the gastrointestinal tract or for feeding. Patients with ileus, intestinal, and gastric outlet obstructions; patients with dysphagia after suffering a cerebrovascular accident; and patients who have undergone a tracheostomy are good candidates for an NG tube.[19] An NG tube is meant to be temporary and can be removed only by a nurse or physician. Patients with NG tubes should not eat or drink anything by mouth, and you may see "NPO" written in the patient's chart (meaning nil per os or nothing by mouth).[19] It is important that if a patient is ordered to be NPO that you do not give them anything to eat or drink; this also may mean mouth swabs and ice chips. You should check with the nurse on duty to clarify the order if you are unsure.

Patients with NG tubes are not contraindicated for therapy, but they may complain of neck pain, and excessive neck motion, including flexion, should be avoided. Additionally, you should avoid any activity that might pull or kink the NG tubing.

A gastric (G) tube is placed through the abdominal wall and directly into the stomach. These can be longer tubes held into place via a balloon and are sometimes called *percutaneous endoscopic gastrostomy (PEG) tubes*

(Figure 7-9).[20] Low profile tubes or buttons do not have the long tubes attached but rather attach for feeding or medications and then disconnect when not in use. These lie flat against the body compared to the PEG tubes.

Like NG tubes, G tubes are used for feeding or medication administration; however, G tubes are typically for more long-term needs. Exercise is not contraindicated for patients with G tubes, but care should be given so as not to disrupt the tube.[20] Placement of gait belts may need to be adjusted to avoid rubbing against or pulling on the G tube.

Intravenous feeding, also known as *parenteral nutrition*, is used when the digestive tract cannot absorb nutrients normally, or when the digestive tract must be kept free from food temporarily, such as with ulcerative colitis.[21] Total parenteral nutrition is needed for patients with a nonfunctioning digestive tract, severe pancreatitis, an intestinal block, birth defects of the intestinal tract, or removal of part of the small intestine.[21] This requires a large tube inserted into a large vein, such as the subclavian vein.

Carbohydrates comprise the majority of the calories, but the different formulas used can include fats, proteins, vitamins, and minerals. The formulas can be customized according to what the patient's diagnosis is and what his or her needs might be.

As with other forms of feeding, therapy is not contraindicated. The tubing should not be removed or occluded, and use of the extremity on the side of the tube may be restricted.

Intravenous infusion lines (Figure 7-10) are the most commonly seen forms of fluid or nutrition infusion in the hospital setting. Medications can also be administered, and blood samples can be taken. The IV needle is inserted into a vein, which connects to a bag or solution container that hangs from a pole or is sometimes connected to an infusion pump. This allows the nursing staff to preset the amount of fluid or medications administered. Typical locations of placement include various areas of the upper extremity, most notably, the metacarpal and dorsal venous plexus of the hand or the antecubital, basilica, or cephalic veins.

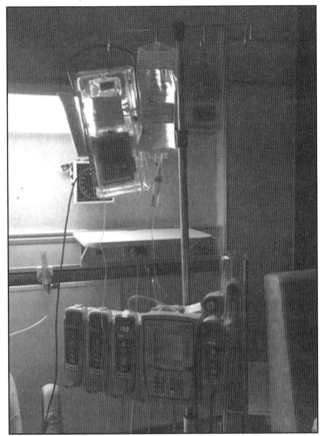

Figure 7-10. An IV pole.

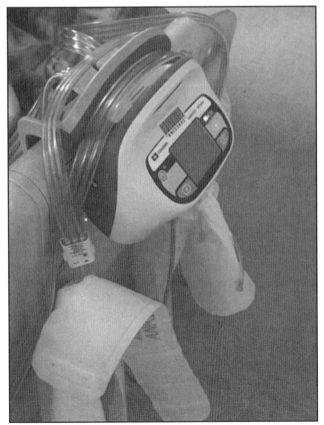

Figure 7-12. Intermittent compression.

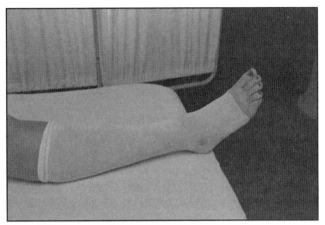

Figure 7-11. A compression garment.

Sometimes it is necessary to place the IV in the lower extremity, such as in the foot, and for infants or the very elderly, a superficial scalp vein may be used. Therapy is not contraindicated, but care should be given at the IV insertion site, avoiding occlusion or removal of the tubing.

DEEP VEIN THROMBOSIS PREVENTION

A deep vein thrombosis (DVT) is a blood clot in a deep vein in the body, typically in the leg. A blood clot manifests as erythema (redness), swelling, heat, and pain in the afflicted limb. Sometimes these blood clots can become dislodged and travel via the bloodstream before becoming lodged in the lungs, heart, or brain. These blood clots are of especial concern to hospitals, as patients who are less mobile after an accident or surgery are at a higher risk for developing a DVT.

Thromboembolic disease (TED) stockings (Cardinal Health) are compression garments generally worn by any patient admitted to the hospital, but are especially recommended for patients who are unable to or have difficulty with getting out of bed or ambulating (Figure 7-11). These are preventative (prophylactic) garments for DVTs, and patients are required to wear these most of the day for days and sometimes weeks or months after hospitalization, per the physician recommendation. These garments provide a certain constant pressure gradient against which the muscles in the legs can contract to replicate normal muscle pump action. TED stockings can go up to the knee or up to the thigh, depending on the patient's needs.

Intermittent compression (Figure 7-12) is another prophylactic method for DVTs. There are various types, but they all have leg wraps that are connected to a compressor that intermittently fills and empties those wraps. The aim is to replicate the normal muscle pump action that occurs when a patient is mobile with the hopes to prevent a DVT from forming.

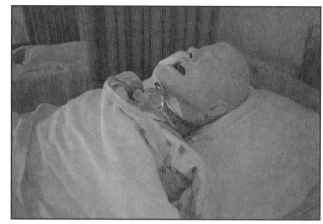

Figure 7-14. A tracheostomy.

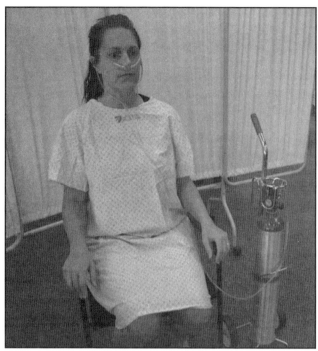

Figure 7-13. An oxygen tank with nasal cannula.

OXYGEN

Patients often need oxygen, and it is important to be aware of the various methods of oxygen delivery and how to overcome obstacles affiliated with patients receiving oxygen. The oxygen comes from oxygen tanks or compressors.

Patients most commonly wear nasal cannulas for oxygen delivery (Figure 7-13). The nasal cannula has 2 tips that rest just below the nose (just above the lip) and blow oxygen up into the nasal passageways. Nasal cannulas are ideal for patients requiring little to moderate oxygen concentrations, and are common for patients who have a temporary need for oxygen.

Sometimes you will see patients wearing an oronasal mask. This type of mask covers the nose and mouth, and is able to deliver higher concentrations of oxygen. These are also used for temporary needs or to help a patient when permanent oxygen delivery is being contemplated.

Oxygen tents cover the patient's head and trunk, and are often for patients who are young or cannot keep a nasal cannula or oronasal mask on. The edges must be sealed to keep the oxygen inside the tent, and the patient's oxygen levels must be monitored more often to ensure oxygen is being delivered.

You may also see a patient wearing a nasal catheter, which is a tube inserted through the nasal passage into the nasopharyngeal junction, or you may see a patient with a tracheostomy (Figure 7-14), which can be either permanent or temporary.

When performing therapy with a patient on oxygen, you should be mindful of the tubing to prevent kinks or tugs, and the oxygen tank should be on a wheeled pulley so it can be carried behind a person ambulating or being pushed in a wheelchair. Aside from monitoring the patient for signs or symptoms of respiratory distress or allowing for rest breaks due to fatigue, patients on oxygen are not contraindicated for therapy interventions.

Oxygen is delivered in terms of liters, and typically the physician sets the amount of oxygen in liters a patient can receive. Sometimes you will look at a patient's chart and it will indicate that the patient is allowed a certain amount of oxygen at rest, but that amount can be increased to another threshold if the patient is active. For example, Mr. Jacobs may be allowed up to 3 L of oxygen at rest, but can go up to 6 L with activity or therapy. Aside from these parameters, physical therapist assistants are not allowed to alter the amount of oxygen delivered. If the physical therapist assistant has followed the set parameters and the patient is demonstrating dyspnea or other signs and symptoms of respiratory distress, nursing staff should be notified. The doctor may be contacted as a result. Document your session and observations, and alert your supervising physical therapist.

TRACTION

When a person suffers from a fracture, sometimes the bones do not align properly. In these cases, the patient will need some kind of traction, which keeps bones in alignment so they will heal correctly. Traction can also assist with soft tissue shortening and muscle spasms. Traction can be applied to the skin or it can be screwed into bones via pins and rods, either internally or externally.

Balanced suspension traction is primarily used to reduce a fracture or dislocation. The traction is set up with a set of bars, pulleys, ropes, and weights to pull on a part (or parts)

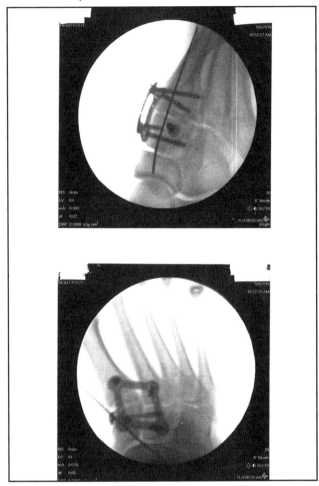

Figure 7-15. Example of an ORIF.

of the body. The body part is then suspended to allow the patient as much mobility as possible without disturbing the healing process. The pull forces must remain constant in the amount and direction until the fragment unites; otherwise, the pull of the muscle will pull the bone out of alignment, and the fracture will not heal correctly.[22]

Skin traction uses tape, moleskin, or specific skin traction strips to align fractures (most commonly those of children or dislocations that only require moderate pulling forces).[22] Skin irritation is a possibility, especially for adults (who take longer to heal from fractures), therefore, skin traction should not be used for fractures requiring more than 5 to 7 lbs of force. It is also not helpful for the control of limb rotation, nor is it helpful for continuous traction that takes 3 to 4 weeks.[22]

Skeletal traction requires the use of pins, wires, screws, cervical tongs, or halos. These tools allow for up to 30 lbs of force for 3 to 4 months, and they control both longitudinal and rotational pulls.[22]

Cervical spine fractures often need Crutchfiled or Vinke cervical tongs drilled directly into the skull to attach to a traction system. These stabilize the vertebrae in order to prevent further spinal injury. A halo traction system includes both a padded vest and upright bars connected to a halo ring or crown, which is screwed into the skull with pins.[22] The setup allows for a patient to be ambulatory while maintaining cervical alignment.

Pelvic fractures use special traction systems with screws inserted into the ilium to maintain alignment.[22] Long bone fractures use Steinmann pins or Kirschner wires, which connect to their respective holders or tractors and the traction force.

External fixation uses pins or wires to provide support for a limb while a bone is healing.[23] The pins and wires are external (thus the name), and they stabilize the joint or bone after trauma. These are beneficial in that they do not require the same amount of damage to soft tissue, and they are temporary. They are ideal for patients have open wounds or skin contusion, skin grafts, poor healing due to diabetes mellitus or peripheral vascular disease, and they reduce the risk of infection.[23] External fixators also allow the alignment of the joint or bone to be adjusted postoperatively. In terms of therapy, a patient with external fixators may be allowed more mobility than those with open reduction internal fixators (ORIFs), although he or she may still have weightbearing restrictions.

Open reduction internal fixators are pins, plates, wires, and screws that are surgically placed internally. The bone fragments are placed in alignment (reduced) and then held together with various implants made from stainless steel or titanium. A patient with ORIFs is more likely to have limitations on mobility, including weightbearing restrictions. The surgeon dictates postoperative therapy protocol, which may include early passive range of motion, followed by advancement to active assistive or active range of motion. Figure 7-15 shows an x-ray with an ORIF placed after a fracture injury.

PAIN CONTROL

Your patient is likely to take something for pain, either intravenously or orally. Sometimes the patient is connected to a patient-controlled analgesia pump system that administers pain medication according to when the patient presses a button. These machines have preset limitations on how often medication can be administered (eg, no sooner than 10 minutes apart) and on how much medication can be delivered in a period of time, but they do allow patients to have some amount of control of their pain and when they receive medication.

DIALYSIS

Some patients' kidneys no longer work properly due to end stage renal disease, so their blood must be filtered via another method. Dialysis cleans the blood of impurities while restoring a normal level of electrolytes and preventing infection.[24] Kidney failure is generally permanent, and the only alternative to dialysis is a kidney transplant.

There are 2 types of dialysis: hemodialysis and peritoneal dialysis. Hemodialysis uses an artificial kidney to remove waste and extra fluid from the blood.[24] A shunt is placed in the patient's arm or leg to provide access, or else a fistula is created by jointing an artery to a vein under the skin. Typical dialysis treatments are 4 hours long and are done 3 times a week, but it depends on the function of the patient's kidneys, how much waste is in the blood, and the kind of hemodialyzer used.

Peritoneal dialysis cleanses the blood inside the body by having a plastic catheter surgically inserted into the abdomen.[24] The treatment involves the abdominal area being filled with dialysate via the catheter, and waste and extra fluid is drawn out into the dialysate.

Patients who have dialysis are often quite fatigued after their treatment, and many times are in no mood to perform therapy the same day as dialysis treatments. You may need to time your therapy sessions for a day the patient does not have dialysis treatments.

CHEST DRAINAGE

Patients with chest tubes require air, blood, or purulent material to be removed from the chest cavity. This may be due to trauma or a disease process, such as pneumonia or cancer. An incision is made between the ribs and a plastic tube is inserted to drain the fluid or air away from the chest cavity and the lungs.[25] The tube is connected to a drainage collection system, sometimes with suction, which measures how much (and what color) fluid is drained. Therapy is not contraindicated for patients with chest tubes, but care should be taken to not tug on the tubing and to keep the collection unit below the level of the chest to assist with drainage.[25] Figure 7-16 shows a chest tube.

LABORATORY VALUES

It has been mentioned before that you should take a moment to consult your patient's chart prior to entering the room or starting a therapy treatment. A patient's laboratory values are worth reviewing because they may determine what kind or how much therapy you can perform (if any) with your patient. These vary according to the patient's medical status, but also according to sex, mental condition, race, etc.

A white blood cell (WBC) count reflects the body's defense mechanism. A patient with a high WBC count may have an active infection (more WBCs are needed to fight off the illness), and he or she may not be a good candidate for strenuous, or any, exercise.[26] On the other hand, a patient with an excessively low WBC count may have an immunosuppressed condition, which would at the very

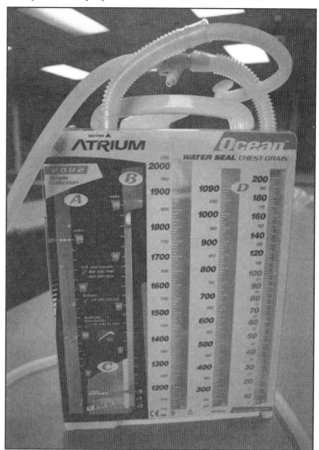

Figure 7-16. A chest tube.

least require the health care worker to maintain universal precautions, including handwashing and personal protective equipment.

Red blood cells (RBCs) bind with hemoglobin (Hgb) and carry oxygen to the tissue's cells. A patient with a low RBC count may have anemia, and may not have a good oxygen supply to the cells. This patient may again be limited in what he or she can do during therapy sessions.

Hematocrit measures the volume of RBCs in a sample of blood; it assesses blood loss and fluid balance.[26] A low RBC count may indicate anemia and that the patient will not tolerate intense exercise. Similarly, Hgb is a protein in the RBC that transports the oxygen in the blood. A measurement of Hgb assesses blood loss, anemia, and bone marrow suppression.[26] A patient with a low Hgb has reduced tolerance of exercise, and a patient with a reading of 6.5 to 8 mg/dL should not participate in therapy at all.

Other values to monitor are a patient's glucose level and international normalized ratio (INR). Glucose is the amount of sugar in the blood, and these values can be used to diagnose diabetes. Too low or too high levels of blood sugar are both dangerous; values below 40 or greater than 500 mg/dL are dangerous and therapy should not be done, but even numbers greater than 200 mg/dL and trending up or less than 70 mg/dL and trending down could indicate a decreased tolerance for activity.[26,27,28]

Table 7-1 Normal Lab Values[30]	
Hemoglobin	Male: 13.5 to 17.5 mg/dL
	Female: 12 to 15.5 mg/dL
Hematocrit	Male: 38% to 50%
	Female: 34.9% to 44.5%
Red blood cells	Male: 25 to 35 mL/kg
	Female: 20 to 30 mL/kg
White blood cells	3.5 to 10.5 billion cells/L
Glucose (fasting)	70 to 105 mg/dL
Creatine phosphokinase	30 to 170 U/L
Oxygen saturation	Greater than 94%
Partial pressure of oxygen	Greater than 80 mmHg
Platelets	150 to 450 billion/L

An INR measures the blood clotting or coagulation; if the number is too high, a patient may be prone to excessive bleeding even with a minor injury. A value greater than 6.0 is dangerous for therapy interventions.

A therapist who works in the ICU should be especially aware of these laboratory values; however, any health care provider should look at these values and understand their meanings, especially when it comes to the type or amount of therapy you plan to administer. Table 7-1 includes normal lab values,[26,29] and Table 7-2 includes critical values for when a therapist should alter or not perform therapy with the patient.

SAFETY/RED FLAGS

Urinary catheters are not contraindications for therapy interventions; however, you should know where the catheter is inserted or attached, and you should be aware of the collection bag. The collection bag should never be above the level of the patient's bladder; gravity assists with the urine draining, and if the bag is placed above the level of the bladder, urine will run back into the urethra and bladder and could cause an infection. Additionally, it is worth your while to assess the collection bag for its fullness. A full catheter bag is at a higher risk to fail or leak; you may want to empty the bag prior to performing therapy interventions with your patient. Just make sure that the nursing staff are not measuring the urine (they often are); if the nursing staff are measuring output, alert them prior to emptying the bag, or find out if you can measure the output yourself. Make sure you wear gloves when emptying catheter bags to prevent infection.

A Foley catheter and a suprapubic catheter can be accidentally removed if caught, pulled, or tangled in other equipment. You should be aware of where the catheter bag and tubing are located to prevent such entanglements. Additionally, a suprapubic catheter is located right where therapists generally place gait belts; you may want to place the gait belt higher to avoid rubbing on or removing the catheter. The tape or strap on external (or condom) catheters should not be so tight as to prevent blood flow, and these catheters come off quite easily (although it does not cause the pain or risk of infection that Foley or suprapubic catheters do when removed accidentally).

Urinary tract infections are common in patients with long-term catheter use. Typical complaints include pain or burning at the catheter insertion site, bloody or cloudy urine, lower back or abdominal pain, or a fever. Cognitive and behavioral changes can be noted in elderly patients. A patient who could follow commands yesterday but seems confused or agitated today may be suffering from an undiagnosed urinary tract infection. You may be the first to notice these changes, so you should report these to the nursing staff, document thoroughly, and alert your supervising physical therapist.

Like catheters, ostomies are also at risk for being accidentally removed. Patients with ostomies are not unable to perform therapeutic activities; however, placement of a gait belt may interfere with the ostomy bag, leakages could be a concern, and accidental removal of the collection pouch could cause discomfort or embarrassment for the patient. If the pouch is full, it would be a good idea to have the patient or nursing staff assist in emptying the bag prior to therapy.

A student physical therapist assistant was scheduled to see a patient in the ICU. This patient had an endotracheal tube to deliver oxygen via the ventilator. Upon sitting this patient up on the end of the bed, the ventilator popped out of the patient's trachea, sounding various alarms from the machine. The student, panicking, was unsure of how to

Table 7-2
Abnormal Lab Values and Their Effects on Therapy

Hematocrit less than 25%	Essential activities of daily living (ADL; assistance for safety)
Hematocrit less than 25% to 35%	Essential ADL, light aerobics or weights (1 to 2 lbs)
Hematocrit greater than 35%	Ambulation and self-care as tolerated; resistance and aerobic exercises
Hemoglobin less than 8 mg/dL	Essential ADL
Hemoglobin less than 8 to 10 mg/dL	Essential ADL, light aerobics or weights (1 to 2 lbs)
Hemoglobin greater than 8 mg/dL	Ambulation and self-care as tolerated; resistance exercises
Platelets less than 10,000 (and temperature greater than 100.5°F)	No exercise (hold therapy)
Platelets 10,000 to 20,000	Therapeutic exercise/bike without resistance
Platelets greater than 20,000	Therapeutic exercise/bike with or without resistance

replace the tube. Thankfully, the ICU nurse was close by and she simply popped the tube back in and walked back to her station. Crisis averted.

Patients on ventilators will need to be monitored first to ensure the ventilator is not kinked or removed. Tubing should also be long enough to prevent problems if the patient is going to transfer to another surface or ambulate. Sometimes tubes pop out with little to no activity; knowing how to handle this situation or knowing who to ask for help will alleviate the panic that comes with alarms ringing all around. Also, signs and symptoms of respiratory distress should be noted if they arise, including tachypnea, dyspnea, hyperventilation, or tachycardia. In these cases, calling a staff emergency and/or alerting the nursing staff are the best solutions.

Patients who need oxygen but are not on ventilators must still be monitored for signs or symptoms of respiratory distress. Get used to the idea of checking oxygenation regularly and looking to ensure the patient is wearing the oxygen device correctly. If a therapist was given a quarter for every time he or she found a patient wearing a nasal cannula incorrectly, well, you get the idea.

Prevent tubing kinks and make sure that the tubing is not pulled out. A therapist once went to a patient's home to work on the patient's endurance. The patient needed oxygen, and she dutifully wore the nasal cannula during the entire therapy session. However, she was still very short of breath, and her SpO$_2$ was 80% when the therapist checked it. A quick inspection revealed that even though the patient was wearing her cannula and the oxygen compressor was on, the cannula was not connected to the compressor so the patient was not receiving any oxygen.

Something else to remember is that oxygen is highly combustible. This may not seem like an issue, until you realize that your home health patient who is on oxygen also goes out on her porch to smoke every 20 minutes (while still wearing the nasal cannula). In hospitals and facilities, oxygen tanks are stored in dry, temperature-controlled areas, and smoking is not allowed on most health care campuses.

Patients who have traction or fixation applied for bone alignment have certain limitations for activity. As mentioned before, the physician or surgeon often provide therapists with a protocol for therapy. Safety concerns include weightbearing (as in do not allow the patient to ambulate full weightbearing if he or she is contraindicated to do so) and infection control. Halos and internal/external fixators have points of entry into the soft tissue; these are all areas where infection can gain entry. Monitor the pin sites or incision locations for signs of infection, including redness, swelling, and warmth.

Be sure to avoid bumping or knocking into the extremity or fixators so as not to disrupt the alignment. Additionally, keep an eye out for signs of a thrombus. Patients who are relatively immobilized are at a higher risk for DVTs, and if a thrombus becomes an embolus, the patient's life is in danger. Nursing staff should be notified immediately if signs or symptoms of a DVT are present, and you should cease all treatment until the situation is resolved.

Patients who have hemodialysis have shunts or fistulas, typically in an arm. It is important to not do excessive activity with that arm, and it is especially key to avoid compression or taking blood pressure in that arm.

A chest tube is held in place with only a couple of stitches, and a tug on it could be very painful. Avoid kinking or pulling on the tubing, and keep the collection unit below the level of the chest. Monitor the patient's response to therapy and provide rest breaks as needed. Alert nursing staff if the collection unit is full or if the tube insertion site is bleeding or especially painful for the patient.

As mentioned before, lab values are very important to consider when performing therapy. Some high or low values influence whether a patient can take part in therapy or how much therapy a practitioner will allow the patient to do. A patient with an INR of 8.2 may start bleeding internally or externally due to decreased clotting. A patient with a low blood sugar level (also known as *hypoglycemia*) may demonstrate signs and symptoms such as heart palpitations, fatigue, shakiness, sweating, irritability, or in the worst situations, confusion, blurred vision, seizures, and loss of consciousness. High blood sugar (hyperglycemia) has its own dangers, including nausea, vomiting, weakness, confusion, and shortness of breath. Too high or too low levels of blood sugar should indicate to a therapist that therapy interventions are not warranted.

Patients with low SpO_2 (less than 60%) are contraindicated for therapy, as are patients with low Hgb, Hct, and potassium. In all of these cases, a patient would be put on hold, with documentation of the patient's lab values. If a patient is still able to participate in therapy, but at a lighter intensity, this should also be documented.

Patients with feeding devices such as NG or G tubes should avoid activities that would disrupt the use of their devices. No tubing should be kinked or occluded, nor should they be removed. A G tube's placement in the abdomen makes it susceptible to pain or disruption with a gait belt application, so the belt may need to be placed superior to the G tube insertion site.

An IV insertion site can be tender to the touch and a therapist should avoid pulling on or occluding the tubing. No compression or blood pressure should be taken on the extremity with the IV, so the proper function of the IV is not disrupted. As a clinician, you should monitor the IV site for signs of infection, including pain, redness, or discharge from the insertion site. Other complications of IVs include phlebitis, thrombophlebitis, air embolism, and allergic reaction. If you observe any of these complications, you should immediately notify the nursing staff. Additionally, if the IV is removed for any reason, you should notify the nursing staff.

DOCUMENTATION

The following examples of documentation include information about the various equipment seen in the patient's room and lab values included on the patient's chart.

O: Patient in bed with HOB elevated. Patient performed bed mobility of rolling to Ⓛ and Ⓡ and supine ←→ sit requiring min Ⓐ for all tasks, with IV pole moved around bed to accommodate length of tubing. Patient is on 3 L of O_2 via nasal cannula and monitor SpO_2; patient at 89% after performing supine ←→ sit transfers so patient allowed time to rest with cues for pursed lip breathing x 5 minutes until O_2 saturation at 95%. Patient performed 5 sit to stands requiring min Ⓐ and

stand pivot transfer to chair mod Ⓐ with gait belt. Patient's Foley catheter full and notified nursing staff.

O: Patient in ICU to receive AAROM. Per patient's chart, patient Hct at 28% so patient only eligible for light exercise. Performed AAROM to shoulder, elbow, knee, and hips; patient complained of fatigue so allowed rest break. Patient requested repositioning in bed so lowered HOB and assisted patient with scooting up in bed. Patient on patient-controlled analgesia and used pump 3 times during therapy session.

REVIEW QUESTIONS

1. List 3 lab values and their abnormal numbers that would limit or prohibit therapy interventions.

2. Discuss the potential concerns or red flags for patients with IVs. What about for patients with Halos?

3. List the types of hospital beds and one advantage and disadvantage of each.

4. You are going to treat a patient with a nasal cannula, an IV, a chest tube, and a urinary (Foley) catheter. What does it mean if his SpO_2 is at 80%? What about if his chart indicates that his WBC count is less than 500 mm^3 and the patient has a fever? What would you need to be mindful of if your daily goal is to perform a sit ←→ stand transfer and have the patient ambulate 20 feet with a walker?

5. Define the following: IV, ORIF, NG tube.

6. If a patient is unable to sit on the edge of the bed for therapy, what other tasks could you perform with this patient?

7. Prior to entering a patient's room, what should you note or do?

8. You are treating a patient in the ICU who is on a ventilator. While performing passive and active assistive exercises with the patient, her ventilator alarm goes off. What should you do?

REFERENCES

1. 965 Wedge Turning Frame: operations and maintenance manual. *Stryker Medical.* https://techweb.stryker.com/Stretcher/0965/0965-001-233E.pdf. Accessed September 5, 2018.

2. Clinitron Rite Hite Air Fluidized Therapy Bed. *Hill-Rom.* http://www.hill-rom.com/usa/Products/Category/Wound-Therapy-Systems/Clinitron-RiteHite-Air-Fluidized-Beds/. Accessed September 5, 2018.

3. RotoRest Critical Care Therapy System. *Arjo Huntleigh.* https://www.arjo.com/DownloadFile?fileId=00000000-0000-0000-0000-000000011235. Published 2015. Accessed November 7, 2018.

4. KinAir IV. *Wound Source.* http://www.woundsource.com/product/kinair-iv. Accessed September 5, 2018.

5. Hill-Rom. Excel Care ES Bariatric Hospital Bed. http://www.hill-rom.com/usa/Products/Category/Hospital-Beds/Excel-Care-ES-bariatric-hospital-bed/. Accessed September 5, 2018.

6. Bariatric hospital bed, medical beds, bariatric bed. *RehabMart.* http://www.rehabmart.com/category/bariatric_hospital_beds.htm. Accessed September 5, 2018.

7. What is an ostomy? *United Ostomy Associations of America, Inc.* http://www.ostomy.org/What_is_an_Ostomy.html. Accessed September 5, 2018.

8. Ventilator modes. *Covidien.* http://www.livingwithavent.com/ventilation-basics/ventilator-modes.html. Accessed November 7, 2018.

9. Modes of mechanical ventilation. *Open Anesthesia.* https://www.openanesthesia.org/modes_of_mechanical_ventilation/. Accessed September 5, 2018.

10. Pulmonary artery catheterization. *Johns Hopkins Medicine.* http://www.hopkinsmedicine.org/healthlibrary/test_procedures/cardiovascular/pulmonary_artery_catheterization_135,392/. Accessed September 5, 2018.

11. Bangalore S, Bhatt DL. Right heart catheterization, coronary angiography, and percutaneous coronary intervention. *Circulation.* 2011;124(17):e428-e433.

12. Intracranial pressure. *Trauma.* http://www.trauma.org/archive/neuro/icp.html. Published 2000. Accessed September 5, 2018.

13. Kawoos U, McCarron RM, Auker CR, Chavko M. Advances in intracranial pressure monitoring and its significance in managing traumatic brain injury. *Int J Mol Sci.* 2015;16(12):28979-28997. Doi: 10.3390/ijms161226146.

14. McConnell EA. Clinical do's & don'ts. Preventing transient increases in ICP. *Nursing.* 2001;31(3):17.

15. Central venous catheters. *American Cancer Society.* https://www.cancer.org/treatment/treatments-and-side-effects/central-venous-catheters.html. Updated February 11, 2016. Accessed September 5, 2018.

16. Hickman catheter care with a needless connector. *UW Health.* https://www.uwhealth.org/healthfacts/vad/4324.pdf. Published November 2015. Accessed September 5, 2018.

17. Care of your Hickman catheter. *Johns Hopkins Medicine.* http://www.hopkinsmedicine.org/kimmel_cancer_center/patient_information/education/treatment/Hickman_catheter_Care_of_Your_booklet.pdf. Published 1999. Updated June 2014. Accessed September 5, 2018.

18. Tegtmeyer K, Brady G, Lai S, Hodo R, Braner D. Videos in clinical medicine. Placement of an arterial line. *N Engl J Med.* 2006;354(15):e13-e14.

19. Nasogastric tubes 1: insertion technique and confirming position. *Nursing Times.* April 24, 2009. https://www.nursingtimes.net/clinical-archive/gastroenterology/nasogastric-tubes-1-insertion-technique-and-confirming-position/5000781.article. Accessed September 5, 2018.

20. Gastrostomy (G) tubes. *Feeding Tube Awareness Foundation.* http://www.feedingtubeawareness.org/tube-feeding-basics/tubetypes/g-tube/. Accessed September 5, 2018.

21. Thomas DR. Intravenous feeding (parenteral nutrition). *Merck Manuals.* http://www.merckmanuals.com/home/disorders-of-nutrition/nutritional-support/intravenous-feeding. Updated March 2018. Accessed September 5, 2018.

22. Zimmer traction handbook: a complete guide to the basics of traction. *Zimmer.* http://www.zimmer.com/content/dam/zimmer-web/documents/en-US/pdf/medical-professionals/surgical-and-operating-room-solutions/zimmer-traction-handbook.pdf. Published 2006. Accessed September 5, 2018.

23. Fragomen A, Rozbruch S. The mechanics of external fixation. *HSS J.* 2007;3(1):13-29. Doi: 10.1007/s11420-006-9025-0.

24. Dialysis. *National Kidney Foundation.* https://www.kidney.org/atoz/content/dialysisinfo. Accessed September 5, 2018.

25. Patient information series: chest tube thoracostomy. *American Thoracic Society.* https://www.thoracic.org/patients/patient-resources/resources/chest-tube-thoracostomy.pdf. Published 2004. Revised August 2012. Accessed September 5, 2018.

26. Laboratory values interpretation resource. *Academy of Acute Care Physical Therapy.* https://cdn.ymaws.com/www.acutept.org/resource/resmgr/docs/2017-Lab-Values-Resource.pdf. Published August 2008. Updated January 2017. Accessed September 5, 2018.

27. Hyperglycemia in diabetes. *Mayo Clinic.* http://www.mayoclinic.org/diseases-conditions/hyperglycemia/basics/symptoms/con-20034795. Updated July 26, 2018. Accessed September 5, 2018.

28. Hypoglycemia. *Mayo Clinic.* http://www.mayoclinic.org/diseases-conditions/hypoglycemia/basics/symptoms/con-20021103. Updated February 16, 2018. Accessed September 5, 2018.

29. Wians FH. Normal laboratory values. *Merck Manuals.* https://www.merckmanuals.com/professional/appendixes/normal-laboratory-values/normal-laboratory-values. Accessed September 5, 2018.

30. Complete Blood Count (CBC). *Mayo Clinic.* https://www.mayoclinic.org/tests-procedures/complete-blood-count/about/pac-20384919. Published January 9, 2018. Accessed October 2, 2018.

Chapter 8

Wheelchair Features and Activities

Memolo J.
Procedures and Patient Care for the Physical Therapist Assistant
(pp 103-122). © 2019 SLACK Incorporated.

KEY TERMS Ascend | Descend | Pneumatic | Popliteal space | Semipneumatic | Restraint

KEY ABBREVIATIONS CVA

CHAPTER OBJECTIVES

1. List and perform the measurements for a wheelchair.
2. Check for wheelchair fit, and discuss the negative effects for a poorly fitted wheelchair.
3. Educate a patient on how to propel and turn a wheelchair, and how to navigate curbs, ramps, and stairs.
4. Name and identify the components of a wheelchair.
5. Identify red flags or safety concerns for users of wheelchairs.

INTRODUCTION

Likely you have seen someone in a wheelchair. Maybe it was the old-fashioned manual kind, the kind that a person has to propel him- or herself. Or perhaps you saw the motorized version with a joystick on the armrest. Surely you have seen the scooters available for use in grocery stores. There are all sorts of wheelchairs out there, and you will interact with a fair amount of them. It is not required or necessary for you to know every single one. In some cases, you may find that occupational therapists have taken over the responsibility of measuring, fitting, and ordering wheelchairs for patients; in many cases, you will bear some, if not all, of the responsibility. Your job will be to constantly assess the patient and the chair to ensure proper use and fit, and to make sure the patient is safe and does not have any complications from using the wheelchair. Box 8-1 includes a list of factors associated with selecting a wheelchair.

TYPES OF WHEELCHAIRS

The following sections discuss the most common types of wheelchairs you might encounter. It is not in any way comprehensive, but it should give you a good idea of what to expect. Your job may include assisting a patient in selecting the right type of wheelchair for his or her needs. You should consider how long the patient will need the chair, the patient's physical abilities, and what the patient plans to use the chair for (or in what environment).[1] You will also need to consider the patient's insurance and other financial resources, as wheelchairs, especially customized versions, can become quite expensive.[1]

Standard Wheelchairs

The most common wheelchair you will see, the one that is in every hospital and therapy gym, is the standard wheelchair (Figure 8-1). It is for patients who weigh under 200 pounds (lbs) and generally for those who are not going

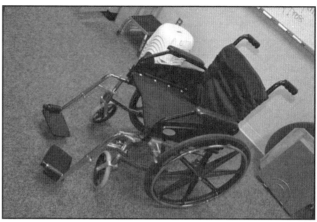

Figure 8-1. A standard wheelchair.

Bariatric Wheelchairs

Bariatric wheelchairs are similar to standard wheelchairs, except they are for patients over 200 lbs and so are made of sturdier materials. This type of chair is also heavier.

Pediatric Wheelchairs

Wheelchairs can also be sized for young adults or children. These pediatric wheelchairs are typically more lightweight and are generally sized to fit a smaller body (Figure 8-2).

Light or Ultralight Wheelchairs

Some wheelchairs are classified as adult but are further classified as lightweight or ultralight; these can vary from 15 to 25 lbs. These can be rigid or collapsible, and legrests may be fixed. The seat back may also be lower so long as the patient has good trunk control.

Sport or Athletic Wheelchairs

Athletes have specialized wheelchairs with angled wheels, low seat backs, and are made with lightweight materials. These are made for patients who play basketball or who race, although they are often preferred by younger patients to get around quickly. These are sometimes called *quickies* (Figure 8-3).[2]

Hemiplegic Wheelchairs

A hemiplegic wheelchair is for patients who have a weak side, often due to a cerebrovascular accident (CVA). These wheelchairs are 2 inches lower to allow the patient to use his or her lower extremities to propel the wheelchair. Some hemiplegic chairs allows for a one-hand drive; in these chairs, instead of using both drive wheels to propel and turn the chair, the chair has a double handrim.[2] This has both handrims on the same side of the wheelchair; the outer rim controls the wheel on that side and the smaller

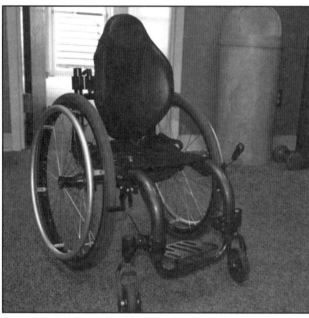

Figure 8-2. A pediatric wheelchair.

to be using the chair for long-term purposes. This chair is propelled manually and is not for use over rough terrain. It is heavier than other chairs, and the seat is a sling seat. The legrests may or may not be removable, and the same goes for the armrests. Generally standard wheelchairs are collapsible, so they can be fit in the trunk of a car for transport.

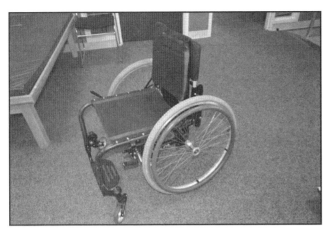

Figure 8-3. A quickie wheelchair.

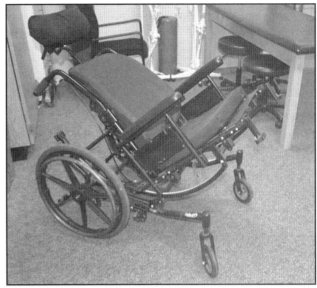

Figure 8-4. A reclining wheelchair.

rim controls the wheel on the contralateral side. Other versions of one-hand drive wheelchairs have a lever driver connected to the rear wheels.[3] The lever has a forward, neutral, and reverse setting, and the patient pumps the lever to move in the direction selected.

Amputee Wheelchairs

An amputee wheelchair has the drive wheels positioned 2 inches posterior to the normal position, which widens the base of support and acts as a counterbalance to the patient's loss of lower extremities.

Reclining and Tilt-In-Space Wheelchairs

Some wheelchairs offer the option to recline or tilt. A reclining wheelchair (Figure 8-4) allows only the back of the chair to tilt back, like a recliner. These can be semi-reclining, in that they only allow the back to tilt to 30 degrees, or fully reclining, in that they allow the back to tilt to horizontal. A tilt-in-space chair (Figure 8-5) tilts the entire chair at different angles. Both of these types of wheelchairs require head rests and elevating legrests. These wheelchairs are beneficial to patients who spend a great deal of time in a wheelchair but may be unable to change positions or shift weight to reduce pressure buildup. Reclining and tilt-in-space wheelchairs can be further customized with lateral trunk support, various seat cushions, and lower extremity supports.

Motorized Wheelchairs

Some wheelchairs are powered by motors, and these are driven by joysticks, chin pieces, or mouth pieces. These chairs function on batteries that must be charged when the chair is not in use. Eventually, the batteries will need to be replaced. These chairs are for patients who cannot operate a manual wheelchair due to a lack of strength or endurance. Some motorized wheelchairs allow the driver to adjust the speed; some systems allow for the speed to be preset. Figure 8-6 shows a motorized wheelchair.

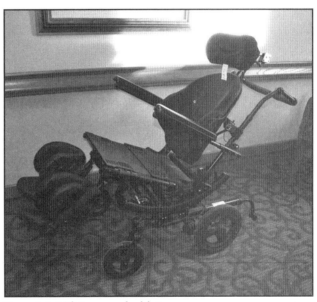

Figure 8-5. A tilt-in-space wheelchair.

Rigid Frame Versus Collapsible Frame Wheelchairs

Wheelchairs can be made of a rigid frame or can be collapsible. Rigid frame wheelchairs are easier to propel and are more compact, but they are more difficult to transport. Collapsible frames allow for easier transport and absorb shock better, but they can be hard to propel and are typically heavier than their rigid-frame counterparts. To collapse a standard wheelchair, one should pull at the center of the sling seat or on the seat rail; to open the chair, push down on the seat rails. Figure 8-7 includes pictures of opening and closing a wheelchair. Some chairs have more complex opening and collapsing systems.

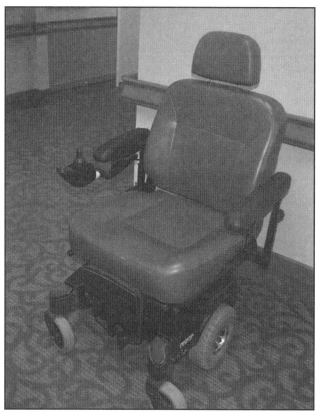

Figure 8-6. A motorized wheelchair.

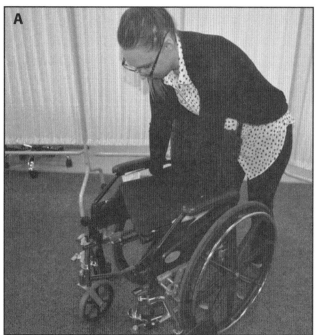

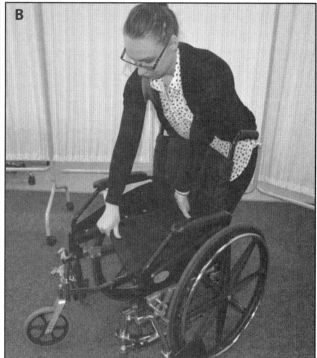

Figure 8-7. (A) Opening and (B) closing a standard wheelchair.

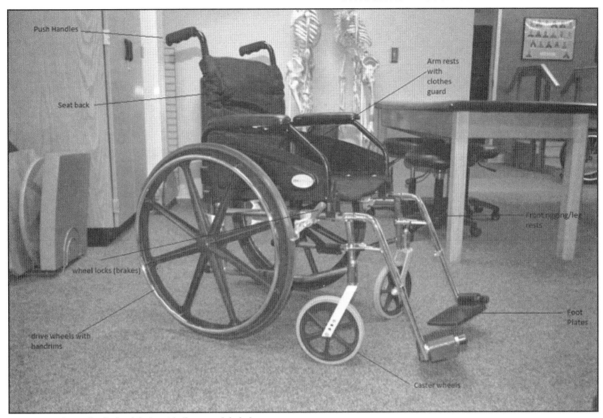

Figure 8-8. A standard wheelchair with the parts labeled.

WHEELCHAIR PARTS

All wheelchairs have basic parts, and although these may vary in type or structure, they serve similar functions. Figure 8-8 shows a standard wheelchair with its parts labeled. Specialization of wheelchairs is not uncommon; the following sections discuss the most common components found on wheelchairs. Wheelchair prescriptions often include the components a patient will need or not need according to his or her needs. It is not unusual for physical therapist assistants to weigh in on wheelchair prescriptions, so you should be familiar with these parts and how they work.

Seating Systems or Options

Standard wheelchairs come with a typical sling seat. This is acceptable for patients who are not planning to use the chair for prolonged periods of time. However, a sling seat promotes internal rotation of the hips and provides no support or cushion for the bony places on a patient's rear end. The ischium, sacrum, and coccyx thusly take a lot of pressure and wounds can appear if pressure relief is not performed regularly. Figure 8-9 shows an example of wheelchair cushions.

Cushions can range in size and type, but all cushions have the main goal of preventing pressure buildup. Basic foam cushions are made from basic or memory foam, and they are flat or contoured. These are the cheapest options for cushions, and they do not prevent pressure buildup as well as other cushions. Some do offer moisture wicking for additional skin protection.

Gel cushions offer a little more support than foam. These can also be flat or contoured, and they also have moisture wicking options. Some of the gel cushions offer a seat well in the back to offer additional pressure relief for the sacrum. Flat gel cushions are less costly but less preventative for pressure buildup. Contoured gel cushions are more costly but are better at distributing weight properly and with positioning the patient.

Air cushions, best represented by the ROHO cushion, consist of air bladders that can be filled or emptied according to the spots where pressure builds up the most. Other versions of air cushions have Comfort Cells, or air-filled packets, that can be added or removed to provide support or reduce pressure. Some air cushions are contoured for additional pressure relief or posture support.

As with all components of wheelchairs, cushions are customizable according to the patient's needs. They also come in various thicknesses, which affects wheelchair

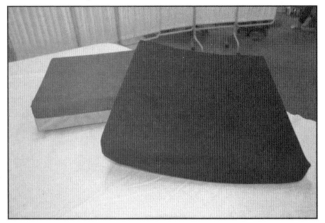

Figure 8-9. Several wheelchair cushions.

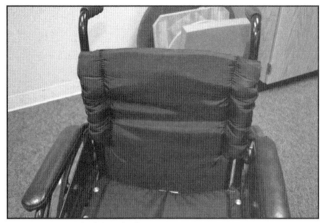

Figure 8-10. A wheelchair backrest.

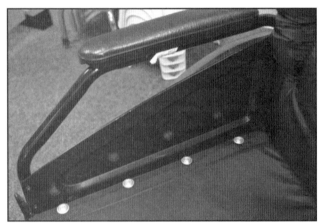

Figure 8-11. A clothing guard.

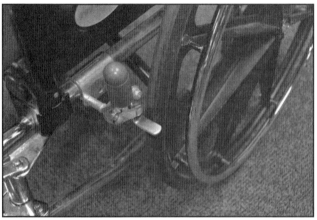

Figure 8-12. A toggle wheelchair lock.

measurements as you will see later in this chapter. Often a patient will undergo pressure mapping, which is a way of measuring the seating pressure and helps a clinician know what cushion would provide the best pressure relief for that person. It is very individualized and can save a patient from pressure injuries in the future.

Backrests

Just as cushions are customizable, so are backrests (Figure 8-10). They can have basic foam or memory foam for support, and most versions offer some measure of lateral trunk support. Specialty versions have more lateral support than generic backrests for those who have less strength or trunk control.

Clothing Guards

Wheelchairs offer clothing guards on either side of the seat (Figure 8-11). These are usually a part of the armrest system, and these protect the patient's clothes or arms from bumping into, being rubbed by, or getting tangled in the drive wheels.

Wheel Locks

One of the most important parts of a wheelchair to identify and become familiar with using is the wheel locks. These prevent the wheelchair from moving, and it is critically important that these are locked when performing wheelchair exercises or transfers. Some people call these the wheelchair brakes, and this is appropriate so long as you do not think of them as something that will slow down a wheelchair, like brakes in a car. They are only for preventing the wheels from moving. If a patient tries to use the brakes to slow down a wheelchair, the chair might tip over.

Wheel locks come in various forms, but the most common is the classic toggle lock (Figure 8-12). You either push or pull a lever until it clicks, and this locks or unlocks the drive wheel. These can also come with extensions for those who cannot reach the shorter levers next to the wheels. It is important to educate your patient (and to recall yourself) that the lock should click to indicate that it is secured.

Scissor locks are for more active patients, but they may require fine motor skills to operate that some patients may lack. A patient needs to lean forward to engage or disengage the locks, so he or she will need good balance or trunk control to operate these locks.

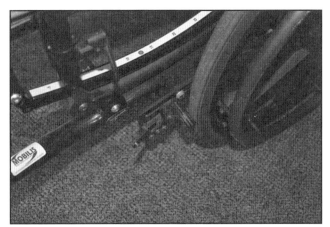

Figure 8-13. A reclining wheelchair lock.

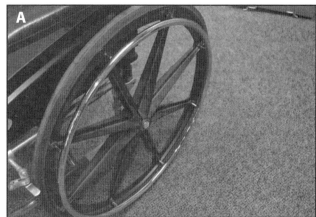

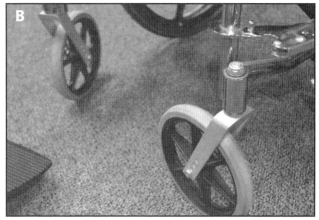

Figure 8-14. (A) The drive wheel with handrims and (B) caster wheels.

Reclining chairs have locks either at the push handles or at the wheels, depending on the make and model (Figure 8-13). Patients are often unable to lock or unlock the wheels themselves unless the chair is motorized; otherwise, the caregiver must lock the wheels.

Wheels and Tires

A wheelchair comes with 2 larger wheels in the back, called the *drive wheels* (Figure 8-14A), and 2 wheels in the front, called *caster wheels* (Figure 8-14B). The drive wheels are used for propulsion, and they can have various types of tires, including pneumatic and solid rubber. The type of tires selected can influence whether the wheelchair is better suited for indoor or outdoor use; solid rubber tires fare better indoors while pneumatic tires may be better for patients who intend to use the wheelchair over various terrains.

The drive wheels have handrims, which are used for propulsion, and the handrims can have a coating on them that increases friction (or reduces slippage) to make propulsion easier for those with reduced hand function, or they can be angled (called a *camber*) to ease propulsion. A new type of wheel, called a *vulcan wheel*, is ergonomically designed to widen the surface area for a patient to push.[4] It combines the handrim and the drive wheel into one, which reduces the risk of hand injuries and allows more force from the user to propel the chair.

The caster wheels are able to turn in all directions and again can be urethane or filled entirely or partially with air. Pneumatic tires do well over rough terrain, while urethane tires do better indoors. Caster wheels also come in different diameters.

Armrests

Armrests assist patients with repositioning, transfers, trunk support, and protection from rubbing on the drive wheels; they can be fixed or removable. Fixed armrests are permanently attached to the chair and are useful for patients who do not need to move the armrests for transfers or other activities. Removable armrests (Figure 8-15) can either completely come off the frame or can swing back and out of the way. This is useful for lateral boost or slide board transfers.

Armrests can be customized as desk or cutout types, allowing a patient to pull the chair up to a desk, table, or sink. Armrests can also be adjustable, meaning that the patient can adjust the armrest height up or down. This is helpful if the patient changes cushion types and is thusly seated higher or lower in the chair.

There are customizable armrests that serve as arm troughs or arm trays. An arm trough is an armrest that has a cushioned groove along its length and prevents the arm from falling off the armrest. An arm trough is useful for patients who lack the muscle tone or strength to keep the arm on the armrest on their own, such as if the person has had a CVA. An arm tray is an armrest with a wider tray that allows the patient to both rest his or her arm, as well as place food, drinks, or reading material on it. See Figure 8-16 for an example of an arm tray. While a trough is meant to hold the upper extremity in position, the tray does not limit or restrict the upper extremity movement. Troughs and trays can often be swung out of the way or angled to better fit the patient.

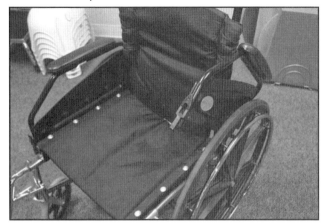

Figure 8-15. Swing away armrests.

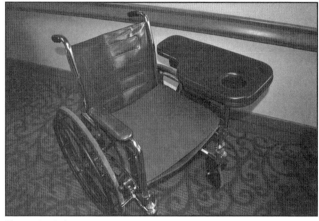

Figure 8-16. An arm tray.

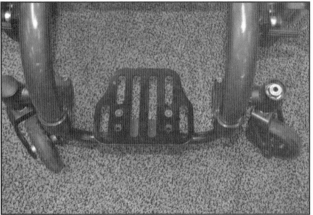

Figure 8-17. Quickie legrests.

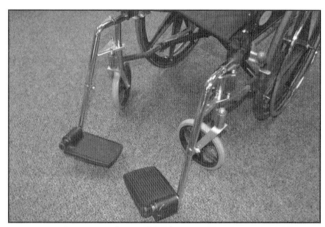

Figure 8-18. Legrests without calf pads.

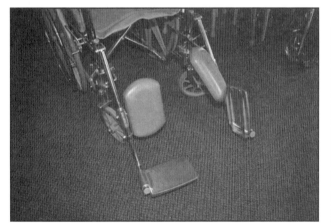

Figure 8-19. Legrests with calf pads.

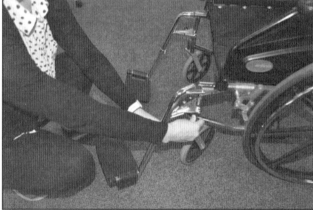

Figure 8-20. Removing legrests and swinging them out of way.

Legrests and Footrests

Legrests, like armrests, can be fixed or removable/adjustable. Fixed legrests are typically for patients who are not and do not plan to be ambulatory, and who transfer via lateral boost or slide board (Figure 8-17). Otherwise, legrests should be able to swing out of the way or be removed so a patient can stand or transfer easily.

To swing the legs rests out of the way, there is usually a lever or pin lock to press or push. To remove the legrests, they generally lift up and off the front rigging of the chair. Figure 8-18 shows typical legrests for a wheelchair without calf pads, Figure 8-19 shows legrests with calf pads, and Figure 8-20 shows how to swing or remove legrests.

Some legrests can be elevated. Elevating legrests usually have calf pads to support the lower leg while it is elevated.

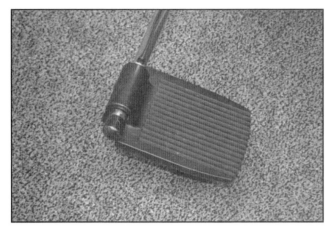

Figure 8-21. Footrests/footplates.

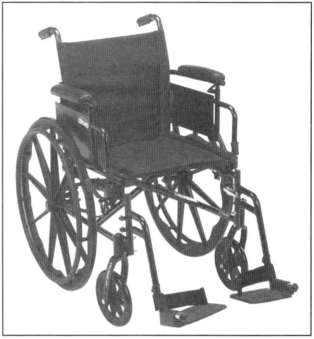

Figure 8-22. Foot rests with heel loops. (Reprinted with permission from Drive Medical.)

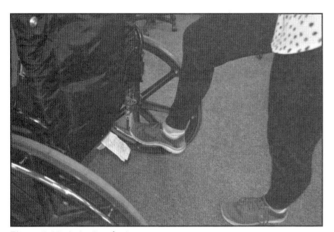

Figure 8-23. A tipping device.

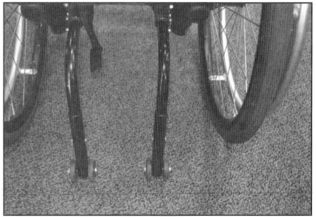

Figure 8-24. An anti-tipping device.

The legrest can be raised into an elevated position, and there is some type of a lever to lower the legrest. These are handy for patients who need one or both lower extremities raised to address edema, or if a patient is unable or contraindicated to flex the knee (such as in a long cast).

Footrests or footplates (not pedals; Figure 8-21) offer a location for the patient's feet to rest so they are not dragging on the floor. These also are able be lifted up and out of the way. Some footrests have heel loops (Figure 8-22) to prevent a patient's foot from sliding off the footrest. More customized wheelchairs have legrests and footrests that are more supportive of the lower extremities if the patient lacks the muscle tone or strength to keep the lower extremities in place. Ultralight or sport wheelchairs have footrests that are one unit, sometimes with a long loop to keep the legs from falling backward off the footplates.

In the case of wheelchair adaptations for patients with amputations, there are custom padded leg pieces that attach to the chair in lieu of a full legrest on the side of the amputation.[5] This allows the residual limb to rest comfortably while preventing injury. The attachment also removes or swings out of the way to make transfers easier.

Tipping/Anti-Tipping Devices

Tipping devices (Figure 8-23) are on the back of the wheelchair and allow a caregiver to tip the wheelchair back in order to negotiate stairs or curbs. Anti-tipping devices (Figure 8-24) are extensions added to the tipping device to prevent a patient from tipping the wheelchair back too far and falling. They also prevent the patient from negotiating curbs or stairs, so they should be removed if the patient is planning to work on or perform these skills. Anti-tipping devices can sometimes be turned up so they are out of the way for curb or stair negotiation.

Table 8-1
Wheelchair Measurements and Rationales

Seat height/leg length	Measure from heel to popliteal fold, and add 2 inches to allow clearance of footrest. Consider the height of the seat cushion if one is present.
Seat depth	Measure from posterior buttock along lateral thigh to popliteal fold, and subtract 2 inches to avoid pressure from seat on popliteal space.
Seat width	Measure widest aspect of buttocks/hips, and add 2 inches to allow for clearance of hips in chair, especially if wearing bulky clothing.
Back height	Measure from seat of the chair to the floor of the axilla with user's shoulder flexed at 90 degrees, and subtract 4 inches to allow the height to be below the inferior angles of the scapulae. Consider the height of the seat cushion if one is present.
Armrest height	Measure from the seat of the chair to the olecranon process with user's elbow flexed at 90 degrees, and add 1 inch to allow correct posture and postural changes while seated. Consider the height of the seat cushion if one is present.

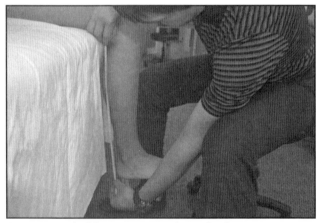

Figure 8-25. Wheelchair measurement for seat height.

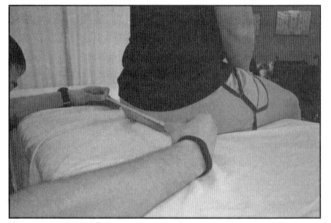

Figure 8-26. Wheelchair measurement for seat width.

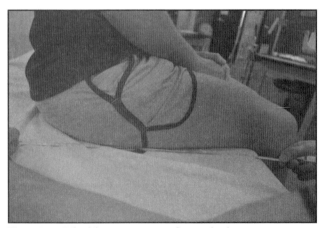

Figure 8-27. Wheelchair measurement for seat depth.

WHEELCHAIR MEASUREMENT

Wheelchair components are only one piece of the puzzle when creating a wheelchair prescription. Another piece is the measurement and assurance of fit of a patient for the wheelchair. Any patient who is going to use a wheelchair for a prolonged or permanent period of time should be measured and assessed for fit.

Measurement of a patient for a wheelchair includes 5 dimensions. Measurements should be taken with the patient not in a wheelchair but on another firm surface. If the patient has a customized cushion, this will add height and seat measurements should be adjusted accordingly. Table 8-1 includes the standard wheelchair measurements.

For seat height (or leg length), measure from the patient's heel to the popliteal fold (Figure 8-25). To allow for clearance of the footrest, 2 inches is added. For seat width, measure along the widest portion of the patient's buttocks or hips, and then add 2 inches to allow clearance of hips in the chair to avoid pressure or friction (Figure 8-26). For seat depth, measure from the posterior buttocks along the thigh to the popliteal fold and subtract 2 inches to prevent pressure from the seat on the popliteal space (Figure 8-27). For back height, measure from the seat of the chair

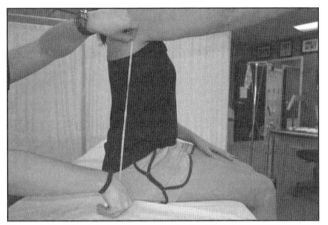

Figure 8-28. Wheelchair measurement for back height.

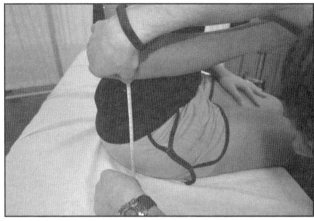

Figure 8-29. Wheelchair measurement for armrest height.

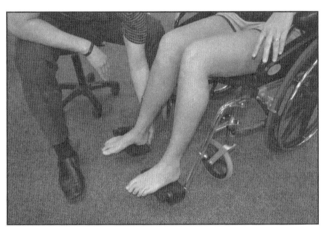

Figure 8-30. Wheelchair fit confirmation for seat height.

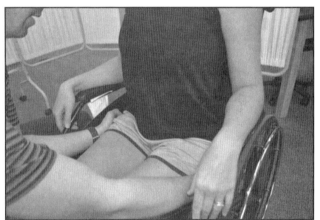

Figure 8-31. Wheelchair fit confirmation for seat width.

to the patient's axilla with the patient's shoulder flexed at 90 degrees (Figure 8-28). Four inches are subtracted from that measurement to allow the back height to be below the scapulae. If the patient has a seat cushion, the patient should be measured while sitting on the cushion to account for the cushion's height. Armrest height is measured from the seat of the chair to the olecranon process, with the patient's elbow flexed at 90 degrees (Figure 8-29). One inch is added to this measurement to prevent the patient's arms from being too elevated or too low, which would affect the patient's posture. Again, if the patient has a seat cushion, the patient should be measured while on the cushion to get an accurate measurement.

Once a prescription has been written and the patient receives the wheelchair, the fit should be confirmed. Seat height/leg length is checked by placing 2 to 3 fingers under the distal thigh to a depth of about 2 inches (Figure 8-30). The footrest should be about 2 inches off the floor to allow for clearance. Vertical placement of the hand between the greater trochanter and the armrest panels/clothing guards should confirm proper seat width (Figure 8-31). Seat depth is confirmed by placing 2 to 3 fingers between the front edge of the seat and the patient's popliteal fold

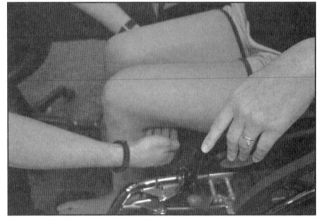

Figure 8-32. Wheelchair fit confirmation for seat depth.

(Figure 8-32). The patient should be positioned in the chair so that his or her bottom is all the way back in the seat. Back height is assessed by placing 4 fingers between the top of the backrest and the user's axilla, with the hands being held vertically (Figure 3-33). To check the armrest height, you should check the patient's posture and ensure that he or she is able to sit upright against the seat back with shoulders level and neither raised nor hunched (Figure 8-34).

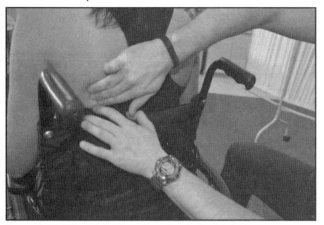

Figure 8-33. Wheelchair fit confirmation for back height.

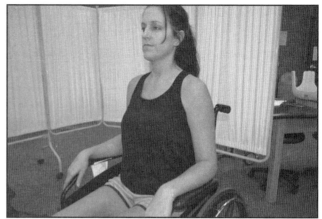

Figure 8-34. Wheelchair fit confirmation for armrest height.

Table 8-2
Wheelchair Fit Confirmation

Seat height/leg length	With user's feet on footrests, 2 to 3 fingers can be placed between user's thigh and seat; bottom of footrests should be 2 inches from the floor.
Seat depth	With user seated back in the chair, 2 to 3 fingers can be placed between the front edge of the seat and the user's popliteal fold.
Seat width	Hands can vertically fit between user's hips and the chair's clothing guards/armrests.
Back height	Four fingers (with hands held vertically) can fit between the top of the back of the seat and the floor of the user's axilla.
Armrest height	Shoulders should be level and position of trunk should be erect. User should be able to rest arms on armrests with no change in posture.

If a wheelchair does not fit properly, several adverse effects are likely. Table 8-2 discusses how to confirm wheelchair fit, and Table 8-3 includes adverse effects of a poorly fitted wheelchair.

WHEELCHAIR OPERATION

Once you have ensured that the wheelchair fits properly to your patient, you need to next work on wheelchair operation and education. The patient, as well as the patient's family or caregivers, should be educated on the parts of the wheelchair and manipulation of those parts. The less functional ability the patient has, the more difficult it will be for the patient to manipulate and propel the wheelchair. Similarly, cognitive deficits make it more difficult with patient education, and this is where education of the family or caregivers is essential.

Propulsion

If a patient is able to use bilateral upper extremities, he or she should hold the drive wheels at the 12 o'clock posi-tion and push forward with both arms pushing at the same time and with the same force.[6] To back up, the patient should pull back on the wheels at the same time. To turn, the patient should push forward on the opposite wheel of the direction he or she wants to turn and pull back on the same side wheel. For example, to turn right, the patient will push forward on the left wheel while pulling back on the right wheel. Figure 8-35 shows propulsion with 2 upper extremities.

If the patient is unable to use both upper extremities, but he or she has function of one or both lower extremities, the upper extremity can be used to push forward (or pull back) while the lower extremity provides additional propulsion and direction (Figure 8-36).[6] If the patient is unable to use either upper extremity, both lower extremities can be used to propel and direct the wheelchair (Figure 8-37).

If the patient is unable to manually propel the wheelchair him- or herself and a caregiver plans to push the wheelchair, the caregiver should be educated on how to lock the wheels, how to use the tipping device for curb or stair negotiation, and how to avoid bumping the patient into walls or corners.

	Table 8-3 Adverse Effects of a Poorly Fitted Wheelchair	
	Too High/Deep/Wide	**Too Low/Shallow/Narrow**
Seat Height/ Leg Length	Insufficient trunk support Difficulty positioning knees under table/desk Difficulty propelling wheelchair (cannot reach drive wheels) Poor posture with forearms on armrests	Difficulty with transfers due to lower center of gravity Footrests may contact items on floor and decrease mobility
Seat Depth	Increased pressure on popliteal space (causing increased pressure and decreased circulation)	Decreased trunk stability due to less support under thighs Increased weightbearing on ischial tuberosities Poor balance due to decreased base of support
Seat Width	Difficulty propelling wheelchair due to inability to reach drive wheels Difficulty performing transfers Difficulty navigating through doorways Postural deviations from leaning to one side	Difficulty changing positions Too much pressure on greater trochanters Difficulty wearing braces or orthoses due to narrow space
Back Height	Difficulty propelling wheelchair due to difficulty using arms Increased pressure/friction on scapulae Decreased balance due to inclined trunk	Decreased trunk stability or postural deviations due to less support
Armrest Height	Difficulty propelling wheelchair due to inability to reach drive wheels Difficulty performing transfers Postural deviations due to raised shoulders Decreased trunk stability due to not using armrests	Postural deviations due to depressed shoulders Decreased balance from leaning forward Difficulty with transfers

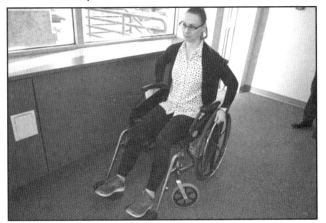

Figure 8-35. Patient propelling wheelchair with 2 upper extremities.

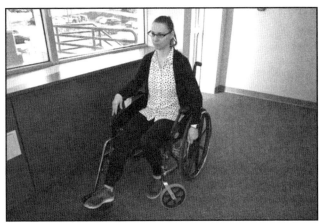

Figure 8-36. Patient propelling wheelchair with one upper extremity and one lower extremity.

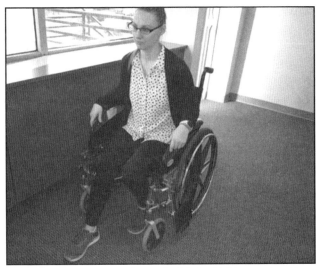

Figure 8-37. A patient propelling a wheelchair with 2 lower extremities.

Some wheelchair companies offer propulsion assist devices. Manual propulsion assist, such as Magicwheels (Magicwheels, Inc), replaces the drive wheel on a standard chair.[7] The handrims multiply the power via a system of gears in the wheel hub, so the same amount of force when a patient pushes yields a 50% decrease in difficulty. Some versions have multiple handrims, which give the patient a choice of speeds. Power assist wheels have motors built into the wheel hubs that assist with propulsion when the patient desires. Each drive wheel is powered separately to allow for forward and backward movement, as well as turning.[7] The power can be turned off to preserve battery or when the patient does not need it.

Motorized wheelchair users also require education. There was once a patient at a skilled nursing facility who requested a motorized wheelchair. Therapy assessed her needs, measured her for fit, and ordered a motorized chair.

When the chair arrived, she was educated on how to drive and how to control speed; however, despite frequent warnings and education, she was always running the chair into walls, taking out corners, and, as the final straw, she ran into another facility resident, knocking him to the ground. Ultimately, the patient was deemed unfit to drive the motorized chair and had to return to using her old manual chair. Patients who cannot manually propel a wheelchair may want or need a motorized chair, but they need to understand how to use it and how to be safe. It is the therapist's job to provide that education and to continue to assess the patient for safety.

Some motorized wheelchairs, such as the one in the above story, are propelled using a joystick. The speed can be set and the patient uses his or her hand to make the wheelchair go forward, backward, or turn.[8] These joysticks can be customized to the person's needs. For example, it can be a carrot joystick, controlled with the thumb and a few fingers; the goal post handle, for those with less hand control; and the ball and dome handle, which offers more contact area and feels different from the column shaped joysticks.[9] Some motorized wheelchairs, however, are made for patients who cannot use their hands or upper extremities. Examples of these include the sip-n-puff, in which the patient puffs or sips in a tube mounted in front of him or her to give commands to the chair; a chin joystick, which is mounted so the patient can use his or her chin to drive the chair; a tongue switch, which is mounted to the roof of the patient's mouth and the patient uses his or her tongue to drive the chair; and the head array, which allows head movement to control the chair.[9] There are even controls that respond to a patient's eye movements on a computer screen. These various controls allow patients of all abilities to still be independent with their mobility.

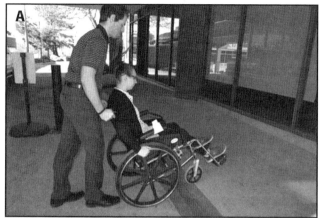 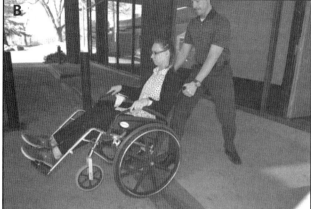

Figure 8-38. Ascending a curb forward and backward.

In regard to documentation, please note that you should reference how much assistance the patient needed with any given wheelchair task. Specific levels of assist are used commonly for gait and transfers; however, the same rules would apply for wheelchair mobility. Please see the specifics on these levels of assist in Chapter 9 (Bed Mobility and Transfers) and again in Chapter 10 (Assistive Devices and Gait). Another way to document wheelchair training can include the number of verbal or tactile cues used during the therapy session.

Curbs

It would be lovely if all streets and shopping centers had curb cutouts for wheelchair access; however, this is unfortunately not so. Patients and caregivers will need to know how to negotiate a curb.

Ascending a Curb

To ascend a curb forward, the caregiver should face the patient toward the curb and tip the patient back onto the drive wheels (using the tipping device). The caster wheels are lifted off the ground and placed up on the curb. Then, the caregiver should lift the chair to put the drive wheels on the curb level (Figure 8-38A).

To ascend a curb backward, the caregiver should first turn the wheelchair around so the patient's back is facing the curb. The caregiver should then tip the wheelchair back onto the drive wheels using the tipping device and carefully lift the drive wheels up onto the curb. Then, the caregiver should pull the chair back and slowly lower until the caster wheels are level on the elevated surface (Figure 8-38B). Box 8-2 provides instructions for ascending curbs.

Descending a Curb

To descend a curb forward, the caregiver should face the patient toward the curb and tip the wheelchair backward onto the drive wheels (using the tipping device). Then, the

> ## Box 8-2
> ### Ascending Curbs
>
> #### Ascending Forward
> 1. Face the patient toward the curb.
> 2. Using the tipping device(s), tip the wheelchair backward to elevate the caster wheels.
> 3. Advance the wheelchair until the caster wheels are on the curb.
> 4. Elevate the drive wheels, and advance the wheelchair until both the drive wheels are on the curb.
>
> #### Ascending Backward
> 1. Face the patient away from the curb.
> 2. Using the tipping device(s), tip the wheelchair backward to elevate the caster wheels.
> 3. Pull the chair over the curb, keeping the caster wheels elevated.
> 4. Pull the wheelchair back until the caster wheels can be placed on the surface; use the tipping device(s) to slowly lower the caster wheels.

caregiver should slowly lower the wheelchair off the curb onto the lower surface and carefully lower the caster wheels to the surface (Figure 8-39A).

To descend a curb backward, the caregiver should have the patient's back facing the curb. First, slowly lower the drive wheels off the curb and then tip the wheelchair back onto the drive wheels (using the tipping device). The caregiver should then back up enough to allow the caster wheels to be lowered to the ground (Figure 8-39B).

The caregiver in these circumstances should be able to assess his or her strength and ability to assist with these tasks; otherwise, the caregiver may want to seek assistance to prevent injury to the patient. Box 8-3 provides instructions for descending curbs.

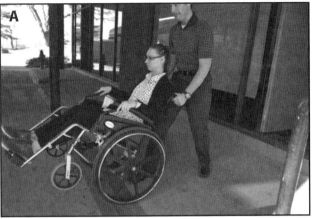 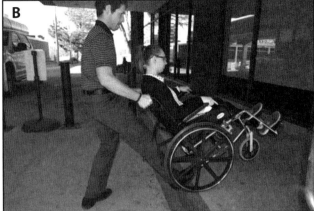

Figure 8-39. Descending a curb forward and backward.

Box 8-3

Descending Curbs

Descending Forward

1. Face the patient toward the curb.
2. Using the tipping device(s), tip the wheelchair to elevate the caster wheels.
3. Advance the wheelchair until the drive wheels descend the curb.
4. Slowly lower the caster wheels, using the tipping device(s) as needed.

Descending Backward

1. Face the patient away from the curb.
2. Slowly lower the drive wheels off the curb.
3. Using the tipping device(s), elevate the caster wheels, and back up the wheelchair until the caster wheels will clear the curb.
4. Slowly lower the caster wheels, using the tipping device(s) as needed.

Independent Curb Negotiation

Additionally, a patient may learn how to negotiate curbs independently. This usually involves popping a "wheelie," meaning the patient lifts the caster wheels off the ground and the patient is able to balance on the drive wheels. To ascend a curb, a patient could face the curb, pop a wheelie, and lift the caster wheels onto the curb before leaning forward and pushing hard with both upper extremities at the same time to lift the drive wheels. To descend a curb, a patient can either pop a wheelie when facing the curb, slowly lowering the drive wheels down, and then lowering the caster wheels to the ground; or, the patient can approach the curb backward and lean forward while backing the drive wheels off the curb and using his or her hands to slow the speed of the wheels.

Stairs

Like curbs, stairs present a potential obstacle for patients in wheelchairs. A caregiver (or multiple caregivers) is needed for a patient to negotiate stairs.

Ascending Stairs

To ascend stairs backward, at least two or possibly three people will be needed to lift the wheelchair. The caregivers should be sure to not lift using any of the removable items on the chair, such as the legrests or the armrests; if these pull loose, the wheelchair and the patient will fall.

The wheelchair should be tipped back onto the drive wheels, using the tipping device. The wheelchair should remain tipped throughout the entire process. One person will be in front of the wheelchair and one person will be behind the wheelchair; one person will be designated the leader. Both people should grab the chair's frame. On the leader's command, both with roll the chair up the stairs one step at a time. A patient could assist by pulling back on the drive wheel at the same time. Once at the top, the chair should be pulled back or turned around, so the caster wheels can be lowered.

Descending Stairs

When descending stairs forward, at least two people will be needed. Again, one will be in front and one behind. The chair should be tipped back onto the drive wheels. The leader will direct the movement, and on the leader's command, both people will slowly lower the wheelchair one step at a time. Once on the ground, the caster wheels should be lowered carefully.

Independent Stair Negotiation

It is very challenging to negotiate stairs independently. A patient can be taught how to do so utilizing a wheelie, but during training he or she should be closely guarded.

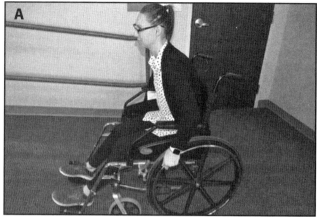

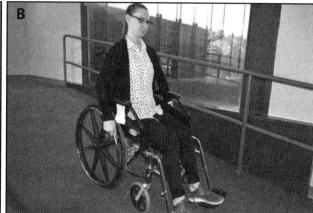

Figure 8-40. Ascending and descending a ramp in a wheelchair.

Box 8-4

Ramp Negotiation

1. To ascend, lean forward in the chair, and push equally with both upper extremities (if able). Reposition the hands as the patient advances the ramp. If the patient has one functional upper extremity, the patient should use that upper extremity and a lower extremity; the patient may need to ascend backward if this is the case.

2. To descend, the patient should lean back in the chair and use both upper extremities to provide friction on the drive wheels to slow the descent. The patient should not stop the chair suddenly, as it could flip forward. If the patient has one functional upper extremity, the patient can use that in addition to the lower extremities to provide friction.

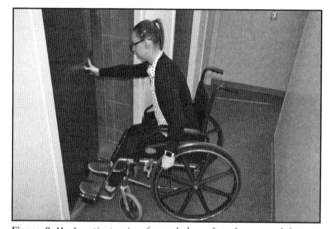

Figure 8-41. A patient going forward through a doorway while in a wheelchair.

Ramps

Patients or the caregivers pushing them should exercise caution with ramps or slopes. Some can be very steep, and it will be necessary to zigzag up or down. To ascend a slope or ramp, it is best for the patient to lean forward, so the chair will not tip backward, and push with the drive wheels at the same time. If the caregiver is pushing the patient, the wheelchair can also be tipped back onto the drive wheels to make the task easier.

To descend a ramp or slope, the patient should lean back in the chair and slowly let the drive wheels slip through the fingers, slowing the momentum. If a caregiver is performing the task, he or she can pull back on the push handles or could also tip the wheelchair back on the drive wheels. Figure 8-40 shows how to ascend and descend a ramp. Box 8-4 provides instructions for ramp negotiation.

Doorways and Elevators

If you are a caregiver pushing a patient onto an elevator, it is best practice to have the wheelchair facing forward.

This way the patient can see out the elevator and other people in the elevator; the patient will not feel like he or she is being put in the corner. If the patient is negotiating the elevator by him or herself, he or she will likely also want to face forward. It can be difficult, however, to back a wheelchair into an elevator. The doors could shut before the patient is fully inside, or the caster wheels could get stuck in the space between the floor and the elevator. Sometimes a patient can turn the wheelchair around once inside the elevator, but not all elevators are large enough to allow this.

Passing through doorways can be another challenge. Doorways in public spaces, if they are up to code, should allow for a wheelchair to pass through. Patients should gauge the distance to ensure the wheelchair will pass and must consider their hands on the drive wheels so they do not injure their fingers. Thresholds may present an obstacle if they are especially raised, and deciding whether to enter the door by going forward or backward can be tricky. The patient should consider whether the door opens in or out. This is especially challenging if the door is a self-close type, such as a public bathroom door. Figure 8-41 shows how to go forward through a doorway.

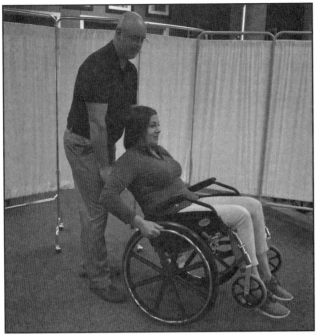

Figure 8-42. A therapist assisting a patient with a wheelie.

Wheelies

A wheelie, sometimes called a *pop-up*, is the elevation of the caster wheels in order to negotiate stairs, curbs, or curb cutouts. It takes a great deal of practice, balance, and skill to pop a wheelie, and the therapist should be very close to the patient when the patient is learning. Initially, you may tip the patient's chair and allow the patient to find the balancing point. Eventually, the patient will be instructed on how to tip the chair back (Figure 8-42). The patient may learn how to pop and maintain a wheelie throughout a curb or stair negotiation. The patient will need to lean forward with his or her trunk and head to prevent the chair from tipping all the way back.

Falls/Return to Chair

If a patient is to learn all there is to know about wheelchair negotiation, then the patient should also learn about what to do if the wheelchair tips and he or she falls out. As much as physical therapists train their patients and aim for safety, a fall is bound to happen, especially if the patient is using wheelies to negotiate the terrain.

If the patient falls backward, the patient should be instructed to cross one arm across the body and grasp the opposite armrest. This will prevent the patient's legs from hitting him or her in the face. The patient should also keep his or her head and trunk forward to prevent injury to the head or neck.

If the patient falls forward, the patient can either hold onto one armrest while reaching forward with the other arm, or the patient can reach forward with both arms to

protect as he or she falls. The patient should attempt to absorb the fall by bending the elbows when the hands hit the floor, and the patient should try to land on his or her side rather than let the knees hit the floor.

In either case, the patient needs instruction on how to return to the chair or to return the chair to upright. How to transfer back into the wheelchair from the floor will be discussed in detail in the chapter about transfers.

To return a chair to upright, the patient should first be in the chair. The wheels should be locked. The patient should reach one arm across the body to the opposite armrest while the other arm is placed behind the patient on the floor. The patient uses this arm and hand to slowly raise the wheelchair up, all while keeping the head and trunk flexed. When the wheelchair has been walked to the length of the arm, one final, strong push should be given while the patient reaches forward with the other arm. Returning a wheelchair to its upright position takes practice, but this should be a part of a patient's therapy session if the goal is to have the patient become independent with his or her wheelchair. Figure 8-43 demonstrates how to get into a wheelchair from the floor both forward and backward.

WHEELCHAIR MAINTENANCE AND CARE

A wheelchair is a tool, and like any tool, it requires regular cleaning and maintenance to keep it working in top condition. Most wheelchairs come with user manuals, and the patient should read and understand these instructions and guidelines. The metal should be cleaned regularly, as should the seat and cushion.[10] Once monthly is a good rule of thumb. If the chair gets wet, it should be wiped dry to prevent rusting. Some areas like the wheel locks, armrest pins, and legrest pins, may need to be lubricated to keep them working properly, and the wheel locks periodically need tightening to effectively secure the wheels. Tires, especially pneumatic tires, should be inspected and checked for proper inflation.[10] The chair should be regularly inspected for damage or wear. If the patient or caregiver does not feel comfortable with certain maintenance tasks, the manufacturer or distributor of the wheelchair can be an excellent resource.

It is important to also keep in mind that wheelchair maintenance varies from a manual chair to a motorized chair. Some chairs also come with warranties or service agreements that may be nullified if the patient works on the machine him- or herself.[10]

SAFETY/RED FLAGS

It is critically important that you lock the wheelchair locks/brakes before a patient performs a transfer. Not doing so will cause the chair to move while the patient is mov-

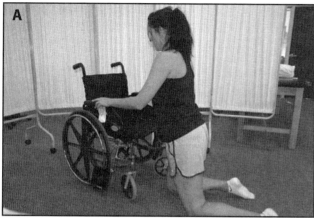 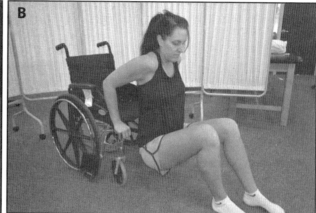

Figure 8-43. A patient getting up in a wheelchair from the floor forward and backward.

ing, which can cause the patient to lose his or her balance. Similarly, you should move the footrests and legrests out of the way before a patient attempts to stand or perform a transfer.

It is important to realize that if a patient cannot remove his or her arm from the trough, the arm trough can be considered a restraint. A restraint can only be ordered by a physician, so you should ensure that the patient can remove his or her arm from the trough before leaving him or her unattended in the wheelchair.

A caregiver who is assisting a patient with wheelchair mobility (either by pushing the chair or by educating the patient) should monitor for safety issues that could result in falls or injuries. For example, a patient with decreased awareness or sensation in an upper extremity may injure his or her hand when propelling through a doorway. Similarly, a patient who is not cognitively able to assess danger may drive too fast or go down a hill too steep. Patients who drive motorized wheelchairs are especially at risk for speeding, and this could cause injury to both the patient and bystanders.

Additionally, a caregiver assisting a patient with wheelchair mobility should be aware of his or her body mechanics. Especially in the cases of assisting patients with curbs and stairs, a caregiver needs to utilize proper body mechanics to avoid injury.

During certain tasks, a caregiver or therapist should guard the patient closely to prevent injury. This is the case when the patient is learning to pop a wheelie, but also when the patient is navigating ramps. The therapist should be behind the patient when he or she is ascending and to the side of or behind the patient when descending to stop a runaway chair.

DOCUMENTATION

When documenting wheelchair measurements, fit checks, and propulsion education, include levels of assist and either number of repetitions or time spent on the task. Indicate how many, if any, verbal or tactile cues the patient required to perform the tasks.

O: Patient measured for wheelchair as follows: armrest height 14 inches, seat back height 21 inches, seat depth 16 inches, seat width 20 inches, and seat height 15 inches. Patient educated on wheelchair propulsion forward and backward, turning Ⓛ and Ⓡ x 20 minutes, requiring supervision. Practiced ascending and descending a ramp x 5 repetitions with supervision and 3 verbal cues to lean forward when ascending and to slow the descent with hands on the drive wheels. Patient practiced popping a wheelie x 5 with CGA on handrims to prevent posterior fall.

REVIEW QUESTIONS

1. Discuss and demonstrate on a classmate how to measure a patient for a wheelchair.

2. Discuss how to assess the fit of a wheelchair and the effects if the wheelchair does not fit properly.

3. List or identify in a picture the most common components of a wheelchair.

4. How would you educate a patient to propel his or her wheelchair up a ramp?

5. Describe the step-by-step process for how you would assist a patient in a wheelchair up a curb.

6. What are 3 safety concerns you should be aware of as a health care provider when educating and training a patient in wheelchair use?

7. Describe how you would educate a patient to negotiate a self-closing door that opens inward.

8. If your patient suffered a CVA and is weak on his or her left side, what type of wheelchair would you recommend? What components would be required or helpful to this patient?

REFERENCES

1. Boninger ML; Model Systems Knowledge Translation Center. Getting the right wheelchair: what the SCI consumer needs to know. *Model Systems Knowledge Translation Center.* http://www.msktc.org/sci/factsheets/wheelchairs/Getting-The-Right-Wheelchair. Accessed September 6, 2018.

2. Quickie all court sport wheelchair. *Quickie Wheelchairs.* https://www.quickie-wheelchairs.com/All-Quickie-Wheelchairs/All-Court-Tennis-Basketball-Wheelchairs/Quickie-All-Court-Sport-Wheelchair/3106p. Accessed November 7, 2018.

3. One arm drive systems. *Mobility Basics.* https://mobilitybasics.ca/wheelchairs/onearmdrives. Accessed September 6, 2018.

4. Spinal Outreach Team and School of Health and Rehabilitation Sciences, University of Queensland. Manual wheelchairs: information resource for service providers. *Queensland Government: Queensland Health.* https://www.health.qld.gov.au/__data/assets/pdf_file/0026/429911/manual-wheelchairs.pdf. Updated August 2017. Accessed September 6, 2018.

5. Swingaway amputee wheelchair. *Karman.* https://www.karmanhealthcare.com/swingaway-amputee-wheelchair/. Accessed September 6, 2018.

6. Denison I. Manual wheelchair skills: guidelines for instructing. *Vancouver Coastal Health.* http://www.assistive-technology.ca/docs/mwcskillsg.pdf. Published 2013. Updated January 30, 2017. Accessed September 6, 2018.

7. Manual wheelchair propulsion assist devices. *Mobility Basics.* https://mobilitybasics.ca/wheelchairs/manualassists. Accessed September 6, 2018.

8. Wheelchairs. *United Spinal Association.* http://www.spinalcord.org/resource-center/askus/index.php?pg=kb.printer.friendly&id=19#p483. Accessed September 6, 2018.

9. Colescot D. Power wheelchair mobility. *University of Washington: Rehabilitation Medicine.* http://sci.washington.edu/info/forums/reports/power_wc_skills_2011.asp. Published November 8, 2011. Accessed September 6, 2018.

10. Cooper RA. The basics of manual wheelchair maintenance. *PNOnline.* http://pvamag.com/pn/article/5810/the_basics_of_manual_wheelchair_maintenance. Published September 12, 2013. Accessed September 6, 2018.

Chapter 9

Bed Mobility and Transfers

KEY TERMS Contralateral | Gait belt | Hemiplegia | Ipsilateral | Paralysis | Paresis

KEY ABBREVIATIONS BOS | CGA | COG | CVA | FIM | HOB | IV | SCI

CHAPTER OBJECTIVES

1. Be able to describe the various levels of assist a patient may need with transfers.
2. Describe and perform bed mobility with a patient.
3. Describe and perform various transfers, including stand pivot, squat pivot, slide board, as well as dependent lifts.
4. Understand under what conditions you should use a mechanical lift to transfer a patient.
5. Describe and assist with chair to floor/floor to chair transfers and how to educate a patient.
6. Understand and demonstrate safety during transfers.
7. Be able to properly document a transfer or bed mobility session.

INTRODUCTION

Perhaps you have heard the adage, "give a man a fish and he will eat for a day; teach a man to fish and he will eat for the rest of his life." How does this apply to transfer training? In the world of physical therapy, therapists often teach patients how to be independent. Physical therapists strengthen, educate, and show patients more efficient ways

of performing a task, and pretty soon the patient graduates and does not need therapy anymore. This is true for transfers. Physical therapist assistants aim to help patients become as independent as possible by teaching them how to perform bed mobility and transfers without help or with as little help as possible.

In light of the need to teach patient's independence, therapists sometimes find themselves asking much from a patient during a therapy session. For example, in the hospital setting, other staff may provide more assistance to the patient during a transfer, whereas a physical therapist assistant may require the patient to work harder to perform the task more independently. However, that staff member's job is not to teach the patient so much as accomplish other goals, such as bathing or linen changes. As a therapist, your goal is to educate the patient and help him or her become as independent as possible during the task, which takes time and patience. Physical therapist assistants are competent in transfer training, and their interventions are skilled interventions. Part of their job also includes training the staff to perform or assist with transfers so that the staff are being consistent with what physical therapy is teaching the patient. The same applies for the patient's family or caregivers; they often need to be educated on how to best assist the patient to allow for independence and strength while preventing injuries.

Memolo J.
Procedures and Patient Care for the Physical Therapist Assistant
(pp 123-143). © 2019 SLACK Incorporated.

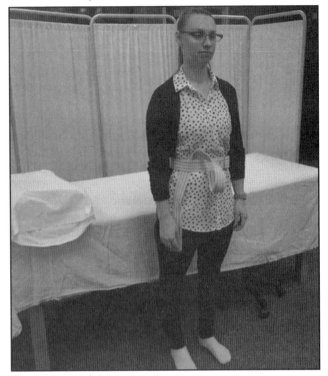

Figure 9-1. A gait belt on a patient.

SAFETY, SETUP, AND PREPARATION

Before performing any type of bed mobility or transfer, it is important that you survey the situation and plan ahead. In Chapter 7 you were encouraged to look at a patient's chart prior to entering the room, and you were educated to look over the room to see what equipment is present so you can plan your activities without disrupting the equipment. The same applies here: look over the patient's chart and peek into the patient's room to see what the situation looks like. This will make your transfer tasks much easier.

The patient's chart should have the previous evaluation or treatment by the physical therapist or physical therapist assistant. This will give you an excellent idea of how much assistance the patient needed last time, and what type of transfer activities were performed. The chart will give you a good idea of the patient's current strength and abilities, so you can plan the best transfer and how much assist to anticipate giving. The physical therapist's evaluation should give you goals, which will also inform your decisions on what activities to perform.

Do not forget the rules of body mechanics when performing transfers, either. You likely will need to raise or lower the patient's bed, use a wider base of support (BOS), lower your center of gravity (COG), get close to the patient, and maintain your normal lumbar lordosis.[1] Following the proper body mechanics protocol will ensure a safer transfer for both you and the patient.

Make sure you also plan ahead for the transfers you intend to perform. Looking over the patient's room will allow you to visualize in your mind what you can or need to move to access the patient best and to easily perform your tasks. For example, if the patient has an intravenous line (IV) and the pole is on the right side of the bed, but you know you want to transfer the patient to the chair on the left side of the bed, you know you will need to move that IV pole prior to performing the transfer.

The planning process will also include considering what equipment you may need for the transfer. You should check that you also have the equipment you need to perform the task prior to entering the patient's room, if possible. You will need a gait belt for safety (Figure 9-1), and you may also need a sliding board, a pivot disc, or a Beasy Board (Beasy Trans Systems, Inc).

If you observe that the patient required a high assist level or is obese, you should also consider your own strength and abilities. Physics and lever arms can be your friend during a transfer, and you will find you can often move a person much larger than you. However, you may find that moving or lifting a patient requires more strength than you possess, in which case the best course of action is to ask for assistance. It is much better to find a second person or to use a mechanical lift than to injure yourself, and possibly the patient, in an attempt to preserve ego or save time.

During the transfer or mobility session, you should explain to the patient what you intend to do and how the patient can and should help. As with all tasks, patient consent is required, and after explaining the task, it may not be enough to simply ask, "do you understand?" The patient may indicate he or she does when he or she does not. Instead, you can ask the patient to repeat back to you the plan of action. When you are explaining the transfer, try to use simple, direct wording. Consider if a therapist says the following: "Okay, first I'm going to get you up to the side of the bed, and then I want you to reach for the rail and scoot forward but be sure to not slide off the bed. We're going to stand up on 3 and then we'll pivot over to the chair where I'll help you sit back in the chair all the way, and make sure you keep your hands on the armrests." Now compare that to a therapist saying, "Let's sit up. Now scoot forward. On 3 we'll stand. Now pivot and sit. Let's scoot back." Patients who have cognitive deficits will especially appreciate a concise set of directions, but everyone will perform better with less fluff. Box 9-1 includes considerations for planning a transfer.

LEVELS OF ASSIST

When you are preparing to transfer or otherwise move a patient, you should consider how much assist the patient will need. You may get this information from the physical therapist's evaluation or from the previous physical therapist's or physical therapist assistant's treatment if you were not the person to treat that patient the last time. It is important to remember that the level of assist refers to how much the patient can do, not how hard it is for the therapist to assist with the task. For example, you may transfer an elderly woman who weighs 89 pounds (lbs). She is so light that you can practically pick her up and throw her over your shoulder. In the next room you must transfer a patient who is 6 feet 8 inches and weighs 235 lbs. You are going to work a lot harder transferring him than the elderly woman. What you need to consider, however, is not how hard you work, but the patient's abilities. Technically, the elderly woman is a maximal assist because she cannot help much with the transfer. The tall man is actually a minimal assist because he can help a great deal with the transfer. Keeping this in mind will allow you to accurately record the level of assist required for the patient, rather than using a subjective assessment based on your personal strength.

These levels of assist will come back to haunt you when you reach Chapter 10; the same rules apply with gait training as with transfers and bed mobility. Remember, too, that these levels of assist are used when documenting wheelchair mobility and training, as discussed in Chapter 8. Table 9-1 includes an explanation of each level of assist. Note that the abbreviations, while common, may not be exactly what you encounter in the clinic. What these terms mean, however, is fairly universal.

Dependent

A patient who is dependent is unable to assist in any way with the transfer. He or she may be unconscious, or perhaps the patient has suffered a spinal cord injury (SCI) and is physically unable to use upper or lower extremities to assist with the transfer or mobility.

Maximal Assist

A patient who is able to perform 25% to 49% of the task requires maximal assist. Remember that this is what the patient can do and not what you can do to help.

Moderate Assist

Moderate assist indicates that the patient is able to perform 50% to 74% of the task.

Minimal Assist

A patient requires minimal assist if he or she is able to perform 75% or more of the activity.

Contact Guard Assist

A patient who is contact guard assist (CGA) requires hands-on only assistance. The therapist must be in physical contact with the patient at all times (during the transfer) utilizing a gait belt. The patient may not need assistance to stand or move, but balance may be an issue.

Box 9-1
Considerations for Planning a Transfer

- How does the patient transfer currently?
- What are patient's limitations/abilities?
- How much assistance does the patient currently require?
- What special equipment does the patient need?
- What is the environment? (eg, stairs, carpet, rails, bathrooms)
- What is the patient's strength?
- What is the patient's pain?
- What is the patient's sitting or standing balance?
- What is the patient's endurance?
- What is the patient's cognitive status or memory?

Supervision/Standby Assist

Supervision or standby assist mean roughly the same thing. The patient is able to perform the task with no assistance and no hands-on guarding, but the therapist feels that he or she must be close to the patient in case the status or situation changes. The patient may need verbal or tactile cues to perform the task correctly.

Modified Independent

Modified independent means that the patient is able to perform the task without assistance, including verbal or tactile cues, but the patient requires the use of an assistive device or equipment, such as a walker, cane, bed rail, or slide board.

Independent

An independent patient is able to perform the task with no assistance from the therapist (neither verbal nor tactile), no hands-on assistance, and with no use of equipment or assistive devices.

Functional Independence Measure Scores

In rehabilitation settings, such as inpatient rehab for stroke or SCI recovery, a patient may have a Functional Independence Measure (FIM) instrument in his or her chart. Therapists are required to record the patient's FIM scores according to the task and how well the patient can perform that task.[2] The FIM instrument is a measurement of disability, or what the patient can actually do, and it records progress on 18 items including eating, bath-

Table 9-1
Levels of Assist

Dependent	The patient is unable to perform the task in any way.
Maximal assist	The patient is able to perform 25% to 49% of the task.
Moderate assist	The patient is able to perform 50% to 74% of the task.
Minimal assist	The patient is able to perform 75% or more of the task.
Contact guard assist	The patient requires hands-on assist only; balance may be an issue.
Supervision/standby assist	The patient is able to perform the task with no hands-on assistance, but the therapist feels the need to be close to the patient, and the patient may need cues (tactile or verbal) to assist.
Modified independent	The patient is able to perform the task with no assistance (verbal or tactile) but requires the use of an assistive device.
Independent	The patient is able to perform the task with no assistance (verbal or tactile) and no use of equipment.

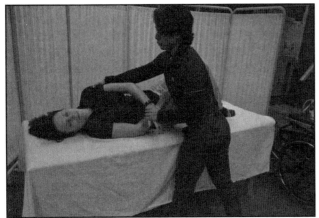

Figure 9-2. A segmental roll.

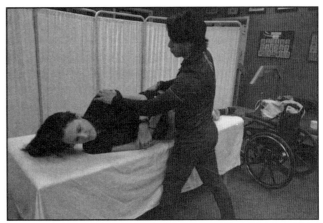

Figure 9-3. A log roll.

ing, dressing, toileting, bed-to-chair transfers, locomotion, problem solving, and memory.[2] Individual task scores range from 1 (meaning the patient requires total assistance for the task) to a 7 (meaning the patient is completely independent with the task).[2] The entire score is tallied up and ranges from 18 (least independent) to 126 (most independent).[2] Scores are gathered at a patient's admission and discharge, but may also be assessed at reevaluation to determine progress and prognosis.

BED MOBILITY

Bed mobility includes any movement in the bed for repositioning or to prepare to get into or out of bed. People take these basic movements for granted when they are healthy; however, simply rolling over or scooting up in bed can be challenging for less mobile patients. As mentioned before, the therapist's goal is to get his or her patients as independent with these tasks as possible.

Rolling

A patient needs to roll in bed to reposition or as a component of getting into or out of bed. Depending on the level of assist the patient requires, and any other safety considerations including recent surgeries or injuries, the therapist can make a decision on how the patient should perform bed mobility in order to avoid injury. A patient can perform a segmental roll (Figure 9-2), in which first the shoulder and upper trunk roll to the side, followed by the pelvis and lower extremities. The other option is the patient can log roll, meaning he or she rolls the entire body at once (Figure 9-3). A log roll is best for patients with lower back pain or who have had recent back surgery. Patients who have had an SCI should also perform a log roll. Your goal as a therapist is to help the patient become as independent as possible with these tasks.

Various Levels of Assist

To roll in bed, the patient should be positioned to the side of the bed opposite of the direction he or she will roll (eg, if the patient will roll to the right, the patient should be positioned on the left side of the bed). To better facilitate a roll, the patient's lower extremities can be crossed at the ankles with the top leg being opposite of the direction he or she is rolling (this is helpful if the patient is dependent or requires significant assistance). The other option is that the patient can bend the knee on the leg opposite of the direction he or she will roll (placing the foot flat on the bed). If the patient is able to bend the opposite knee with the foot flat on the bed, the patient can use that foot to push during the roll.

Make sure that your body is lowered, and your lever arms are short. You may need to raise the height of the bed, and your hips and knees should be flexed. Position your feet in the direction you are moving the patient. No matter the level of assistance the patient needs, you should be positioned so that the patient will roll toward you. Otherwise the patient could roll off the bed. If the patient is able, you can instruct the patient to reach for the opposite side of the bed or the bed rail. Use of a bed rail is not encouraged for long-term use, but it can be a useful introductory tool while the patient is gaining strength and skill. If the roll is segmental, the patient (or you) will roll first the shoulders and upper trunk. If the roll is a log roll, the entire body will roll together.

To roll a patient from supine to prone, cross the patient's legs and position the patient as mentioned earlier. You will help the patient roll or the patient will roll him- or herself in the direction wished, but the patient will continue beyond the sidelying position. It is easiest if the patient's arm (the one being rolled over to reach prone) is either with the elbow straight and the arm along the patient's side or the elbow straight with the shoulder flexed. The same procedure would be reversed if returning the patient from prone to supine.

If rolling the patient to sidelying so the patient will stay in that position for a while, it is important to recall the rules for sidelying positioning discussed in Chapter 3.

It is also worth noting if the patient has precautions or restrictions; for example, if they had a total hip arthroplasty, crossing the legs or bending the hips beyond a certain point will be contraindicated.

Scooting

When I worked at the hospital, nearly every time I walked into a patient's room to see them for therapy I found the patient in bed with his or her feet bunched up at the foot of the bed and his or her head practically in the middle of the bed. Patients tend to slide down in bed, especially as they raise and lower the head of the bed (HOB), and it is necessary sometimes to reposition them. Scooting also plays a role in rolling (see the section on rolling) and preparing for transitions of supine to and from sitting.

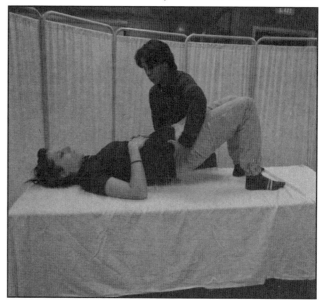
Figure 9-4. Moving a patient up and down in bed.

Up or Down

If your patient is supine, there are several ways to move the patient up or down in bed. To prepare for the movement, it is best to lower the HOB so the bed is flat and to remove the pillows, covers, or blankets so the movement can be unrestricted. It is also necessary to take every effort to reduce friction or shear on the patient's buttocks, so there is a reduced risk of injury to the skin. If the patient is toward the side of the bed, shorten your lever arm so the effort is easier for you. Regardless of how much assistance the patient needs, it is best for the patient to move in short increments rather than attempting the mobility in one big move. Figure 9-4 shows how to move a patient up or down in bed.

Sideways

To move a patient laterally in bed, you have several options. This may be in preparation for a transfer or to roll the patient in the bed. As with rolling, your goal as a therapist is to ultimately help the patient to become as independent as possible with these skills. It is still a good idea to lower the HOB so the movement can be easier. Figure 9-5 shows how to move a patient sideways in bed.

Various Levels of Assist

If the patient is unable to assist (if they are dependent or maximal assist), you can use a draw sheet and 2 clinicians to slide the patient up in bed. A draw sheet is a folded sheet under the patient that assists with bed mobility. It typically reaches from the buttocks to the mid back. One clinician on either side of the patient grasps the draw sheet and at the same time pulls the patient up in bed. The same applies if moving the patient down in bed. It is important that the 2 clinicians lift and pull at the same time. There are various

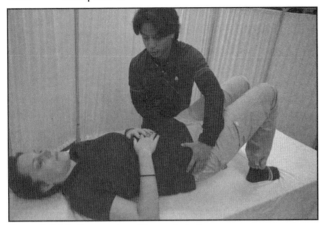

Figure 9-5. Moving a patient sideways in bed.

draw sheet alternatives you can find in supply catalogs or in facilities that reduce friction or make the process easier for clinicians. A patient may be dependent or require maximal assist for this task currently, but your job is to strengthen and educate the patient. You should still ask the patient to participate as much as possible in these movements, with the hope that the patient will grow stronger and more mobile in the future.

If the patient is able to assist with the movement, you will cue the patient to perform a bridge. The patient will bend both knees so that both feet are flat on the bed, and a bridge involves lifting the buttocks off the bed. To move up in bed, the patient will press down with his or her elbows to assist with lifting the buttocks and the back, and the patient will push up with the lower extremities. Short movements should be encouraged to decrease the risk of friction. Once the patient moves up, the legs should be repositioned closer to the body, and if necessary, the patient can bridge and press down again with the elbows to move again.

To move down in the bed, the same kind of movement will happen. The patient will bridge and use his or her elbows to lift, except this time the patient will lift and move down in bed.

For either moving up or down, the therapist can assist with facilitation of this. If you get close to the patient (to shorten the lever arm) and support the patient's head and shoulders, you can reduce the amount of body weight the patient has to overcome to move in the bed. Alternatively, you can position yourself at the patient's feet (with the knees bent) and assist with lifting the buttocks while the patient moves. It may be difficult or too much of a strain to lift the patient in these ways, in which case you should call for a second clinician and use the draw sheet method.

In order to move the patient to the left or right in bed, you again need to assess how much help the patient can contribute. If the patient is dependent, you can position yourself close to the patient, placing your arms under the patient's head and upper back. Slide the upper body toward you (toward the side of the bed), and then reposition yourself to the patient's trunk to do the same. Finally, you will

position yourself at the patient's lower extremities and slide them toward you. In this way you are segmentally moving the patient to the side of the bed. You will want to maintain a low COG and a short lever arm. You may need to raise the bed to reduce strain on your back.

Another dependent option is to use the draw sheet. You can pull the patient to the side using the draw sheet, but you will need to be careful to avoid friction or shearing on the skin and should use your body to block the patient from sliding off the bed. With the use of the draw sheet, the patient cannot assist as much; if you can facilitate mobility while also allowing the patient to assist, this is the best option.

If the patient is more mobile, you can cue the patient to perform a bridge as described in the section about moving up or down in bed. The patient will push with his or her elbows and lift the back and buttocks while moving them to the side. The head can then be repositioned, and the patient can reposition the lower extremities.

In these cases, the patient may be able to perform a great deal of the work, but you may still be required to assist. Remember that any level of assist at or above CGA requires your hands on the patient and potentially some assistance from you to perform the task.

Supine to/from Sit

The human body is not made to be horizontal. Bones, musculature, and organs all thrive in upright positions, so a significant goal for patients is to get them sitting up. This may be just on the edge of the bed to start, and eventually the goal may be to transfer the patient to another surface or to begin gait. Whatever the intention, transitioning from supine to sit and back again is an important mobility skill that takes practice.

Various Levels of Assist

As with the other bed mobility tasks, a patient can be more or less helpful depending on strength and endurance. If the patient is dependent or requires maximal assist, you should first move the patient to the edge of the bed (Figure 9-6). The patient should then be rolled to the side, and you should use your body to block the patient from rolling off the bed. Stay close to the patient, use short lever arms, and use one arm to hook behind the patient's knees while the other arm comes underneath the patient's shoulders. At no time should you pull on the patient's arms or legs to perform this task, as you may dislocate something. As you lower the legs down, you will lift the shoulders and trunk up. This will work well because the buttocks serve as a pivot point. At this point, the patient should be sitting on the edge of the bed.

Alternatively, you could have the patient near the edge of the bed but supine. The patient bends both knees so his or her feet are flat on the bed. You can reach under the patient's shoulders and scapulae and lift the patient upright into a long-seated position. From there, the patient can be

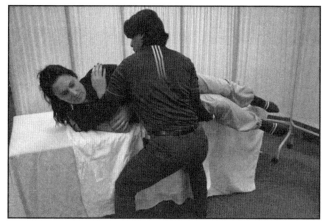

Figure 9-6. A patient moving from supine to sit dependently.

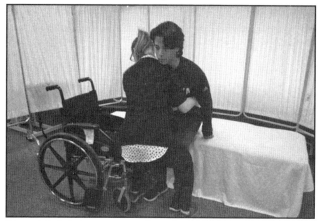

Figure 9-7. A sitting one-person dependent transfer.

pivoted so that the legs hang off the bed in a short-seated position. Figure 9-7 shows how to perform this task with a more dependent patient.

Remember you should not leave a patient sitting unattended. He or she could lose his or her balance and fall, either due to dizziness or lack of strength, causing significant injury.

If your patient is able to assist, you will cue the patient to roll or scoot to the edge of the bed. The patient should be in sidelying near the edge. The patient will then lower his or her lower extremities to the floor while using his or her upper extremities, especially the elbow of the lowermost arm, to push into an upright position on the edge of the bed.

Alternatively, the patient can bend both knees with feet flat on the bed, lift his or her trunk and head into a long-seated position, and then pivot on the bed until his or her legs are on the floor. Depending on the patient's strength, you may still need to offer varying degrees of assistance. Figure 9-8 shows how to perform supine to and from sitting with a patient who can assist.

Cerebrovascular Accident

A patient who has suffered a stroke will likely have decreased strength or mobility on one side of his or her body. In this case, you will need to gauge how much assistance the patient will need while also protecting the side of the body that has been affected. In some cases, the affected side is flaccid, meaning there is no muscle tone. Additionally, some patients who have had a cerebrovascular accident (CVA) lose awareness of or forget about the affected side of the body. Patients with this neglect may accidentally injure themselves because they are not paying attention to their affected side.

In cases of rolling, the patient may not be able to use the affected upper or lower extremity. The physical therapist may need to have the patient roll to the unaffected side, especially if the patient is going to sit up on the edge of the bed. It is easier for the patient to push up using the unaffected upper extremity than the affected side. The physical

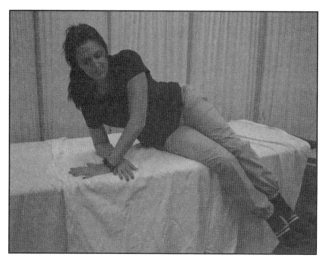

Figure 9-8. A patient moving from supine to sit independently.

therapist or caregiver should avoid pulling on the involved or affected limbs as the patient is at risk for subluxation or dislocation, especially at the shoulder. Be aware, too, that patients who have suffered a stroke often have pain when they roll onto or lie on their affected limbs.

Amputation

When a patient has had an amputation, the patient may have significant pain that limits mobility. Also, the residual limb must be attended to in order to prevent bumping or otherwise injuring the area. The patient may have difficulty moving in bed because one or several extremities could be missing; for example, it is much harder to bridge with one leg than two.

Joint Replacement

A patient who has had a joint replacement surgery will have pain and reduced strength, which will limit the patient's ability to move in and out of bed. As mentioned earlier, some patients who have had joint replacements also have movement restrictions or limitations. For example, a

Table 9-2 Types of Transfers	
Standing dependent pivot	Patient required to bear weight on at least one lower extremity; do not attempt unless physically able; use a mechanical lift if available (dependent stand pivot transfer not recommended).
Standing assisted pivot	Patient provides 25% to 75% of the effort.
Standing standby/supervision pivot	Patient is able to stand, pivot, and sit with cues (tactile or verbal) or close guarding.
Standing independent pivot	Patient is able to perform the transfer safely without physical assistance or cueing.
Sitting or lateral assisted	Patient is able to move from one surface to another in sitting or squat position, providing 25% to 75% of the effort; patient may need sliding board or other equipment.
Sitting independent	Patient is able to move from one surface to another safely and without assistance or cueing but may use assistive equipment.
Sitting dependent	One, two, or three persons required to lift the patient from one surface to another while the patient is sitting/squatting; may use mechanical lift also. Patient is unable to assist.
Recumbent dependent	One, two, or three persons required to transfer patient; patient is in recumbent position; may use mechanical lift, draw sheet, or transfer board as needed. Patient is unable to physically assist.

patient who has had a total hip arthroplasty will be unable to flex the hip past 90 degrees, internally or externally rotate the hip (no internal rotation for posterior-lateral approach; no external rotation for anterior-lateral approach), or cross the legs at the knees (hip adduction).[3] Otherwise the hip is at risk for dislocation. These restrictions can limit what the patient can do in the bed during mobility activities, and you and the patient should be aware of positioning so the patient does not break protocol.

Spinal Cord Injury or Low Back Pain

Patients with SCIs are under certain restrictions when the injury is acute, and mobility is limited by the location and severity of the injury. Acute injuries require log rolls for patients in bed to prevent disruption of surgical repair and to also prevent additional injury. Once the injury is healed, the patient will have to adapt to his or her limited strength and mobility, but transfers and bed mobility will still be doable and necessary for the patient to become independent.[4]

Similarly, if the patient has had lower back surgery or has low back pain, the restrictions usually include no lifting, no bending (past 90 degrees), and no twisting of the spine. This again requires the patient to use a log roll technique to get into and out of bed.[5]

TYPES OF TRANSFERS

Transfers are the movement of a person from one surface to another. There are many types of transfers: bed to wheelchair, bed to bedside commode, wheelchair to shower, wheelchair to car, etc. There are also many methods of transferring a patient depending on the patient's abilities. Table 9-2 includes the types of transfers, and Box 9-2 includes transfer principles to keep in mind before performing and during transfers with your patients.

Description of Types

The type of transfer used depends on the patient's strength and endurance. As with bed mobility, the physical therapist's goals are to help the patient be as independent as possible with transfers, so the patient may begin with a less difficult transfer and slowly graduate to a more complex transfer.

Dependent Transfers

Dependent transfers are for patients who are unable to participate in the transfer. As with bed mobility, this may be a patient who has had an SCI or is unconscious. Any time you are transferring a dependent patient, you should be very aware of your body mechanics and strength. Any time you are uncertain of your ability to transfer a patient on your own, you should consider either bringing in a second person or using a mechanical lift. If you are able to perform the lift on your own, lower your COG and widen your BOS. Get very close to the patient to shorten the lever arm.

Sitting One Person

A sitting one-person transfer requires the transfer surface (eg, a wheelchair) to be very close to the surface the patient is being transferred from. The wheelchair should be at a 45-degree angle and in contact with or very close to the other surface. The patient should be sitting on the edge of the bed or chair. You may have to assist the patient into this position if the patient cannot do it alone. You can have the patient lean forward, resting his or her head on your shoulder, while you lift under his or her buttocks first on one side and then the other to scoot the patient forward. You could alternatively cue the patient to slouch in the seat, which will scoot the patient's buttocks forward, and then assist the patient with sitting upright. If using a wheelchair, either to transfer to or from, the wheels should be locked, and the armrest closest to the transfer surface should be removed or lifted out of the way. Legrests should also be removed or swung out of the way to prevent entanglement.

You should apply a gait belt to the patient prior to attempting the transfer. You could also use a transfer sling, towel, or sheet to assist with the transfer, but you should still always have a gait belt on the patient. Stand in front of the patient and flex at the hips and knees to lower your COG. You should also widen your BOS. The patient should be flexed forward at the hips, so the patient's head is resting on your shoulder. At no time should the patient grab you around the shoulders or neck, as this could cause injury to you if the patient begins to fall. Instead, encourage the patient to cross his or her arms across the chest. The patient's head should be on the side opposite of the direction you are transferring the patient, so you have an unobstructed view.

Using the gait belt (or other transfer device), lift the patient forward and quickly pivot the patient to the other surface. The patient (and you) will not come into an upright position. A standing dependent lift is not recommended due to the increased risk of injury. Figure 9-7 shows a sitting one-person dependent lift.

An alternate method for a single person lift is to use a rolling stool. The patient is positioned the same way at the edge of the bed/surface. The physical therapist sits on the rolling stool and holds onto the gait belt. The patient is leaned forward so his or her head is resting on the physical therapist's shoulder, and the patient's feet are positioned on the rolling stool's legs or squeezed between the therapist's knees. The patient is pivoted forward and

Box 9-2
Transfer Principles

- Determine the patient's ability to assist and weightbearing status.
- Ensure the patient is wearing appropriate clothing and footwear.
- Mentally prepare for the transfer.
- Arrange the room/area as needed to accommodate patient movement.
- Use simple language to educate the patient on transfer components or plan.
- Acquire equipment needed (eg, gait belt, sliding board).
- Use gait belt for transfer (not patient extremities or clothing).
- Appropriately position yourself to guard or block as needed.
- Adhere to proper body mechanics during the transfer.
- Ensure the patient is safe and secure at the conclusion of the transfer.

quickly transferred to the other surface. This is sometimes a transfer method used that is slightly safer than the standing version, but it is still not recommended.

Sitting Two Person

There are 2 ways to transfer a patient in sitting with 2 clinicians. The first method requires one clinician to be at the patient's head and the other to be at the patient's feet. The clinician at the patient's head is the leader and will dictate when the lift will occur. The leader will ask the patient to cross his or her arms, and a gait belt should be applied. The leader will reach from behind the patient and wrap his or her arms around the patient, grasping the gait belt on each side. The clinician at the feet will place his or her arms under the distal lower extremities, just distal to the knee and proximal to the ankles. When the leader indicates (the leader may say "on 3," "1-2-3-now," or "1-2-3-lift"), both clinicians will lift the patient and transfer the patient to the other surface. If transferring to or from a wheelchair, the wheels should be locked. Figure 9-9 shows the front and back version of a 2-person lift.

The other method involves a clinician to be positioned on either side of the patient. The patient will still have a gait belt. Each clinician will place on hand on the gait belt and the other under the thigh just proximal to the knee. The patient can sling his or her arms around the clinicians' shoulders for support. Again, one person is the leader and

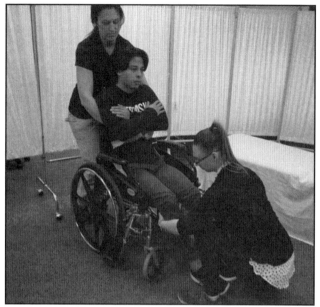

Figure 9-9. A 2-person lift from the front and back.

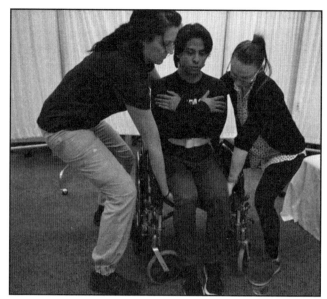

Figure 9-10. A side-to-side 2-person lift.

indicates when the lift should occur. Both clinicians should lift at the same time. Then the patient is moved to the next surface, avoiding the wheelchair. Figure 9-10 shows the side-to-side 2-person lift. Box 9-3 provides the instructions for both 2-person lift options.

If you have a bariatric patient, 2 persons can lift that patient manually, if a mechanical lift is not available, by using a sheet under the patient. The sheet is used like a cradle to support the patient during the transfer. The patient should still wear a gait belt during this transfer. Physical therapists should know and respect their limitations on strength, to both protect themselves and the patient from injury.

Supine Three Person

In some cases, a patient needs to be moved quickly, such as in an emergency situation requiring cardiopulmonary resuscitation or evacuation from a building. In this case, the clinician may not be able to wait for a mechanical lift. In a supine 3-person lift, 3 clinicians will lift a patient while in supine and move the patient from one surface to another. One clinician will be at the patient's head, with his or her arms under the patient's neck and shoulders. This clinician is also the leader of the lift. The second clinician will support the patient's lower back and upper thighs, and the third clinician will support the patient's lower thighs and lower legs. The leader should indicate what command or cue on which the 3 will simultaneously lift. First, the clinicians first must roll the patient toward them before lifting. If they are unable to roll the patient toward them or if they are unable to fully reach their arms under the patient prior to the lift, the lift should not be attempted.

The transfer surfaces need to be perpendicular so that the head of one surface is at the foot of the other surface. This will allow the clinicians to more easily move the patient from one surface to the next without getting tangled up with each other. Figure 9-11 shows the 3-person lift. Box 9-4 provides the instructions for performing a 3-person lift.

Assisted Lifts

If your patient is able to participate in the transfer, the lift is considered assisted. The levels of assist depend on how much the patient can participate during the lift. As a general rule, it is a good idea to transfer the patient toward his or her strongest side, unless the therapeutic intervention dictates that you will work on strengthening the weaker side. Also, transfer surfaces should be relatively close to one another to reduce the risk of falls. A gait belt should always be used during transfers, even if the patient is independent with the task. Wheelchair armrests and legrests may need to be removed or swung out of the way to facilitate the transfers. All assisted and independent transfers work best if both surfaces being transferred to and from are level with each other. Just because the patient can assist with the transfer does not mean that you should not be mindful of your body mechanics. You should still have a low COG and wide BOS, and you should educate the patient to not grab you around the neck or shoulders.

Sit to/from Stand

A sit to stand is the precursor to a transfer, and the patient should be a participant if possible. In assisted lifts, especially, a patient can and should participate as much as possible.

Box 9-3

Sitting Two-Person Lifts

Two-Person Lift From the Front and Back

1. Position the wheelchair parallel to the transfer surface.

2. One physical therapist (typically the stronger of the two) positions him- or herself behind the patient. This person is also the leader. The other physical therapist positions him- or herself at the patient's feet.

3. Ensure the wheelchair is locked, and remove the legrests as well as the armrests for clearance.

4. Apply a gait belt to the patient, and have the patient cross his or her arms.

5. The leader leans forward and reaches under the axillae, grasping the gait belt around the rib cage/umbilicus.

6. The other therapist squats at the patient's feet, assisting the patient in keeping his or her knees extended, and supporting under the distal thighs and calves.

7. When the leader indicates, both therapists lift at the same time and move together, using short steps, to place the patient on the new surface. Keep in mind the therapists will have to lift the patient up and over the push handles of the wheelchair and/or the drive wheel.

Side-to-Side Two-Person Lift

1. Position the wheelchair parallel to the transfer surface, but ensure there is enough room for the therapist closest to the transfer surface.

2. The therapists position themselves on either side of the patient.

3. Ensure the wheelchair is locked, and remove the leg and armrests to provide clearance.

4. Apply a gait belt to the patient.

5. The therapists stand at the patient's sides. The therapists instruct the patient to put his or her arms around their shoulders for support. The therapists cross their arms behind the patient and grasp the gait belt, while their other arms support the patient under the distal thighs.

6. When the leader indicates, the therapists lift at the same time. Keep in mind that the therapists will have to lift the patient over the drive wheel and walk around the chair to access the transfer surface. The therapists will have to back the patient up to the transfer surface in order to complete the transfer safely.

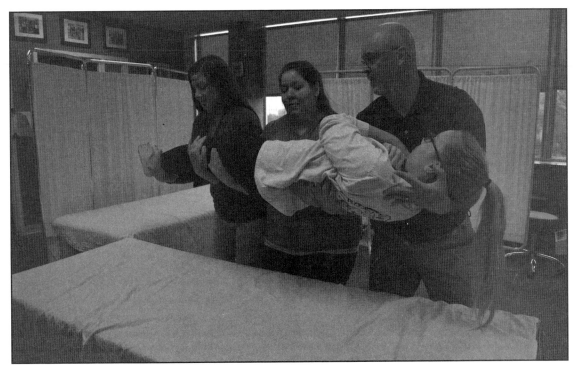

Figure 9-11. A supine 3-person lift.

Box 9-4

Supine Three-Person Lift

1. Determine which clinician will be the leader. This person will be at the patient's head.

2. Position the patient's bed/surface perpendicular to the transfer surface.

3. The leader will assume a position at the patient's head and upper trunk. The second clinician will be just above and below the pelvis, and the third clinician will be under the upper thigh and lower legs, keeping the patient's knees straight.

4. The leader provides the commands; the other 2 lifters should follow the commands, and the leader needs to be clear on the command that indicates lift.

5. Move the patient close to the edge of the bed.

6. When the leader indicates, the clinicians roll the patient toward them.

7. When the leader indicates, the clinicians all lift at once and move together using short steps to move the patient from one surface to the next.

8. When the leader indicates, the clinicians will all slowly lower the patient to the new surface, and then assist the patient with positioning in the bed to ensure safety.

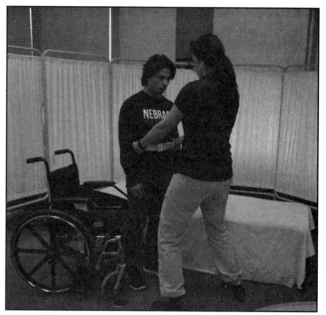

Figure 9-12. A stand pivot transfer with assist (wheelchair to mat).

The patient should be cued to scoot forward to the edge of the chair or bed. You may need to assist the patient, as described earlier in the dependent lift section. However, you should encourage and educate your patient on how to scoot forward as much as possible. The patient should push from the chair or bed with one or both extremities (as able), and the patient should also lean forward ("nose over toes") to unweight the buttocks and make standing easier. Consider the patient's assist level, and do not help the patient more than he or she needs. Let the patient do as much of the work as possible.

To go from stand to sit, the patient needs to back up to the transfer surface until he or she feels the seat on the back of his or her legs. The patient should then reach back for the surface with one or both hands while leaning forward and slowly lowering the buttocks toward the surface. The descent should not be a plop, but rather an eccentric, controlled lowering.

Stand Pivot

A stand pivot transfer is for patients who have relatively good strength and balance. The patient will stand fully upright, pivot, and sit on the other surface. The physical

therapist should be in front of or to the side of the patient, depending on the level of assist the patient needs; a weaker patient will need the therapist to be in front to better facilitate the transfer, while a stronger patient may only need incidental assistance or cues to perform the task and the therapist can be off to the side.

As the physical therapist, you will need to give cues to the patient to make the transfer go smoothly. The patient should be cued to scoot to the edge of the chair or bed, and the patient should position (or you should position) the feet so they are underneath the patient, flat on the floor. The patient should also be cued to assist as much as possible with the transfer (so cueing the patient to push from the armrests will help with those stand or squat pivot transfers). To stand up, patients should lean forward (nose over toes). Once the patient is standing, he or she should be given a moment to regain balance before being asked to move. The patient may need additional cues, either tactile or verbal, to move the feet. Figure 9-12 shows the stand pivot transfer with assist. Box 9-5 provides instructions for a stand pivot transfer.

Squat Pivot

A squat pivot transfer is much like a stand pivot transfer, except that the patient will not fully stand up. This is a good transfer for a patient who is not as strong or lacks the endurance to stand upright. The therapist is positioned in front of the patient and assists with the patient standing up, but the patient maintains a squat or knees bent position. The patient then pivots and sits on the other surface.

Box 9-5
Stand Pivot Transfer

1. Position the wheelchair so that it is parallel or at a 45-degree angle to the transfer surface. Transfer toward the patient's stronger side unless you are working on a different skilled intervention.

2. Lock the wheelchair brakes, and remove the legrests.

3. Apply a gait belt to the patient.

4. Instruct the patient to scoot forward in the seat; if he or she cannot do so independently, you may provide assistance. Alternatively, you can instruct the patient to slouch in the seat and then sit up (effectively sliding the buttocks forward so they are at the edge of the seat).

5. Cue the patient to assist as much as he or she can by pushing from the armrests and leaning forward (nose over toes).

6. Depending on the level of assist, you may position yourself either in front of the patient or to the side; use the gait belt to assist with the transfer.

7. Once the patient is standing, allow the patient to steady him- or herself before taking steps.

8. The patient may need verbal and/or tactile cues to move his or her feet or to shift weight.

9. Do not allow the patient to reach around your neck for support. If the patient feels unsteady, you can cue the patient to use your forearms for support.

10. Once the patient has turned and is backed up to the transfer surface, cue the patient to feel for the surface on the back of his or her legs and to reach back for the surface with one or both upper extremities.

11. Once the patient is seated, ensure he or she is safe.

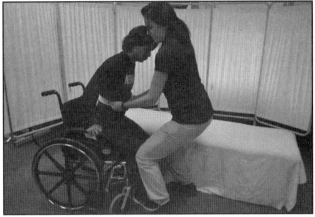

Figure 9-13. A squat pivot transfer with assist.

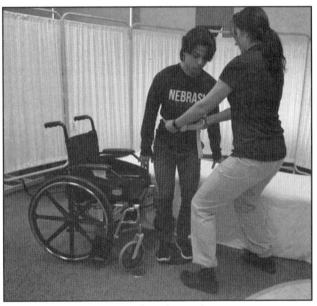

Figure 9-14. A squat pivot transfer with pivot disc.

The therapist may or may not need to move the armrest out of the way, depending on how low the patient squats. As with the stand pivot transfer, the patient should scoot forward to the edge of the seat (or be assisted with that motion), and the feet should be under the patient flat on the floor. The patient should assist as much as possible during the transfer.

If the patient is able to stand but not easily move his or her legs, the physical therapist may choose to use a pivot disc. The patient's feet are placed on the disc, and the patient can then rotate on the disc with the therapist's assistance.

The same cues of scooting forward and helping as much as possible still apply to squat pivot transfers; remember, you want the patient to do as much of the work as possible. Figure 9-13 shows the squat pivot transfer with assist, and Figure 9-14 shows the squat pivot transfer with the use of a pivot disc.

Slide Board

Some patients lack mobility or strength in one or both lower extremities. If the patient is unable to stand, even in a squat position, a sliding board may be useful. This may be the case if the patient has weakness in both lower extremities or has suffered an SCI resulting in paralysis of the lower extremities. The patient still requires fair sitting balance and fair strength in one or both upper extremities to assist with the transfer. A slide board is a long piece of sanded and finished wood that is beveled on each end. The physical therapist will need to assist the patient in placing the board under the buttocks, at least initially. Be sure that the board is not just under the buttocks, but is actually under the proximal thigh and well under the ischial tuberosities; otherwise, the patient is at risk for sliding or falling off the board. Ultimately, the goal is for the patient to become independent with this task; often patients progress from needing this tool to being able to laterally boost without it.

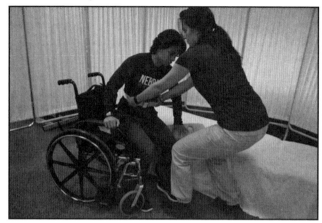

Figure 9-15. A slide board transfer with assist.

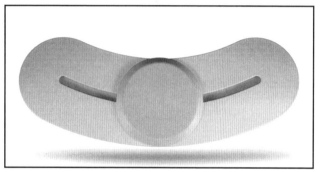

Figure 9-16. A Beasy Board. (Reprinted with permission from Beasy Trans Systems, Inc.)

Box 9-6
Slide Board Transfer

1. Position the wheelchair so that it is parallel to the transfer surface and as close to it as possible. Position so the patient is transferring toward his or her stronger side, unless you are working on a different skilled intervention.

2. Remove the legrest and armrest on the transfer side; lock the wheelchair brakes.

3. Apply a gait belt to the patient.

4. Depending on the level of assist, have the patient lean away from the transfer side, and slide the board under the buttocks so that it is secure and will not slide/move during the transfer. The other end of the board should be on the transfer surface.

5. Cue the patient to lean forward and use both upper extremities to lift and move buttocks across the board. Remind the patient to not wrap his or her fingers around or under the board, or they will be pinched.

6. Guard and assist the patient as needed, until the patient is completely on the new surface.

7. Ask the patient to lean away from the board so it can be removed from under the buttocks. Ensure the patient is safe.

The patient will use the board as a bridge to get from one surface to the next. The transfer surfaces should be close to one another to reduce the risk of falling. If using a wheelchair, the armrest on the transfer side will need to be removed or swung out of the way, and the wheels should be locked. The legrests should also be removed or swung out of the way. Initially the patient will be unable to do this on his or her own, and the therapist will need to assist. The same rules apply when determining the level of assist; it depends on what the patient can do. A gait belt will still need to be used, and if the patient requires CGA or more, the therapist should always be in contact with the patient. The patient should be cautioned to not put his or her fingers under the board lest they be squished, and the patient should aim to boost and move, rather than slide, to prevent friction and shearing on the buttocks. This is best facilitated by the patient leaning forward and pushing down with extended upper extremities (like in a chair push-up) to lift the buttocks. Some patients use pillow cases over the board to decrease friction and allow for easier movement along the board. Figure 9-15 shows a slide board transfer with assist. Box 9-6 provides instructions for a slide board transfer.

There are other types of boards that can be used for slide board transfers; the Beasy Board comes in several shapes.

It has a disc that glides in a groove along the length of the board.[6] The patient can use his or her arms to pull the body along the board from one surface to another. Since the seat moves along a track, the patient has less friction and shear. Figure 9-16 shows a transfer using a Beasy Board.

Lateral Boost

A lateral boost (Figure 9-17) is for patients who are unable to use their lower extremities but have very strong upper extremities and good upper trunk balance. Similar to the slide board method, the physical therapist positions the transfer surfaces close to one another at 45-degree angles. If using a wheelchair, the wheels should be locked, and the armrest and legrests should be removed. The patient will boost or do a seated push-up to move from one surface to the next, and this is easiest if the patient leans forward a bit to unweight the buttocks. It will take several boosts to get across, and it is especially difficult to lift up and over the drive wheel. The patient will need assistance when first trying out this transfer method, and it will take much practice to master. Sometimes patients who start off with a slide board transition to a lateral boost as strength and balance improve. A gait belt should always be used during transfer training.

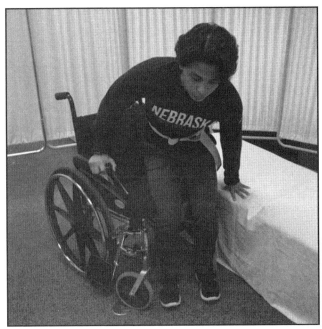

Figure 9-17. A lateral boost transfer.

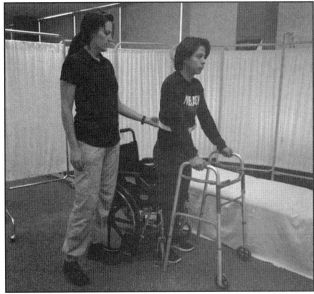

Figure 9-18. A stand pivot transfer with a walker.

Independent Transfers

Eventually your patient may become independent with his or her transfers. This is the hope of every physical therapist and patient, and it only comes from much practice and education. Keep in mind that any of these transfers can also be done using an assistive device. The use of an assistive device means that the patient can be no better than a modified independent on the assist level scale or FIM scoring. If the patient plans to use a cane, walker, or other device, transfers should be practiced while using the device. More about using assistive devices during transfers will be discussed in Chapter 10.

Stand Pivot

An independent stand pivot transfer requires the patient to be able to manipulate the wheelchair or bed while maintaining safety during the process. The transfer surfaces should be close together and at a 45-degree angle, and if using a wheelchair, the patient will need to lock the wheels and remove the legrests. If the patient is using an assistive device, the patient will need to manipulate that independently as well. The patient also needs to remember to have both feet pulled back underneath his or her body and to have nonslip socks or shoes. Remember that transfers can be from bed to wheelchair, but also from recliners, bedside commodes, toilets, showers, and cars. The rules are the same no matter the surface. The patient will perform a sit to stand as detailed earlier. If the patient is independent, he or she will be able to scoot to the edge of the chair, lean forward, and push from the armrests without assistance or cueing. If the patient is modified independent and uses an

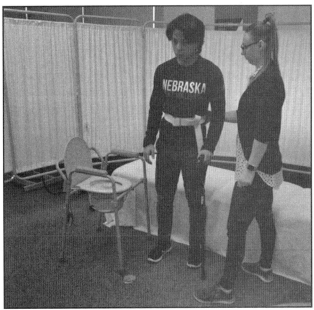

Figure 9-19. A stand pivot transfer to a commode with a cane.

assistive device, he or she will need to remember to not pull on or use the device to stand. This will be covered in more detail in Chapter 10, but Figures 9-18 and 9-19 show a stand pivot transfer using a walker and a cane, respectively.

Squat Pivot

A patient can be independent with a squat pivot transfer. The transfer surfaces should be close together, and the patient will need to follow all safety rules, including locking wheelchair brakes and moving legs rests and armrests out of the way. The patient will pivot as with a stand pivot transfer, but he or she will not come to a fully upright posture.

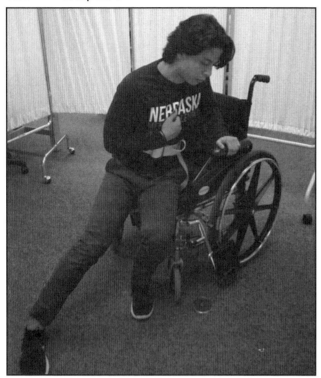

Figure 9-20. A transfer from the wheelchair to the floor with one weak side.

Slide Board

Sliding boards (or Beasy Boards) can be used independently by patients after education and practice. The patient will need to prevent fingers from being caught under the boards, and legrests and armrests will need to be removed from the wheelchair. Wheelchair locks should be engaged and transfer surfaces should be close together and at a 45-degree angle.

Lateral Boost

A patient can also perform a lateral boost independently with practice. Wheelchair or surface positioning follows the 45-degree angle rule and should be in close proximity. The wheelchair should be locked, and armrests and legrests should be removed or moved out of the way. The patient will push with the upper extremities to boost across from one surface to the next.

Floor Transfers

In therapy, physical therapists always practice for the worst-case scenario. Of course, physical therapists hope that a patient will not fall; however, they know that in reality, a fall is quite possible. It is best, then, to prepare and educate the patient on how to return to the chair after a fall, especially if the patient is alone. Additionally, some patients may want to transfer to the floor intentionally; a grandfather may want to play with his grandchildren; a woman may want to sit and pet her dog. In all these cases, a patient should be able to safely transfer from the wheelchair to the floor and back again. Your job is to perform the training incrementally, so the patient gradually builds up strength and confidence in the skill. You must guard the patient carefully to avoid injury during the training. The patient should ensure the wheels are locked and that the legrests or front rigging are out of the way.

Forward

As with all transfers, you must consider the patient's strength and abilities when training. If the patient is weak on one side, as in the case of a CVA, the patient must learn to lock the wheels, remove feet from the legrests or foot plates, and then move forward in the chair (as if preparing to stand). The patient should lead with the strong side, bearing weight on the strong leg and leaning forward until the strong arm is on the ground. The patient can then lower the body to the floor using the strong arm and leg to slow the descent (Figure 9-20).

To return, the patient should ensure the wheelchair is locked and position him- or herself so his or her stronger side is facing the chair. The patient then bends both knees and hips and reaches to the back of the seat with the strong upper extremity until he or she is kneeling. From there, the patient will move to a half-kneeling position (strong lower extremity being up) and push up using that strong leg. The patient may either partially stand or fully stand, depending on strength.

If the patient has strong upper extremities but weaker or paralyzed lower extremities (as in the case of an SCI), the patient can transition to the floor forward by preparing in the same way described previously: lock the wheelchair and scoot to the edge of the chair. In this case, the patient reaches with one upper extremity toward the floor while maintaining contact with an armrest on the chair (to prevent tipping). The patient should let go of the armrest once the other hand is in contact with the floor. Then the patient will have both hands on the floor and be in a hands-and-knees position (Figure 9-21).

An alternate option is for the patient to scoot forward in the seat with the lower extremities straight in front. Then the patient performs a push up to the clear the buttocks from the seat using the front rigging of the chair (with the legrests swung out of the way) and slowly lowers the buttocks to the floor.

To return to the chair in a forward position, the patient will face the wheelchair while on hands and knees. Ensure the chair is locked, and then the patient should place one hand on the armrest and the other on the seat and perform a push up until the hips are above the level of the seat. The patient will then turn and sit one hip on the seat, reposition hands on both armrests, and then sit with both hips in the seat (Figure 9-22).

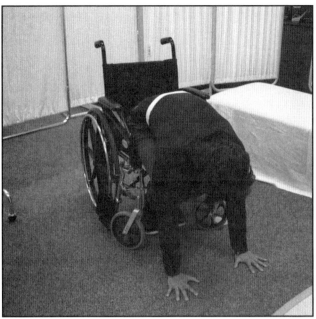

Figure 9-21. A transfer from the wheelchair to the floor with 2 weak lower extremities (hands and knees).

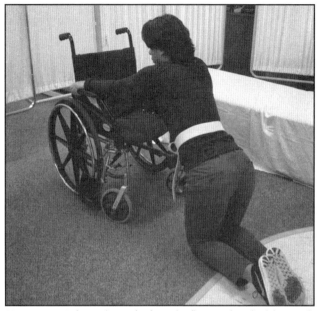

Figure 9-22. A forward transfer from the floor to the wheelchair with weak lower extremities.

Sideways

To perform a sideways transfer from the wheelchair to the floor, it would be as described earlier, except that instead of the patient facing the chair while on hands and knees, the patient will be sitting with one hip close to the chair (sitting sideways) with both knees and hips bent.

Backward

To transfer from a wheelchair to the floor backward, the patient will lock the wheels and then move to the front of the chair. The patient then pivots onto one hip and then rotates the body so both arms are holding onto the armrests. If the patient is on the left hip, the left hand would be on the right armrest and the right hand would be on the left armrest. The patient would perform a push up to clear the buttocks from the seat and further rotate until the knees are on the floor in a tall kneel position. Then the patient can lower all the way down into the most comfortable position.

To transfer from the floor to the wheelchair backward, the patient will lock the wheels and remove the legrests. The patient then backs up to the chair, facing away from the chair. The patient uses the front rigging (with the legrests removed) to push up until the pelvis is above the level of the seat (using the lower extremities if possible) and then lowers the buttocks into the seat. This requires a great deal of strength and balance. Figure 9-23 depicts how to transfer from the floor to the wheelchair backward.

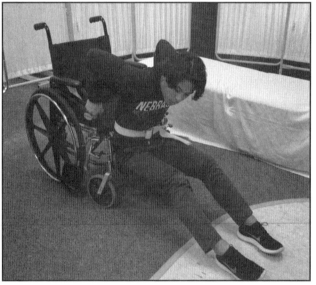

Figure 9-23. Transferring backward from the floor to the wheelchair.

Car Transfers

A transfer to a car (presumably from a wheelchair) is the same as earlier described transfers. The transfer could be a stand pivot, a squat pivot, it could use a sliding board, or have the patient boost. The transfer setup also depends on how much assistance the patient needs. There is some limitation of space with a car transfer because a car door only opens so far and there must be room for you to assist the patient. You should always use a gait belt, and the wheel-

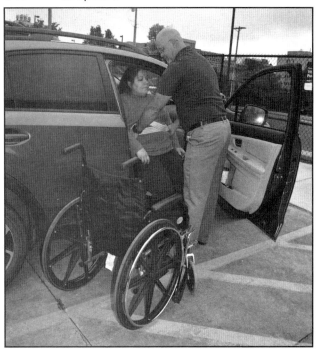

Figure 9-24. A car transfer with a wheelchair.

chair will need to be as close to the car as possible. If the patient is using an assistive device, there must be enough room for that to fit in the space. The general rule of thumb when transferring a patient from a wheelchair to the car is to sit the patient first in the seat, and then pivot so the legs are placed inside the car. The reverse is true for a car-to-wheelchair transfer: pivot the legs out first, and then have the patient stand or perform the transfer. Figure 9-24 shows a car transfer with a wheelchair.

Cerebrovascular Accident

As with bed mobility, there are some special considerations for patients who have had a CVA. Because these patients have one side that is weaker than the other, it may be necessary to guard or protect the weaker side. Sometimes during a stand or squat pivot transfer, the physical therapist must use his or her knee to block the patient's knee. This will keep the knee from buckling when the patient comes to a full or partial stand. Direct knee-on-knee contact tends to be uncomfortable, so it is best to have your knee on the inside or outside of the patient's knee.

Similarly, since patients who have had a stroke sometimes neglect or forget about the affected side and both upper and lower extremities are often very weak, you may need to assist with the patient's hand placement or with the movement of the foot or leg during the transfer. This does not mean the patient is not able to perform the transfer, but it does affect the level of assist the patient needs.

Amputation

A patient who has had an amputation, especially one who has not yet received or is not wearing a prosthetic, will need some additional assistance because balance and strength will be affected upon standing. The patient will need to lean toward the intact side to maintain balance, and if the transfer is a stand or squat pivot, the patient will need to hop rather than step to make the turn to sit. Once the patient has a prosthetic limb, the patient will better be able to perform a transfer due to regained balance.

Joint Replacement

A patient who has had a hip replaced is usually restricted from bending at the hips greater than 90 degrees. This may make a sit to stand more difficult, since the general rule of thumb is to cue the patient to lean forward before standing. To solve this problem, you should cue the patient to kick out the affected leg (so that it is more or less straight out in front of the patient) and to lean forward only a little and on the unaffected side to stand. The patient can also make sit to stand easier by scooting forward in the chair or seat. To sit, the patient will again straighten out the affected limb first before sitting. This will decrease the amount of flexion at the hips.

A patient with a hip replacement also needs to adhere to other surgical precautions. Always follow the surgeon's protocol. Typically, an anterolateral approach dictates that the patient should not perform external hip rotation, no flexion greater than 90 degrees, and no hip adduction. A posterolateral or posterior approach requires no flexion past 90 degrees, no internal hip rotation, and no hip adduction.

This also would apply for a patient who is nonweightbearing, either due to a joint replacement or another injury. The patient will kick out the affected leg without putting any weight on it, and your job will be to protect that affected limb to prevent the patient from accidentally bearing weight on it.

This concept of standing and sitting with a straight leg also applies for a patient who has had a knee replacement. Eventually, of course, you will want the patient to flex the knee to sit and stand, as patients with knee replacements do not have the same restrictions as patients with hip replacements. Initially, however, flexing the knee is quite painful, so you may allow or educate the patient to extend the knee with sitting or standing to decrease pain.

Spinal Cord Injury

A patient with an SCI will need a great deal of training for transfers. Ability and type of transfer depends on the patient's level of injury and recovered strength and balance. Immediately after the injury, the patient will have less strength and balance, and will need much more assistance. He or she may even be dependent. However, if the level of lesion is low enough that the patient has some use of the upper extremities and/or trunk, the patient can eventually learn how to transfer, sometimes achieving full independence with this task. The American Physical Therapy Association's clinical summary on SCIs recommends bed mobility tasks such as supine to/from sit and supine to/from prone; the transfers recommended include in and out of bed, on and off the floor, and on and off various surfaces such as couches, toilets, etc.[7]

Immediately after an SCI, great care should be taken to avoid moving the injury site; transfers will be necessary, but multiple people should be involved to protect the patient and avoid further injury.

Hoyer/Mechanical Lifts

Mechanical lifts come in different forms. A Hoyer lift, or a full-body sling lift, is a hydraulic lift that uses a sling to raise the patient up into the air. The lift rolls on wheels so the patient can be moved or repositioned as needed. A sit-to-stand lift also rolls on wheels and a patient can either be lifted via remote control or manual lever. The patient is strapped into place and then lifted into a standing position. The patient can then either be moved to another surface and lowered back into sitting, or the patient can stay in standing for a period of time to help with off-loading pressure and increasing weightbearing in the lower extremities.

A Hoyer lift uses a sling that must be appropriate for the patient's height and weight. The patient is rolled to be positioned on the sling, or if the patient is in a wheelchair, the patient must lift and move around in the chair to get the sling under the body. Then the lift is positioned so that the sling bar is over the patient and lowered so the sling can be attached to the bar.[8] The lift's wheels need to be locked to prevent injury.[9] The patient's head and back should be supported by the sling. The sling is then slowly raised until the patient is off the surface and hanging from the lift. The patient should be educated to keep arms inside the lift at all times.[9] In a Hoyer lift, the patient can never be left unattended in the sling. The patient should be lowered slowly onto the transfer surface.[8] The sling is then unhooked from the bar, being mindful to not hit the patient in the head with the bar, and the sling should then be removed from under the patient. It is tempting to leave the sling under the patient, especially when the patient is in a wheelchair, because it is a hassle to get it back under the patient correctly; however, leaving the sling under the patient increases the risk of wounds.

Some patients have lift chairs in their homes. Sometimes the entire chair raises, and sometimes the patient has an insert in the seat that raises. Either way, this lift raises the patient from sitting to an almost fully upright position, which eliminates the lifting portion of the transfer on the physical therapist's or caregiver's part. Likewise, when the

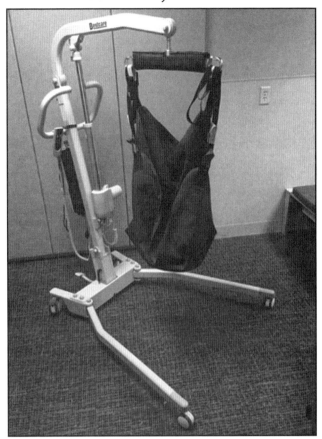

Figure 9-25. A mechanical lift.

patient returns to that chair to sit, the patient can be lowered into the raised seat without as much effort required from the caregiver.

There are also standing frame or standing lifts in hospitals or facilities that can get a patient into a standing position either for transferring or to simply allow the patient to be upright, promoting better respiration, circulation, and weightbearing through the lower extremities. These can be either raised and lowered by hand or by remote control, but they all require the patient to be first transferred to the standing lift seat before being stood up. These lifts often are on wheels, so the patient can be moved from one location to another. These are good options for patients who are dependent or require maximal assist to stand; those patients will benefit from standing but doing so manually is challenging and potentially unsafe. Figure 9-25 shows a mechanical lift.

Hospital Safety and Lifts

As mentioned in Chapter 2, more and more facilities are encouraging the use of mechanical lifts to do the work of transferring dependent or maximal assist patients from one surface to another. Repetitive lifting, especially when proper body mechanics are not performed, leads inevitably to therapist injuries and lost time from work. In worst case scenarios, physical therapists who suffer from these work-related musculoskeletal disorders either change their practice setting or leave the field of physical therapy altogether. As a result, most facilities have some kind of lifting protocol, and more facilities are integrating technology, including mechanical lifts, to reduce injuries. Education is also key to ensure physical therapists and other clinicians know how to use the equipment or what the protocol is for lifting. The American Physical Therapy Association created a statement to notify physical therapists and physical therapist assistants regarding its status on patient handling, stipulating that physical therapists and physical therapist assistants should lead by example and should also play a role in educating patients and other caregivers regarding patient handling practices.[10] Physical therapist assistants can and do have the critical problem-solving skills to safely handle (ie, transfer or move) patients.

SAFETY/RED FLAGS

There are many safety concerns when it comes to bed mobility and transfers. Thankfully, there are many considerations and changes you can make to create a safe environment for your patients.

First and foremost, you need to follow the rules of proper body mechanics. Use a wide BOS, and lower your COG. Get close to the patient, and maintain normal lumbar lordosis as you lift with your legs and not your back. Enlist the help of another person, if needed, or utilize a mechanical lift if one is available. Remember to make your patient do as much work as possible, and avoid simultaneous trunk flexion and rotation.

Remember, too, that gait belts must be used during transfers. You may go to a clinic and see physical therapists not use gait belts on their patients. Perhaps it is an outpatient clinic and most of the patients are young and relatively healthy. It does not matter. If you are a good clinician, you will be challenging a patient's strength and balance, which means that no matter how strong or healthy the person may be, they are still at a risk for falling. As a part of that conversation, you should only use the gait belt for assisting a patient up or out of a bed or chair. You should never grab the patient's clothing or extremities; if a patient begins to lose his or her balance, the clothing will not help, and you could dislocate an arm.

There was once a patient on the inpatient rehabilitation floor who was getting ready to graduate from therapy. He was relatively young and had suffered a stroke. He was doing really well with therapy, and the physical therapist had him working on dynamic balance tasks by hitting a beach ball back and forth with a technician. All of a sudden, he lost his balance and fell. He was not injured, but

an incident report had to be filed. In this case, the physical therapist could honestly report that the patient was wearing a gait belt, even if it did not stop the patient's fall. This example shows that the best practice is to always apply a gait belt. If the patient falls, you can indicate in your incident report that the patient was wearing a gait belt. It is always better to be safe than sorry.

When transferring a patient, you should look at the patient's shoes. Slippers or slick-soled shoes are hazards and may cause the patient to get tripped up or slip on the floor. The patient should absolutely not be wearing only socks, unless they are the hospital-provided socks with the nonslip bottoms.

When transferring from a hospital bed, be sure to have all tubes and lines moved to prevent pulling or tugging. Make sure the IV pole and the catheter bag are on the side you are transferring the patient to. Make sure the ventilator tubing has enough slack to allow the patient mobility. You would not want to find out the hard way that you did not plan ahead well or have enough length to perform the task safely. Make sure to move all other equipment and furniture out of the way in order to perform the transfer without tripping hazards.

If you are transferring a patient to or from a wheelchair, do not forget to engage the wheel locks. Make sure also that the legrests are out of the way, and if you are performing a lateral boost or slide board transfer, you will need to remove the armrest on the transfer side to allow a safe transfer to happen. Whether you are transferring to a wheelchair or not, you should always make sure the wheels on the bed are locked.

As mentioned earlier, you should know when or if you need a second person or a mechanical lift, so you can avoid injury to yourself or your patient. Body mechanics are also vital when performing transfers or bed mobility. Review Chapter 2 regarding body mechanics and lifts. Raise the height of the bed, if needed, so you can assist with the task without injuring yourself. When the transfer is completed, you should never leave a patient unattended unless the patient is in a safe, stable, and supported position.

In all transfer cases, you should consider the patient's comorbidities. Is the patient a diabetic? You should monitor blood sugar or the patient's symptoms that might indicate low blood sugar. Low blood sugar manifests as fatigue, shakiness, sweating, irritability, or in worse situations, confusion or loss of consciousness.[11] You should not attempt a transfer with a patient who has low blood sugar due to the possible injury the patient may incur.

Similarly, the patient's blood pressure should be monitored. If the patient suffers from orthostatic hypotension, or a sudden drop in blood pressure with position change, the patient may lose consciousness or fall.[12]

DOCUMENTATION

When documenting transfers, remember to include the type of transfer performed, the level of assist required, whether another person (and how many) were needed to assist, and the transfer surfaces. You can also include any verbal or tactile cues that the patient needed.

O: Performed rolling with patient to the Ⓛ, requiring min Ⓐ and 3 verbal cues to perform the task correctly. Supine to sit mod Ⓐ with some additional assistance for balance required once patient sitting EOB. Patient transferred from EOB to chair in hospital room. Chair positioned close to bed's surface with bed lowered so patient's feet could touch the floor. Patient attempted stand pivot transfer but unable to come to full stand. Transferred squat pivot mod Ⓐ with patient requiring tactile assist to move Ⓡ LE due to weakness.

REVIEW QUESTIONS

1. Describe what it means for a patient to require maximal assist for bed mobility or a transfer. What about CGA?

2. What is the difference between independent and modified independent?

3. Describe how you would perform supine to sit with a patient who requires a log roll.

4. Describe how you would perform a stand pivot transfer for a patient who has suffered a left-sided CVA (with right side affected).

5. What is a safety concern with using a mechanical lift for a transfer?

6. What is one way a patient could transfer from the wheelchair to the floor if both lower extremities are weak, but both upper extremities are fairly strong?

7. Why should a patient wear a gait belt during all transfers?

8. You perform a supine-to-sit bed mobility and a transfer from bed to wheelchair for a patient who requires 25% assistance. What level of assist is this patient, and how would you document your activities?

REFERENCES

1. Venema DM, Hassel J, Jones KJ. Best practices in safe transfers and mobility to decrease fall risk. *University of Nebraska Medical Center.* https://www.unmc.edu/patient-safety/_documents/safe-transfers-mobility-handout.pdf. Published August 20, 2013. Accessed September 7, 2018.

2. Functional Independence Measure. *Rehabilitation Measures Database.* https://www.sralab.org/rehabilitation-measures/fimr-instrument-fim-fimr-trademark-uniform-data-system-fro-medical. Updated October 6, 2015. Accessed September 7, 2018.

3. Activities after hip replacement. *American Academy of Orthopaedic Surgeons.* http://orthoinfo.aaos.org/topic.cfm?topic=a00356. Updated 2014. Accessed September 7, 2018.

4. Transfer techniques for patients with spinal cord injury: level surfaces. *Good Shepherd Rehabilitation.* http://www.good-shepherdrehab.org/sites/goodshepherdrehab.org/files/documents/TRANSFER%20TECHNIQUES%20-%20updated.pdf. Accessed September 7, 2018.

5. Healthwise Staff. Log roll method for safe movement. *UPMC.* http://www.upmc.com/patients-visitors/education/rehab/Pages/bed-transfer-log-roll-method.aspx. Updated July 11, 2017. Accessed September 7, 2018.

6. Beasy premium transfer boards. *Beasy.* https://beasyboards.com/. Accessed September 7, 2018.

7. Somers MF, Bruce J, Cohen ET, Csiza L, Karpatkin HI. Spinal Cord Injury (SCI) in Adults. *PT Now.* http://ptnow.org/clinical-summaries-detail/spinal-cord-injury-sci. Published January 15, 2014. Accessed September 7, 2018.

8. Patient lifts: safety guide. *US Food and Drug Administration.* https://www.fda.gov/downloads/MedicalDevices/ProductsandMedicalProcedures/HomeHealthandConsumer/HomeUseDevices/UCM386178.pdf. Accessed September 7, 2018.

9. Wagman V. Best practices for using patient lifts. *US Food and Drug Administration.* https://www.fda.gov/downloads/forhealthprofessionals/ucm362873.pdf. Published 2013. Accessed September 7, 2018.

10. The role of physical therapy in safe patient handling. *APTA.* http://www.apta.org/uploadedFiles/APTAorg/About_Us/Policies/Practice/SafePatientHandling.pdf. Updated August 22, 2012. Accessed September 7, 2018.

11. Hypoglycemia. *Mayo Clinic.* http://www.mayoclinic.org/diseases-conditions/hypoglycemia/basics/symptoms/con-20021103. Updated September 7, 2018. Accessed September 7, 2018.

12. Orthostatic hypotension (postural hypotension). *Mayo Clinic.* http://www.mayoclinic.org/diseases-conditions/orthostatic-hypotension/home/ovc-20324946. Updated July 17, 2017. Accessed September 7, 2018.

Chapter 10

Assistive Devices and Gait

KEY TERMS Ambulation | Bilateral | Bridging | Concentric | Eccentric | Flaccid | Hook lying | Lofstrands | Prone | Quad cane | Rollator | Unilateral | Walker

KEY ABBREVIATIONS BOS | BWST | CGA | CVA | DGI | FWB | FWW | NWB | PWB | SPC | TDWB/TTWB | TUG | WBAT

CHAPTER OBJECTIVES

1. Describe the pre-gait or developmental postures and when they are useful for patients.
2. Describe the gait cycle, including all its parts and what muscles or joint positions are used in each phase.
3. Select and fit patients for the correct assistive devices.
4. Identify weightbearing status for a patient, and understand how it applies to gait training.
5. Educate patients on how to use assistive devices correctly, including the general gait patterns and stair/curb negotiation.
6. Understand and administer gait assessment tests for patients.
7. Identify safety concerns or red flags for patients to avoid injury.

INTRODUCTION

Transfers are one of the most common therapeutic interventions a clinician will perform with a patient; this may only be outweighed by gait training and the use of assistive devices. Your patient may lack the strength or the balance to walk without assistance. The patient may have permanent or temporary limitation on weightbearing or

use of extremities. Whatever the limitation, a patient often needs corrective assistance with gait, and the patient may need to be fitted for and educated on the use of an assistive device. Your job will be to ensure these things happen, so the patient can be functional and safe.

PRE-GAIT

Sometimes a patient is not ready to just stand up and walk. Maybe the patient has been immobilized for quite some time. Muscles have atrophied, and blood pressure issues associated with a prolonged recumbent position may be an issue. The patient may need to be gradually introduced to upright postures and gait activities, so pre-gait activities provide that segue.

Developmental Postures

Developmental postures offer the chance to strengthen certain muscle groups while also challenging balance in order to prepare the patient for fully upright gait training. These can be done on a mat or floor, progressing to the use of parallel bars or tables. While in these positions, a patient's balance or strength can be further challenged with perturbations or isometric holds. It is worth noting that a patient can benefit from these positions at any time during gait training; these positions do not need to only be used

Memolo J.
Procedures and Patient Care for the Physical Therapist Assistant
(pp 145-173). © 2019 SLACK Incorporated.

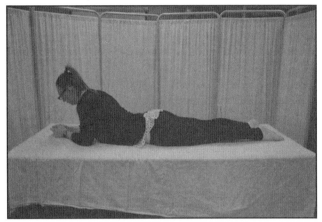

Figure 10-1. Prone on elbows.

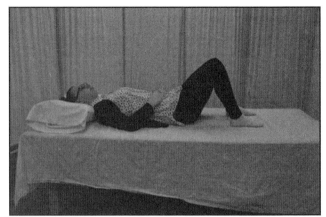

Figure 10-2. Hook lying.

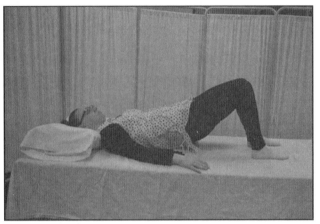

Figure 10-3. Bridging.

during pre-gait sessions. Also, these positions do not need to be done in any particular order. You can move a patient in and out of each position as you see necessary.

Prone on Elbows

A patient in prone is very stable. There is little chance the patient can fall or injure him- or herself when in a prone position. In this position, the patient can push up to his or her elbows, elevating the upper trunk, head, and neck, and in doing so, the patient can strengthen the muscles of the shoulders, arms, and neck to prepare for being more upright. In this position, the patient can also perform mini push-ups or can progress to pushing up on the hands rather than the elbows. A physical therapist can offer perturbations to the patient that the patient must hold against. A patient will need strong upper extremities to use an assistive device or to push up from sitting to standing, so this position assists the patient in being ready for those activities. Figure 10-1 shows a prone-on-elbows position.

Hook Lying/Bridging

In hook lying (Figure 10-2), a patient is on his or her back with knees bent and feet flat on the mat or bed. Like prone, this is a very stable position, and the patient can have his or her lower extremity strength or balance challenged. In hook lying, the patient first may struggle to just hold the lower extremities in the knee flexed position. Additional resistance can be offered by the therapist giving perturbations, or requiring the patient to hold a ball between the knees. The patient may be asked to lift one leg and then the other alternately, and to progress, the patient can attempt bridging. From the hook lying position, the patient can lift his or her buttocks off the bed or mat in a bridge position (Figure 10-3) while keeping the knees bent and the feet flat on the mat. The patient can also work on pelvic tilts, both anterior and posterior. Initially, the patient may be challenged just to hold this position; however, as strength improves, perturbations can be offered, and the patient can perform bridging in sets and repetitions as a concentric/eccentric exercise.

Quadruped

A patient in quadruped is on all fours, which is less stable than prone or hook lying and requires more strength and balance to maintain the position. The position may begin as an isometric hold, but the patient can progress to lifting one arm or leg, or opposite arms and legs at the same time. You can offer perturbations to the patient from the side, forward, or backward; the patient can practice weight shifting; and you can even have the patient practice crawling, which facilitates the reciprocal arm/leg movement that must happen during gait. Figure 10-4 shows a quadruped position.

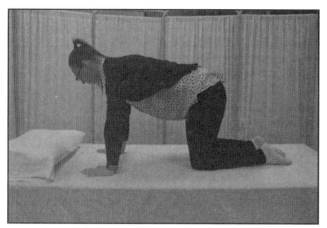

Figure 10-4. Quadruped.

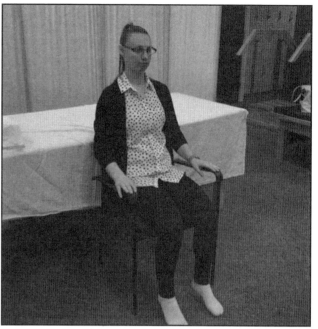

Figure 10-5. A seated position.

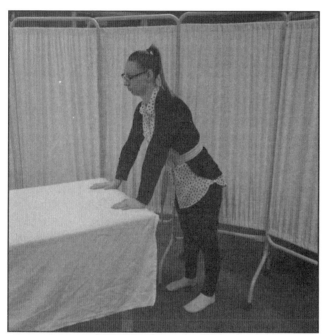

Figure 10-6. Modified plantigrade.

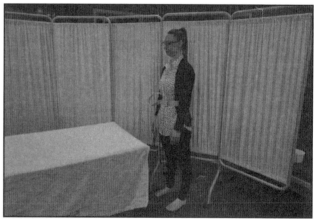

Figure 10-7. Plantigrade.

Seated

A patient in sitting is more stable than in standing, and the patient can be challenged more in this position due to a more narrow base of support (BOS). In sitting, the patient can practice lifting one leg, which further narrows the BOS; shifting weight left to right, which prepares the patient for the weight shifting required during gait; scooting laterally, forward, or backward; reaching in different planes; or resisting perturbations given by the therapist. From sitting, a patient can practice sit to stand, which progresses the patient to standing postures. Figure 10-5 depicts a patient in a seated position.

Modified Plantigrade

A patient who is able to be more upright but still needs support can practice modified plantigrade (Figure 10-6).

The patient is on 2 feet and fully upright, but the patient may use the parallel bars or a table top to support the upper extremities. In this position, the patient is working on holding an upright posture while being able to work on lower extremity activities, such as weight shifting; marching in place; stepping forward, backward, or to the side; or performing heel or toe lifts. The patient feels supported by having hands on a stable surface, but the patient is being challenged at the same time. Many of these movements prepare the patient for more complex gait activities, such as backing up to open a door or sidestepping to get through a narrow bathroom entrance with an assistive device.

Plantigrade

Plantigrade is when the patient is fully upright without upper extremity support (Figure 10-7). Activities in plantigrade may still be done in the parallel bars or with other

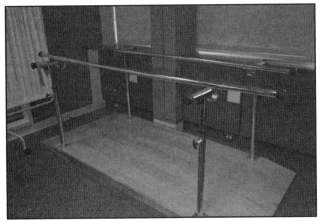

Figure 10-8. Parallel bars.

upper extremity support as needed, but the goal is for the patient to practice standing upright with little to no support in preparation for gait. Again, the patient can practice standing exercises for the lower extremities, such as marching; leg kicks; heel raises; or stepping forward, backward, and to the side.

Equipment

As mentioned earlier, there are several pieces of equipment that patients can use to practice these pre-gait activities. These devices offer the patient some security against falls and allow the patient to become more confident with gait activities as they progress.

Tilt Table

A tilt table is a table that starts in the horizontal position and then can slowly be raised so the patient is at a 90-degree angle to the floor. The patient is initially strapped to the table when it is horizontal to prevent the patient from falling out when the table moves to upright. There is also a foot plate at the bottom of the table so the patient's feet can rest on it as he or she moves to a more vertical position. A tilt table is used for patients who suffer from orthostatic hypotension or who have otherwise been immobilized for a prolonged period of time and need to slowly become acclimated to upright positions.[1] Many times the table is used for a tilt table test, which measures the heart rate and blood pressure response to changes of position. The table is usually run via remote control, and the table has a scale to measure how many degrees the patient is from upright.

If the patient's heart rate increases significantly or blood pressure drops, the patient should be lowered back to a more horizontal position and retested for vital sign changes.[1] Then the patient can be raised again, and the physical therapist should always monitor patient's vitals and response or reaction. The patient may feel dizzy, nauseated, and even may lose consciousness, so it is important the clinician monitor the patient closely. Other patient complaints may be vision changes, pallor, edema in the lower extremities, and excessive perspiration. If you note any of these signs or symptoms, lower the patient back to a level where he or she stabilizes and allow the patient to recover. The next attempt at raising the table may require you to do so at a slower pace or smaller increment. Some patients wear compression stockings or abdominal binders to help keep blood flow up toward the brain, decreasing the signs or symptoms listed previously.

Parallel Bars

Parallel bars are 2 metal bars that are parallel to each other, which allow a patient to have something to hold on to while working on static standing or short distances of gait (Figure 10-8). The height of the bars can usually be raised or lowered to accommodate the patient's height, and chairs, step stools, or other exercise or training devices can be used inside the bars while the patient stands and holds on. The bars offer a nice segue from sitting to standing, offering stability and the allure of short distances before the patient graduates to more advanced activities.

One activity a patient can perform in the parallel bars is shifting weight from side to side (weight is shifted this way during normal gait). The goal is to keep the shoulders and pelvis in line and the trunk upright. The patient can also practice lifting one hand at a time (alternating) from the bars to work on balance; eventually, the patient could attempt lifting both hands. To improve strength, the patient could practice push-ups on the bars. The patient could also alternately lift the opposite upper and lower extremities to simulate normal gait. Eventually, specific gait patterns (detailed later in this chapter) can be practiced in the parallel bars, as well as moving in differing directions (sidestepping, backward, and turning to the right or left).

Therapists also use the parallel bars to assist with measuring and fitting patients for assistive devices. The methods for measuring and fitting are discussed later in this chapter, but a general rule to follow is that you never have the patient stand unattended while adjusting an assistive device. In the parallel bars, you can have the patient stand while you fit for axillary crutches or a cane, and then have the patient sit while you make the necessary adjustments.

During parallel bar activities, you may need to stand behind or in front of the patient depending on if the patient needs knee blocking or general guarding. Either way, you should remain inside the bars with the patient to ensure patient safety.

Body Weight Supported Treadmill

A body weight supported treadmill (BWST) uses a harness system, to suspend a patient from upright, and cross bars so the patient can practice gait on a treadmill without the fear of falling (Figure 10-9). The patient's weight is fully supported by the harness system, allowing the therapist to be more involved in assisting the patient with the proper phases of gait or the specific movements needed in the lower extremities instead of worrying about holding the patient up against gravity. The amount of weight taken off the patient can be varied, so the patient can progress from having all or most of his or her weight removed to less and less as time goes by. Sometimes these harness systems are suspended from overhead tracks in the ceiling, while other versions are stand-alone devices that roll on wheels, so the patient can walk across the ground as well as on the treadmill. The patient can then practice all the necessary elements of proper gait without the fear of falling, although care should be given when setting the patient up in the harness to avoid pinching or pain.

Research has shown that patients who use the BWST system improve with balance, spatiotemporal gait, and lower extremity range of motion, especially for patients who have recently suffered a stroke.[2] As technology changes, the systems have become more advanced. Overhead track systems, such as SafeGait (Gorbel Medical) or FreeStep (Biodex), are the newer versions of this technology, and these allow the patient to walk anywhere the track is installed.[3,4] Larger rehabilitation clinics often have these systems, as they can be very pricey.

ASSISTIVE DEVICES

Once your patient is ambulatory, he or she may need an assistive device to facilitate proper gait, as well as to ensure safety and balance. Assistive devices are classified according to how restrictive they are and how much balance they require. When assigning a patient an assistive device, the physical therapist assistant should be sure to consider the patient's strength, endurance, and balance, as well as home setup (eg, width of doorways, number of stairs, and accessibility of bathrooms) and how much caregiver assistance will be provided. A physical therapist will then need to educate the patient and caregivers on how to use the device properly when navigating the home and the outside community. The therapist will also need to fit the device properly to the patient. There is no counting how many times a therapist witnesses someone walking in the community with an assistive device either using it incorrectly or without the correct fit, and the therapist cringes. You will be that way too after reading this chapter and practicing these skills.

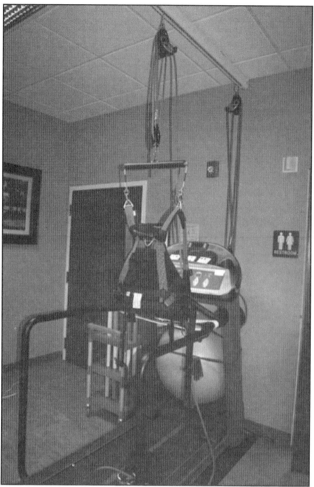

Figure 10-9. A BWST.

Additionally, your job includes knowing if or when to progress a patient to a less restrictive and more functional assistive device. The patient may start therapy with a walker, but by the end of the patient's tenure in rehab, he or she may only need a single-point cane (SPC). Working with your supervising physical therapist and the patient's physician, you get to make these clinical and skilled decisions about what the patient needs (or does not need).

Walkers

Walkers come in several different styles, and each offers certain benefits and drawbacks. Walkers are the most restrictive form of assistive device because they take up more room, are typically heavy, and are more difficult to transport. Additionally, walkers are difficult to use on stairs, and a patient cannot have normal reciprocal arm swing when using a walker. However, walkers are also the most supportive assistive device, offering a wide BOS to patients who have poor balance.

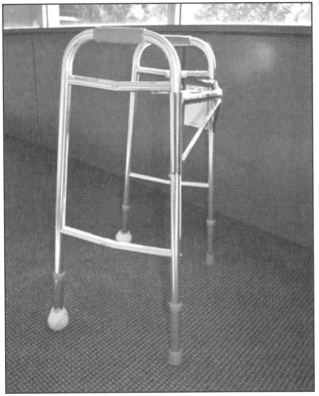

Figure 10-10. A standard walker.

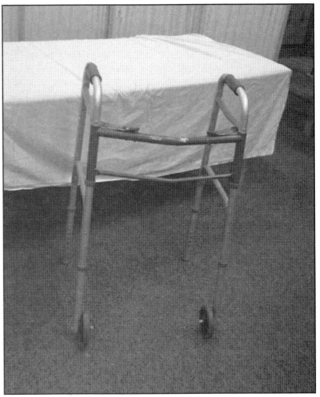

Figure 10-11. A front-wheeled walker.

A patient requires a certain amount of upper extremity strength to hold him- or herself upright when using a walker, and it is important to educate your patient to be mindful of his or her posture when using a walker. A walker is adjustable for height, and the patient should aim to walk inside the walker's frame and avoid excessive flexion of the trunk or hips. Most walkers are collapsible to some degree, so they can more easily fit in the trunk or back seat of a car. Some walkers have wheels, some have seats, and some have baskets to hold tissues or purses. Walkers can have various attachments to customize for the patient. A platform can be used on a walker if the patient is nonweightbearing (NWB) on the forearm or wrist or if he or she has difficulty with hand grip. Walkers, with the exception of the hemi-walker, are ideal for patients who are NWB or partial weightbearing (PWB).

Standard Walker

A standard walker (Figure 10-10) has 4 solid legs in contact with the ground. The patient supports him- or herself on the crossbars and must lift the walker to advance it. This is most beneficial for a patient with very poor balance; the wider BOS and because the walker does not roll allows the patient a certain security from falling. On the flip side, the patient must have the strength and balance to lift and advance the walker. Sometimes patients will place skis, or gliders, on the front legs to facilitate sliding the walker rather than lifting it, and you will often see tennis balls cut and placed over the walker feet to assist with gliding.

Front-Wheeled Walker

A front-wheeled walker (FWW; Figure 10-11) has 2 solid legs in the back and 2 wheels in the front. The wheels are not caster wheels, and so do not allow for easy turning, but the wheels do allow the patient to push the walker rather than lift it, as the standard walker requires. The rear legs may have skis, or the patient may place tennis balls on the rear legs, to reduce friction when pushing the walker. This walker requires a bit more balance from the patient in order to be safe, but patients who do have sufficient balance find the FWW to be a little easier to maneuver.

Four-Wheeled Walker/Rollator

A 4-wheeled walker, sometimes called a *rollator* (Figure 10-12), has 4 wheels, and the 2 front wheels are caster wheels. This allows for significant freedom in movement, but as you can imagine, the patient must have good balance to use this walker safely. These walkers, unlike the standard or FWW, have hand brakes that can be used to temporarily stop or lock the wheels on the walker for transfer safety.

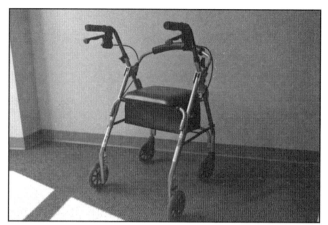

Figure 10-12. A 4-wheeled walker or rollator.

These walkers often have baskets or seats in the middle for the patient. These seats are handy for when a patient is fatigued and needs a quick rest break, and patients like the baskets because they can keep their belongings in them. However, the patient needs to understand that the wheels should be locked before sitting. Also, it is fairly common to see a patient sitting on the walker seat and using his or her legs to push him- or herself down the hallway; this is not a safe or intended use for the 4-wheeled walker, and the patient should be educated against doing this. The seat is only for a rest break and should not act as a wheelchair supplement. As a general rule, 4-wheeled walkers are heavier than standard or FWWs, and they do not collapse as compactly either. A patient may need another walker for transportation or for the top/bottom of stairs if the patient needs to use the device in the house, or the patient may need to rely on a caregiver to transport the walker. This walker is also not safe for use on stairs and can be challenging on curbs.

Three-Wheeled Walker/Rollator

Some versions of the rollator have only 3 wheels, making them slightly smaller, more lightweight, and easier to collapse (Figure 10-13). These can also come with a basket, but it is less common to see a seat with the 3-wheeled walker. These walkers are also not safe for use on stairs.

Hemi-Walker

A hemi-walker is sometimes called and classified as a *hemi-cane*, but here, it is designated in the walker category (Figure 10-14). A hemi-walker looks like a triangle when opened; it is used only on one side (unlike the other walkers that utilize both upper extremities), and it is most often used for patients who have suffered a cerebrovascular accident (CVA) or otherwise have an affected upper extremity that makes use of a bilateral device difficult or impossible. After a stroke, a patient often has weakness or flaccidity in

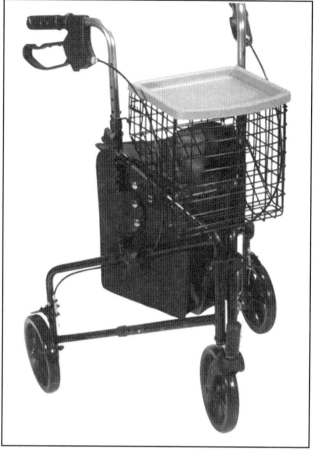

Figure 10-13. A deluxe 3-wheel aluminum walker or rollator. (Reprinted with permission from Drive Medical.)

one upper extremity. This makes pushing or manipulating a traditional walker difficult. A hemi-walker is placed on the patient's unaffected side to still offer a wide BOS while eliminating the difficulty of using the affected upper extremity. The patient must be educated on how to lift and advance the walker safely (to avoid tripping on it), being sure to keep the flat side against the body. It is relatively lightweight (compared to traditional walkers) and easy to collapse and fit in a trunk or back seat. It is not appropriate to use a hemi-walker on the stairs unless it is collapsed.

Fit

As mentioned earlier, it is very important to fit the assistive device selected to your patient. It is easiest to fit a patient while standing, but the patient could also be supine if unable to maintain a standing position long enough to fit the device. As mentioned earlier in this chapter, you could have the patient stand in the parallel bars to offer upper extremity support while measuring the fit, but remember that no matter what the patient's balance or strength status, you should always have the patient sit while you are adjusting the fit of the device.

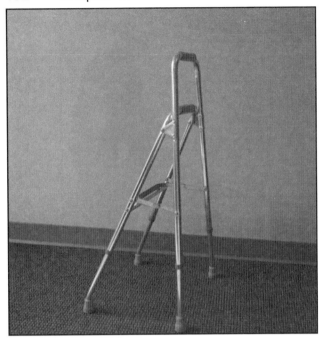

Figure 10-14. A hemi-walker.

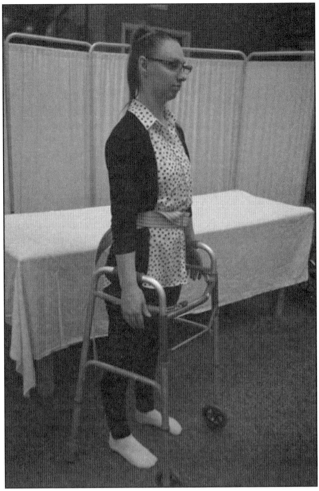

Figure 10-15. Fitting a walker.

For all walker types, the hand grips should be at the patient's wrist crease or greater trochanter, and when the therapist assesses the fit, the patient should be standing inside the walker. The patient's elbows should be flexed approximately 20 to 30 degrees when holding on to the hand grips; the elbows should not be fully extended, nor should the patient be flexed at the hips or knees when assessing the walker fit.

If fitting for a hemi-walker, the flatter side of the device should be against the body and the flared side away from the body; this ensures the patient will not trip over the device. The hand grip should still come to the wrist crease or greater trochanter. Figure 10-15 depicts how to fit a walker to a patient.

Axillary Crutches

Axillary crutches can be wooden or aluminum, and they are most often used for temporary purposes, such as if a patient breaks his or her leg and needs the crutches until the fracture heals (Figure 10-16). Axillary crutches offer good lateral support for a patient while allowing slightly easier mobility in tight spaces or on stairs. However, proper fit and good education on use are necessary, as a patient can injure his or her brachial plexus in the axillary region, causing damage to both blood vessels and nerves. Additionally, a patient requires good standing balance and coordination to use axillary crutches, and the patient also needs enough strength and endurance to use the crutches on a daily basis. It is unusual to see elderly patients with axillary crutches due to this need for strength and balance. Patients who are NWB or PWB can use axillary crutches to ambulate while still maintaining their weightbearing restrictions.

Axillary crutches are adjustable for height, and some come with preset height numbers to help the therapist with approximate fit. However, there are more accurate methods of ensuring proper fit.

Fit

There are several methods to measure and fit a patient for axillary crutches (Figure 10-17). As mentioned previously in the walker fit section, a patient should not be standing while the therapist makes height adjustments on the crutches. If the patient can stand to measure, position the crutches so that the tips are 4 to 6 inches anterior and 2 inches lateral to the patient's toes. The axillary pad should not be in contact with the axilla; rather, the therapist should be able to fit 2 to 3 fingers between the axillary pad and the patient's axilla. This ensures the patient does not damage the superficial nerves and blood vessels in the axilla.

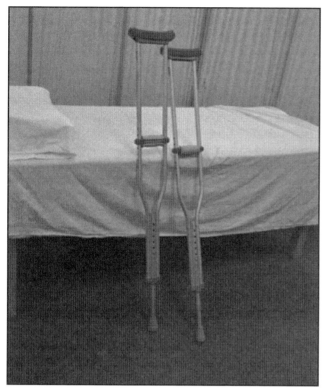

Figure 10-16. Axillary crutches.

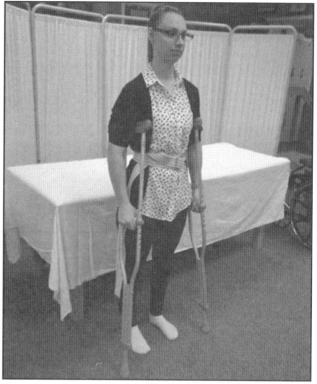

Figure 10-17. Fitting axillary crutches in standing.

If the therapist already knows the patient's height, the height in inches can be multiplied by 77% (68 inches x 0.77 = 52.3, or 52 inches). Another method is to subtract 16 inches from the patient's height (68 inches - 16 inches = 52 inches). Either of these calculations would produce the necessary height of the crutch (from tip to axillary pad), or at least give you a starting point.

If the patient cannot stand and you do not know the patient's height, you can measure for fit with the patient supine or seated. In supine, measure from the axillary fold to approximately 6 to 8 inches lateral of the patient's heel to determine the crutch length. In sitting, have the patient abduct the upper extremities at shoulder level with one elbow extended and one flexed to 90 degrees. Measure from the olecranon process of the flexed elbow to the tip of the long finger of the other upper extremity.

No matter what method you use to determine crutch height, fit should be confirmed once the patient is standing and adjustments can be made if necessary.

Axillary crutches also have hand grips, and these can also be adjusted for the patient. The hand grips should come to the patient's wrist crease or greater trochanter when the arm is resting at the patient's side.

Forearm Crutches (Lofstrands)

Forearm crutches or Lofstrands are often used for patients who will need the assistive devices on a more permanent basis (Figure 10-18). It is not uncommon to see patients who have neurological disorders use one or two

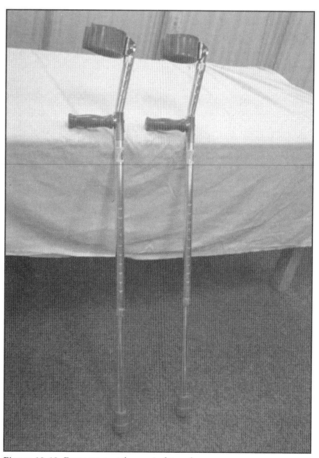

Figure 10-18. Forearm crutches or Lofstrands.

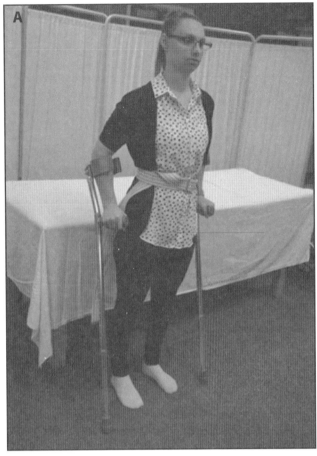

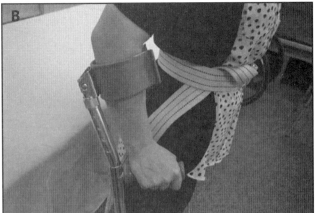

Figure 10-19. Fitting Lofstrands (leg and cuff).

Lofstrand crutches. Like axillary crutches, Lofstrands can be wooden or aluminum. They offer some lateral support, but not as much as axillary crutches. Because Lofstrand crutches do not come up as high, the risk for injuring the axillary blood vessels and nerves is eliminated, but so is the additional balance that axillary crutches afford. Lofstrands also have forearm cuffs which allow the patient to let go of the crutch to perform a task without the risk of dropping the crutch to the floor; however, these cuffs can be difficult to remove. Lofstrands are less restrictive than axillary crutches, but they also require even more balance and strength to manipulate them. Unlike axillary crutches, Lofstrands are not functional for patients who are NWB or PWB.

Fit

Lofstrands are ideally measured with the patient standing. The cuff should be 1 to 1.5 inches distal to the olecranon process, and the hand piece should come to the patient's wrist crease or greater trochanter. If necessary, you can attempt an initial fit for the patient in supine, but final fit will need to be assessed in standing. Figure 10-19 shows how to fit Lofstrands to your patient.

Canes

Canes come in many forms so that they can accommodate a patient's needs. Again, canes can be aluminum or wooden, and they are adjustable. The handles can be curved, a *T*-shape, or a pistol grip. Some canes can collapse so that they can more easily fit in a car. Canes can have one or multiple points, depending on the patient's balance. A cane is the least restrictive device (and least costly), meaning that it is lightweight and easy to transport, especially in small spaces or on stairs; however, it also requires the most balance and strength from the patient due to its unilateral use and narrow BOS. Canes are not appropriate for patients who are NWB or PWB. Additionally, some canes cannot stand on their own, so like axillary crutches, the patient must be sure to not drop the cane lest the patient risk falling.

Single-Point Cane

An SPC is exactly as it sounds; it has one point in contact with the ground (Figure 10-20). The patient uses it for incidental balance needs, but it is not appropriate for patients who need more support than that.

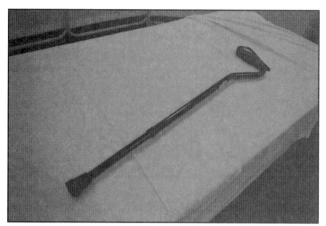

Figure 10-20. An SPC.

Quad Cane

A quad cane, so called because it has 4 points in contact with the ground, offers a slightly wider BOS than an SPC. There are 2 typical varieties: the small-based quad cane and the wide-based quad cane. Both have 4 points; however, the base is smaller or wider, depending on the type. The wider the BOS, the more restrictive the cane becomes; however, the can is more supportive with a wider BOS.

There are canes with 3 points or canes with a solid wider base that can stand on their own, such as the Hurrycane (HurryWorks LLC). These offer the safety of a wider BOS and also allow the patient to stand the cane somewhere without the concern of the cane falling to the floor.[5] Figure 10-21 shows various types of quad canes.

Fit

Fitting a cane is somewhat dependent on the type of cane used. An SPC is measured with the patient standing, if possible. The handle should reach the patient's wrist crease or greater trochanter. Also, the curve of the handle should point backward when the patient is fit for and uses the device. No matter the cane type, it should always be used on the side opposite of the affected or weaker limb.

When fitting a quad cane, the handle should also point backward, and the handle should reach the wrist crease or greater trochanter. The base of the cane is more flared on one side and flatter on the other; the flat side should go against the body when fitting for and using a quad cane. Figure 10-22 shows how to fit a cane or quad cane to your patient.

Bariatric

Patients who weigh over 200 to 250 pounds (lbs) may need to use a bariatric assistive device. These devices are made of more heavy-duty materials, and the dimensions are wider and taller than those of typical assistive devices (Figure 10-23). These devices are costly, heavy, and more

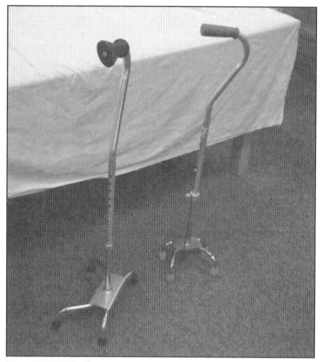

Figure 10-21. Quad canes.

difficult to transport or manipulate, especially the walkers. Bariatric devices can hold between 400 to 700 lbs, depending on the brand.

Pediatric

Pediatric patients need assistive devices that fit their needs and dimensions. Pediatric devices are smaller and more lightweight. Pediatric walkers are often the kind that pull behind the patient rather than requiring the patient to push from the front, which allows the patient more mobility and freedom. Pediatric walkers also usually have 2 or 4 caster wheels to ensure greater mobility.

Platform Attachments

Sometimes a patient lacks good hand grip strength, or placing weight on one or both forearms, wrists, or hands is contraindicated due to injury. In these cases, the patient may need a platform attachment to the assistive device being used. Platforms can be attached to walkers, axillary crutches, Lofstrands, and canes. They act as a shelf for the forearm, wrist, and hand. These are ideal for patients with weightbearing restrictions or strength problems, but platforms can be difficult to apply, and it becomes more difficult to transport the assistive device with platforms attached. A walker may not collapse as easily, may not fit as well in a car or trunk, or may be heavier to transport. Using an assistive device with platforms on stairs is also a challenge. Prolonged use of a platform attachment may also result in atrophy or weakness of the triceps or

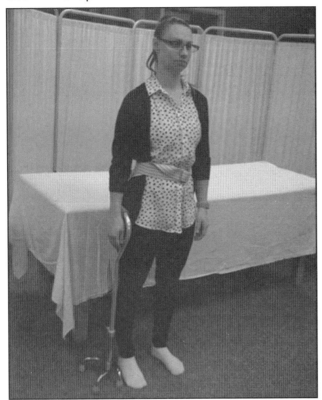

Figure 10-22. Fitting a cane.

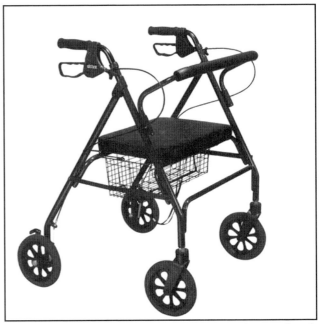

Figure 10-23. A Go-Lite bariatric steel rollator. (Reprinted with permission from Drive Medical.)

biceps muscles. Figure 10-24 shows a walker with a platform attachment, and Figure 10-25 shows a cane with a platform attachment. Table 10-1 lists the devices and how to confirm fit for each.

WEIGHTBEARING LEVELS

A patient may be limited on how much weight he or she can place on an extremity. The patient's weightbearing status is determined by the patient's physician, and it is based on what interventions the physician or surgeon performed on the patient. For example, a patient with a fractured femur will likely be NWB on that extremity for a certain period of time until the fracture heals. A patient's weightbearing status is important for a therapist to consider. It determines what assistive device the patient will need, and it affects the education provided to the patient to avoid disrupting the repairs made to the patient's extremity.

There was once a patient who was only allowed to put 50% of weightbearing on her left leg. However, every time she walked, she obviously put full weight on that extremity. The therapist attempted to educate the patient that she was not maintaining her weightbearing status, but the patient assured the therapist that of course she was following the restrictions. The therapist then applied a weightbearing monitor attached to the outside of the patient's shoe. The monitor served as a biofeedback system that sounded an

alarm whenever the patient put too much weight on the extremity. Sure enough, as the patient again ambulated with the monitor now attached, every time she stepped on the left leg the monitor beeped loudly. "Well what do you know?" the patient said. "I guess I *was* putting too much weight on that leg!"

Sometimes patients are unable to maintain their weightbearing status and often do not believe the therapist when they are told they are not following the rules. In these cases, a weightbearing monitor can be helpful. Examples of this include the PedAlert (Planet LLC) and the SmartStep, which sound an alarm or otherwise alert the patient if the weightbearing status is not being followed.[6,7] These biofeedback systems allow patients and therapists to better measure the patient's weightbearing during standing and ambulation. If this equipment is not available or the patient is still unable to maintain the proper weightbearing status, the physical therapist assistant should converse with the physical therapist and possibly the surgeon. Often the therapist will encourage the patient to ambulate as if NWB in order to avoid disrupting the healing process.

Note that the following abbreviations, although common, may not reflect the abbreviations used in your specific clinical setting.

Full Weightbearing

Full weightbearing (FWB) indicates that the patient is able to put the full amount of weight on the extremity in question. There are no restrictions for this patient. Additionally, this patient can use any assistive device that meets his or her mobility needs.

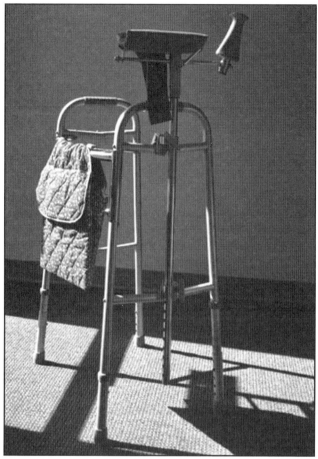

Figure 10-24. A walker with a platform.

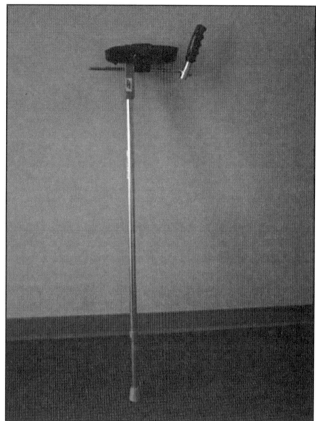

Figure 10-25. A cane with a platform.

Table 10-1	
How to Confirm the Fit of Assistive Devices	
Walkers	Position the walker so the patient is standing inside.
	The handgrip should come to the greater trochanter or wrist crease.
	When the patient grasps the handgrips, elbow flexion should be 20 to 30 degrees.
Axillary crutches	Position the tips 2 inches lateral and 4 to 6 inches anterior to toe of shoes.
	The handgrips should come to the greater trochanter or wrist crease.
	When the patient grasps the handgrips, the wrists should be straight and elbow flexion should be 20 to 30 degrees.
	There should be about 2 inches between the axilla and the top of the axillary rest (2 to 3 fingers).
Forearm crutches (Lofstrands)	Position the tips 2 inches lateral and 4 to 6 inches anterior to toe of shoes; the arms should be in the cuffs.
	When the patient grasps the handgrips, elbow flexion should be 20 to 30 degrees.
	The cuff should be 1 to 1.5 inches below the olecranon process.
Canes	With the patient in a standing or supine position, the handgrip should come to the greater trochanter or wrist crease.
	When the patient grasps the handgrip, elbow flexion should be 20 to 30 degrees.

Table 10-2
Weightbearing Restrictions and Definitions

Full weightbearing	The patient is allowed to place full weight through the extremity and is not limited by pain.
Weightbearing as tolerated	The patient is allowed to put as much weight as possible through the extremity and is only limited by his or her pain tolerance.
Partial weightbearing	The patient is allowed to bear some weight on the extremity, but the amount is often dictated by the physician.
Toe-touch/touch-down weightbearing	The patient is allowed to only put weight through the tippy toes, sometimes limited to 10% of weight or less, to maintain balance only.
Nonweightbearing	The patient is not allowed (generally due to physician orders) to bear any weight on the extremity.

Weightbearing As Tolerated

Weightbearing as tolerated (WBAT) indicates that the surgeon or physician has not limited the patient's weightbearing due to medical reasons. The patient, however, may be suffering pain or discomfort with FWB and may self-limit how much weight is put on the extremity. The patient should be encouraged to place as much weight as possible on the extremity, but it may be a gradual process. Patients who are WBAT can use any of the listed assistive devices; the only restriction is the patient's pain and mobility.

Partial Weightbearing

Partial weightbearing indicates that the patient can only put a certain amount of weight on the extremity. This is where the physician or surgeon steps in, dictating what that weightbearing percentage should be. The physician will also determine how long the patient must maintain that status before progressing. Patients who are PWB will not be able to use canes, hemi-walkers, or Lofstrands because these devices will not allow the patient to maintain his or her weightbearing status.

Toe-Touch/Touch-Down Weightbearing

Toe-touch weightbearing (TTWB) or touch-down weightbearing (TDWB) means that the patient can literally only place the tip of the toes or the heel on the ground. This is not so much to bear weight on the limb as it is to offer incidental balance correction. Some physicians indicate that TTWB or TDWB is a 10% or less weight bearing status. This is not a functional weight bearing status for long term, but again, it is based on the physician orders. Patients who are TTWB/TDWB cannot use canes, hemi-walkers, or Lofstrands because these devices will not offer enough support for the patient.

Nonweightbearing

Nonweightbearing is designated for patients who are not allowed to place any weight whatsoever on the extremity in question. Again, the physician determines this status. Patients who are NWB cannot use canes, hemi-walkers, or Lofstrands because these devices are unable to support the patient sufficiently. Table 10-2 lists the various weightbearing restrictions.

ASSIST LEVELS

In Chapter 9, the various levels of assist were described. Refer to Table 9-1 for a refresher on those levels of assist, as they once again apply to gait training. You should consider what the patient can do, and not how much work you have to do, to complete the task. Remember too that if the patient requires contact guard assist (CGA) or more assist, you should have a hand on the patient at all times to maintain safety.

USE OF ASSISTIVE DEVICES WITH TRANSFERS

Although transfers were discussed in detail in Chapter 9, it is worth revisiting the topic because assistive devices often play a role in safe and functional transfers.

When a patient stands from a chair or bed and is using axillary crutches, the patient should hold both crutches in one hand (Figure 10-26). If the patient has one upper extremity stronger than the other, he or she should hold the crutches in that hand. The patient can use the empty hand to push from the surface to stand. Once standing, the patient should move one crutch over and then progress with the transfer (or ambulation). The reverse is true if the patient sits; the patient will back up to the surface, and once

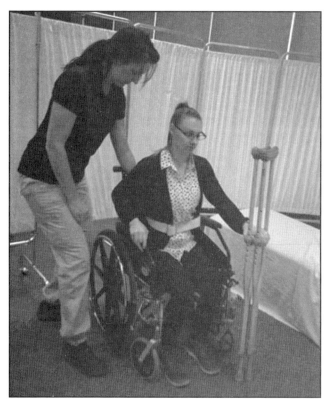

Figure 10-26. Standing/sitting with crutches.

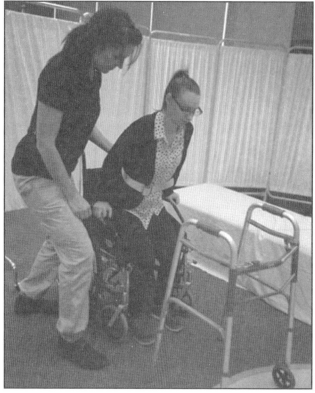

Figure 10-27. Standing/sitting with a walker.

close enough to sit, the patient will move one crutch over so that one hand is holding both crutches, and the other hand reaches back and assists with lowering safely to the surface.

If the patient uses a walker, the tendency for some patients is to reach for and pull on the walker to stand or to keep hands on the walker to sit, but these are not safe practices. The patient should be cued to push from the chair or bed, come to a standing position, and then put hands on the walker. The same applies for sitting; the patient should reach back for the transfer surface rather than keep his or her hands on the walker. If the patient is unable to do this, the walker should be removed from the patient's reach before he or she sits or stands (Figure 10-27).

For other assistive devices, such as an SPC, the cane can simply be propped within reach and used once the patient is standing. Quad canes and hemi-walkers can stand to the side, but these should only be used once the patient is standing. Lofstrands, like axillary crutches, can be held in one hand while standing or sitting (Figure 10-28).

GAIT

Gait is a person's manner of walking, stepping, or running. When a person who is healthy and without restrictions walks, the body is working at its most efficient level. However, once a person acquires an injury or adopts poor posture, the entire gait pattern can change and the body becomes less efficient. Injury begets injury, and the process can become a cyclical problem until corrections are made.

Gait Cycle and Muscles

Just as it will become impossible to ignore a person using an assistive device incorrectly, it is impossible to ignore a person's gait pattern, especially an abnormal pattern once you learn what is normal.

Gait (or a gait cycle or stride) is defined as the moment from initial contact (heel strike) of one lower extremity to the initial contact (heel strike) of the same lower extremity.

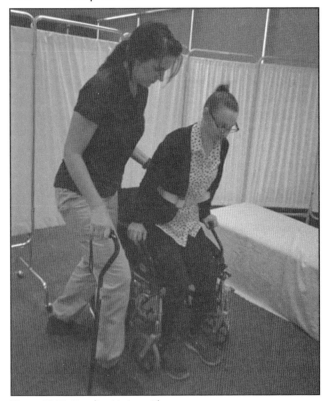

Figure 10-28. Standing/sitting with a cane.

It is divided into stance and swing phases. The stance phase is when one lower extremity is in contact with the floor; swing phase is when the lower extremity is not in contact with the floor. While one lower extremity is in the stance phase, the other is in the swing phase; this is why it is important for you to document which lower extremity you are referencing when talking about stance or swing phase. Stance phase composes approximately 60% of the gait cycle, while swing phase composes approximately 40% of the cycle. The brief period when both lower extremities are in contact with the ground is called *double support*.

In addition to the gait cycle, a therapist can talk about a patient's stride length, which is the distance of the gait cycle, or a patient's step length, which is the distance between the initial contact (heel strike) of one lower extremity and the initial contact (heel strike) of the other lower extremity. The faster a person walks, the less double support the person has. When a person is running, he or she may even have a moment of nonsupport, when no lower extremity is in contact with the ground.

The stance phase is divided further into subphases. This book uses both the traditional terms (found in parentheses)

as well as the newer Ranchos Los Amigos labeling. You should be familiar with both because you will likely see both depending on the clinical setting. The subphases of the stance phase include initial contact (heel strike), loading response, midstance (midswing), terminal stance (heel off), and preswing (toe off). The subphases of the swing phase include initial swing (acceleration), midswing, and terminal swing (deceleration).

There are many ways to assess a patient's gait, including analysis of each of these subphases. You can measure the time it takes for a patient to perform a stride or a step, or you can measure the distance of strides and steps. The University of Oklahoma Health Sciences Center determined that the average stride length is approximately 62 inches for men and 52 inches for women.[8] You can also measure the width of a patient's step laterally; a 2- to 4-inch distance is considered a normal width for the lower extremities.

It is important to consider what muscles are used during the different phases of gait; this will better assist the therapist in knowing what is weak or tight, and therefore what needs to be strengthened or stretched to improve gait. For example, a patient with weak dorsiflexors will be unable to fully clear his or her foot from the floor. Weak hamstrings could yield knee hyperextension during the stance phase of gait. Table 10-3 includes a list of muscles used during each phase.

More information about the gait cycle can be found in textbooks specific to the topic. Additionally, more information can be found regarding abnormal gait patterns, such as ataxic, antalgic, Parkinson's, and Trendelenburg. Table 10-4 includes a table with some common gait deviations, their causes, and their presentations.

Gait Patterns

When educating your patients on how to use their assistive devices, you will need to know and understand the various gait patterns and when they are appropriate to use. Each pattern lends itself to certain assistive devices or weightbearing statuses, so you need to keep this information in mind also when prescribing a pattern for your patient. As with selecting assistive devices, your goal as a patient's therapist is to select the appropriate pattern for the patient's needs. You should also always consider if and when it is appropriate to advance the patient to a less restrictive and more functional gait pattern as the patient heals and progresses with therapy. Figure 10-29 depicts each gait pattern.

Table 10-3

Muscles Used in Stance and Swing Phases

	Gluteus Maximus	Gluteus Medius/ Minimus	Hip Flexors/ Adductors	Quadriceps	Hamstrings	Tibialis Anterior/ Peroneals	Gastrocnemius	Erector Spinae
Initial Contact	✓				✓	✓		✓
Loading Response	✓			✓		✓		✓
Midstance	✓					✓	✓	✓
Terminal Stance		✓					✓	✓
Preswing		✓	✓			✓	✓	✓
Initial Swing			✓			✓		✓
Midswing			✓		✓	✓		✓
Terminal Swing					✓	✓		✓

Table 10-4

Gait Deviations, Causes, and Presentation

Deviations	Causes	Presentation
Trendelenburg Gait	Weak gluteus medius/minimus	Hip drop on side opposite of weak muscle during swing
Genu Recurvatum	Weak hamstrings	Hyperextension of the knee during stance phase
Foot Slap/Foot Drop	Foot slap: poor or no eccentric control of dorsiflexion during heel strike	Foot slaps on ground due to weakness at heel strike
	Foot drop: no neurological control of dorsiflexion	Foot hangs during swing phase and ball of foot hits first (vs heel)
Circumduction	Knee fusion or prosthetic limb that does not fit	Lower extremity circles around to accommodate for lack of clearance during swing phase
Ataxic Gait	Lack of coordination; cerebellum affected	Wide BOS, abducted lower extremities, jerky, uncoordinated movements, staggering
Antalgic Gait (Sore Foot Limp)	Pain in lower extremity	Shorten stance phase on affected limb; shortened step length on uninvolved side, decreased arm swing
Parkinsonian Gait	Parkinson's or other neurological disease that presents as such	Shuffling gait, festination, forward head, rounded shoulders, decreased arm swing, decreased/no heel strike, decreased trunk rotation
Hemiplegic Gait	Cerebral palsy or CVA	Affected lower extremity internally rotated, ankle plantar flexion, walk on inside and ball of foot, decreased arm swing, possible circumduction on affected lower extremity

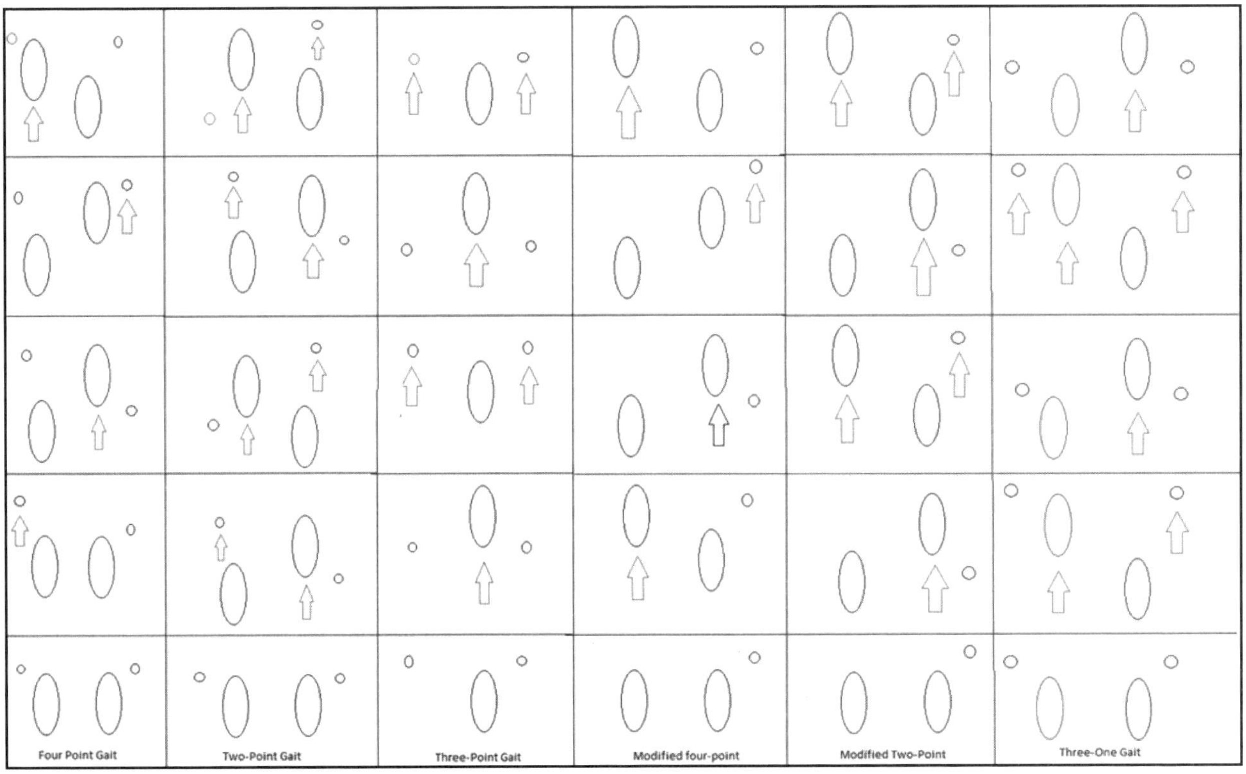

Figure 10-29. Diagram of all the gait patterns.

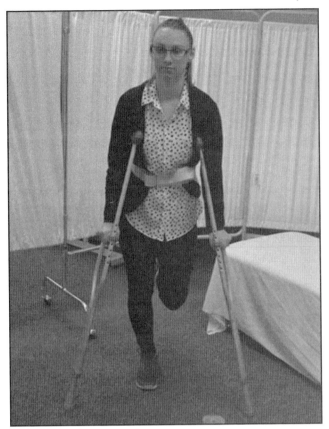

Figure 10-30. Three-point gait pattern.

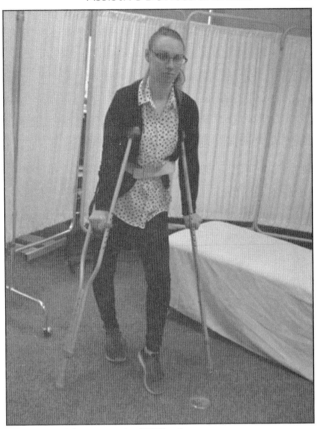

Figure 10-31. Three-one point (PWB) gait pattern.

Three-Point Gait Pattern

A 3-point gait pattern (Figure 10-30) is used for patients who are NWB or who have had a lower extremity amputated and do not have a prosthetic. The best assistive devices for this pattern are axillary crutches or a walker. These are the only devices that will allow a patient to ambulate safely with one lower extremity.

In a 3-point gait pattern, the patient advances the assistive device (crutches or walker) first, and then the patient steps to or through with the intact lower extremity. Step to means the patient only swings the lower extremity to the point where the crutches or the walker tips are located on the ground; Step through means the intact lower extremity advances a bit beyond the tips of the assistive device. Stepping through when NWB may prove dangerous, so a step-to method is usually encouraged.

A 3-point gait pattern requires a great deal of strength and balance on the patient's part because it is more difficult to ambulate with one lower extremity. The patient will need enough upper extremity and shoulder strength to hold him- or herself up with the crutches or walker.

Three-One Point and Modified Three-Point Gait Pattern

A 3-1 point gait pattern (Figure 10-31) assumes the patient is PWB or TDWB/TTWB as prescribed by the physician. The patient will have a specific percentage of weight allowed on that lower extremity. Sometimes this pattern is also used for a patient who has pain in a lower extremity, even without a specific PWB prescription from the doctor. If the patient has pain, he or she can still only want to put partial weight on the extremity (also known as WBAT). As with the NWB patient, patients using a 3-1 point gait pattern should use either a walker or axillary crutches.

In a 3-1 point gait pattern, the patient advances the assistive device first. Then the painful or PWB extremity is advanced, with only the prescribed or tolerated amount of weight placed on that extremity. The patient will then quickly advance the intact lower extremity. Alternatively, the patient can advance the assistive device and the PWB limb at the same time and then quickly advance the intact limb.

This pattern is a bit more stable than the 3-point gait pattern, but it still requires a fair amount of strength and balance to sustain.

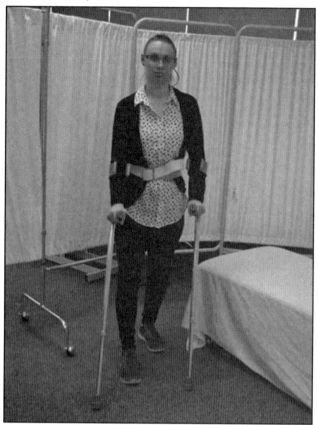

Figure 10-32. Four-point gait pattern.

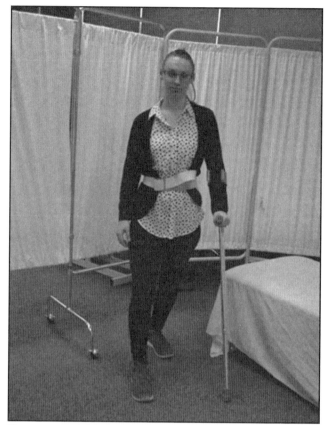

Figure 10-33. Modified 4-point gait pattern.

Four-Point and Modified Four-Point Gait Pattern

A 4-point gait pattern (Figure 10-32) attempts to be like normal gait, but it is broken down into individual movements. The patient is WBAT to FWB, and the patient must use a bilateral device: 2 axillary/Lofstrand crutches or 2 canes (although it is generally not advised to use 2 canes). The patient first advances one assistive device, then advances the opposite lower extremity (not simultaneously). Then the other assistive device is advanced, and then the opposite extremity (again, one at a time). This gait pattern is very stable but quite slow. It is helpful because it resembles normal gait with reciprocal arm movement. The patient may be able to quickly advance to the more functional 2-point gait pattern.

The modified 4-point gait pattern (Figure 10-33) is similar to the 4-point gait pattern, except that the patient only uses one assistive device, such as one cane or one crutch. The cane or crutch goes on the opposite side of the injury (eg, if the patient was healing after a right tibia fracture, the cane or crutch would go on the patient's left side). Using the assistive device on the opposite side of the injury widens the patient's BOS and improves stability. The patient first advances the assistive device, then the affected lower extremity, followed by the intact lower extremity (all one at a time). This is a bit slower, but it is still very stable and still allows for reciprocal arm swing. The patient may quickly progress, however, to using the modified 2-point pattern.

Two-Point and Modified Two-Point Gait Pattern

A 2-point gait pattern (Figure 10-34) is used for patients who are WBAT to FWB. Patients using this gait pattern can use axillary crutches, Lofstrands, or bilateral canes. A 2-point gait pattern requires the use of bilateral assistive devices. The patient moves one assistive device and the opposite lower extremity simultaneously; then the patient moves the other assistive device and opposite lower extremity at the same time. This gait pattern best reflects normal gait with opposite, reciprocal arm swing. It is very stable and requires less strength and balance to sustain. However, the patient does need some coordination, but once the pattern is learned, the patient can move fairly quickly.

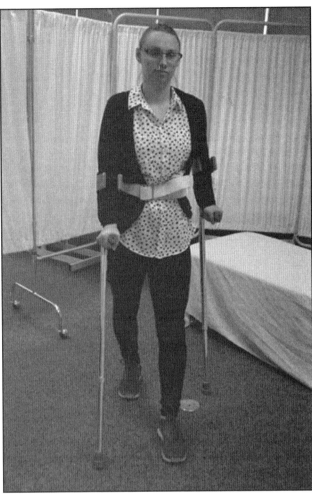

Figure 10-34. Two-point gait pattern.

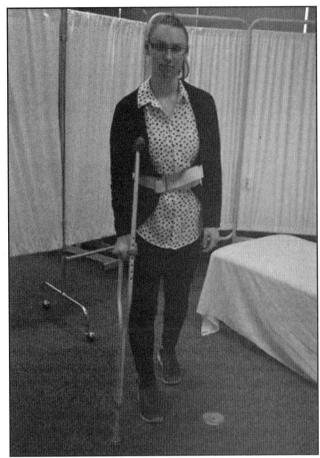

Figure 10-35. Modified 2-point gait pattern.

A modified 2-point gait pattern (Figure 10-35) also is for patients who are WBAT to FWB. The difference is that the modified 2-point gait pattern requires the use of only one assistive device: one axillary crutch, one Lofstrand, one hemi-walker, or one cane. The patient uses the assistive device on the opposite side of the injured or affected lower extremity. The patient simultaneously advances the assistive device and the opposite (affected) limb, followed by the intact limb. This is similar to the modified 4-point gait pattern, but it better reflects normal gait and arm swing. Table 10-5 provides descriptions of each gait pattern, and Table 10-6 lists the gait patterns, appropriate assistive devices for each pattern, and weightbearing statuses.

Curbs

Negotiating a curb with an assistive device depends on the device. In an ideal world there would be curb cutouts everywhere, but that just is not so. In these cases, you need to educate your patient on how to negotiate a curb safely.

When assisting your patient, it is best practice to position yourself behind the patient when he or she is ascending the curb and in front of the patient when he or she is descending. The therapist can also guard the patient by placing a hand over the shoulder girdle (either in front or from behind) to help correct minor losses of balance; the therapist should never grab the patient by the arm for fear of dislocating the shoulder. The patient should also always wear a gait belt with curb training, and you need to consider what level of assist the patient requires during your training sessions. If the patient is CGA or higher (meaning the patient requires hands-on assist or more), you should always have at least one hand on the patient at all times. Otherwise if the patient falls, you are potentially liable for that person's injury.

If the patient is using a walker to ascend a curb, the patient steps up close to the curb and then lifts and places the walker (all 4 tips) on the higher surface. The patient then steps closer, if needed, and first steps up with the stronger lower extremity followed by the weaker. The reverse happens in descending; the patient first advances the walker to the lower surface, and then the patient steps down with the weaker lower extremity, followed by the stronger (Figure 10-36A).

Table 10-5
Gait Pattern Descriptions

Three point	Nonweightbearing; assistive device advances simultaneously with NWB lower extremity and then unaffected lower extremity advances.
Three-one point (modified three point)	Partial weightbearing; assistive device advances, followed by PWB lower extremity (or can be done simultaneously); unaffected lower extremity advances next.
Four point	Full weightbearing or WBAT; assistive device and opposite lower extremity alternately advance.
Modified four point	Full weightbearing or WBAT; utilizes one assistive device; assistive device and opposite (affected) lower extremity alternately advance.
Two point	Full weightbearing or WBAT; assistive device and opposite lower extremity advance simultaneously.
Modified two point	Full weightbearing or WBAT; utilizes one assistive device; assistive device and opposite (affected) lower extremity advance simultaneously.

Table 10-6
Gait Patterns, Weightbearing Statuses, and Assistive Devices

Patterns	Weightbearing Statuses	Assistive Devices
Three Point	NWB	Walker, axillary crutches (bilateral)
Four Point, Two Point	WBAT, FWB	Axillary or forearm crutches (bilateral)
Three-One Point (Modified Three Point)	PWB	Walker, axillary crutches (bilateral)
Modified Four Point, Modified Two Point	FWB, WBAT	One crutch (axillary or forearm), one cane

If the patient is using axillary crutches and is NWB, the patient pushes on the crutches to lift the intact leg up, followed by bringing up the crutches. Going down, the patient lowers the crutches first and then steps down with the intact leg.

If the patient is using crutches but is PWB to FWB, the patient still pushes on the crutches and advances the stronger lower extremity. Then the weaker lower extremity follows along with the crutches. To go down, the patient will lower the crutches first, then step down with the weaker leg followed by the stronger. Sometimes the patient will lower the crutches and the affected limb simultaneously (Figure 10-36B).

If the patient is using a cane, the patient will advance with the stronger leg first, followed by the cane and the weaker leg. Going down, the affected leg and cane will descend first, followed by the intact leg.

Stairs

Negotiating stairs is similar to curbs except that the patient has more than one step to traverse. The same safety rules apply; the patient should wear a gait belt when stair training, and the therapist should have at least one hand on the patient if the patient is CGA or greater. The therapist still guards the patient from behind when the patient ascends or from the front when the patient descends, and the therapist can offer additional support at the shoulder girdle (either from behind or in front).

Additional education of the patient includes asking whether the patient has stairs at home, and if so, how many. It is also important to know if the patient has railings on the stairs and on which side they are located. If the patient has rails, stair training should also include the use of rails to mimic home life. The patient should practice with rails

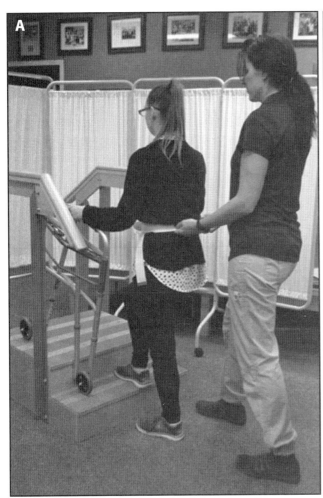 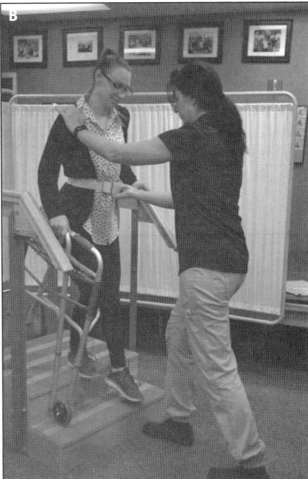

Figure 10-36. Ascending and descending stairs with a walker.

on both or one side, and on different sides, to plan for all situations. In a patient's home, the stairs up to the house may have a rail on the right side, but the stairs to the basement may only have a rail on the left side. In some cases, the patient's home, especially the outside steps, may have no rail. Training will need to accommodate that situation, and additional education can be offered in terms of whether the patient can have rails installed. Community organizations, churches, and fixed-rate handy-man companies can be options for rail installation, as rails (properly installed) will always be safer than an assistive device.

If the patient is using a walker, the best practice may be to have the patient collapse the walker and carry it up the stairs. The patient will have to advance the collapsed walker up a step ahead, either parallel to the step or perpendicular to it, but the patient should not rely on the walker for balance. The patient may be too weak to do this, and this method only works if the patient has a rail on one side of the stairs to use as support. Another method is to have the patient turn the walker sideways and advance

it up the stairs, but again, the patient needs to have a rail for this. Ascending stairs with an open walker presents its own concerns with tripping over the legs or otherwise losing one's balance, so this method is not recommended. Sometimes patients have two walkers, one for the top of the stairs and one for the bottom, to avoid having to carry their walkers up and down stairs frequently. Other patients have caregivers who can carry the walkers for them. You will need to speak with the patient about what help they have at home (if any), how many stairs they have, and where rails are located, and then use this information to determine your training sessions.

When ascending the stairs, the patient will step up with the intact lower extremity first. The affected limb will follow as the patient also advances the walker. It is not safe or recommended for a NWB patient to use a walker on stairs, as the weight bearing status cannot be maintained and the patient is likely to fall. To descend, the patient will step down with the affected limb while also lowering the walker to the next step, and then follow with the intact limb.

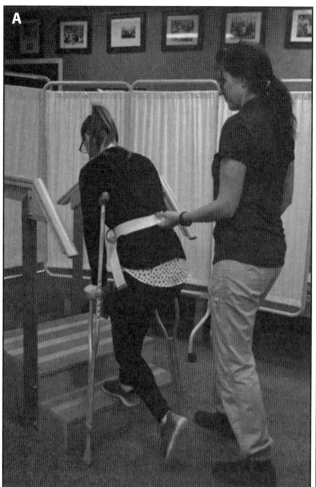
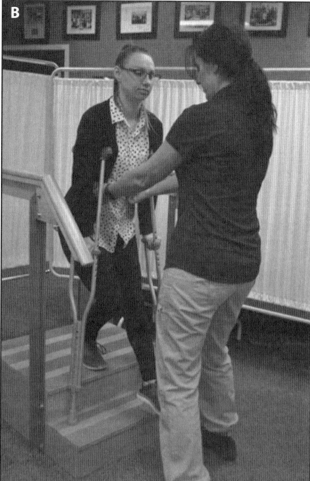

Figure 10-37. Ascending and descending stairs with crutches.

If the patient is using crutches, the procedure is the same as with curb negotiation. Be advised that NWB patients will need significant strength, endurance, and balance to negotiate a flight of stairs with axillary crutches. The same rules of going up with the unaffected leg and descending with the affected leg apply. If the patient has a rail, the patient can move both crutches under the axilla opposite the side of the rail. If the patient has a caregiver helping him or her, the caregiver can also hold one crutch while the patient uses one and the rail to negotiate the stairs.

If the patient is NWB while using crutches, you should educate the patient to keep the affected limb flexed and behind the patient when he or she is ascending the stairs and extended and in front of him or her when descending. This prevents the patient from having the limb catch on the stairs and trip him or her. Figure 10-37 shows ascending and descending stairs using crutches.

When using a cane, the patient will ascend and descend just as with a curb. If the patient has a rail, he or she can hold onto that with the other upper extremity. If the rail is on the side the patient typically uses the cane (eg, the patient has an affected left lower extremity, which means he or she uses the cane on the right side, but the rail is also on the right), the patient can switch the cane to the other side for stair negotiation only and use the rail and the cane.

In all of these cases, the methodology may need to be adjusted for each patient's individual needs or home setup. A patient's medical status, home situation, and other factors can significantly affect the stair training provided. There was once a patient who after surgery was prohibited from putting weight on her left lower extremity and was only TTWB on her right. Of course she had a full flight of stairs to navigate in the home. Another patient had bilateral amputations above the knee and had 6 stairs to enter the home and another 12 to get to his room upstairs. In these cases, physical therapists had to improvise, so patients could be functional in their homes while also being safe. Perhaps the education includes scooting up the stairs on the buttocks, or in some cases, the patient is educated to stay on the main floor until the weightbearing status changes. Box 10-1 provides instruction on negotiating stairs (and curbs) with various devices.

Floor Transfers

Floor transfers using assistive devices typically involves moving the device out of the way enough so the patient does not injure him- or herself. If the patient has crutches, the patient should move them so that both are in one hand while using the other upper extremity to lower him- or herself to the floor. If the patient is using a walker or cane, the patient likely will be safer not using the device to lower him- or herself to the floor. The patient and therapist should consider the patient's weightbearing status; if the patient is PWB the patient should be sure to bear the majority of the weight on the intact or unaffected limb.

If the patient is alone and starts to fall, he or she should be educated to move the assistive device(s) out of the way. Landing on crutches or a walker will not feel good. If the patient falls backward, he or she should be educated to flex the trunk and bring the chin to the chest to avoid a head injury. A forward fall should also indicate the patient first releasing the assistive device, and then using the upper extremities to break the fall. Falls can be practiced in the clinic, but the therapist should use a floor mat to avoid patient injury.

If the patient ends up on the floor accidently, he or she should be educated to first self-assess. Is anything broken or bleeding? If everything is okay and the patient is able to move, the following methods can be attempted to rise from the floor. If the patient cannot use the assistive device(s), the patient can always crawl over to a piece of furniture and pull up on it to at least get off the floor. If the patient determines he or she is too injured to get up, he or she should call for assistance. Therapists often educate their patients to keep their cell phones or cordless phones on them in case falls occur.

To rise, the patient again can hold the assistive device(s) in one hand while using the stronger upper extremity to push up from the floor. The patient can begin from side sitting or half kneeling, depending on strength and ability. Alternatively, the assistive device(s) can be within easy reach and utilized once the patient is more upright.

TESTS AND MEASURES

The gait cycle and normal vs abnormal gait were discussed earlier in this chapter. As you become a more seasoned practitioner, you will observe abnormal gait patterns on your own. However, for proper documentation, it is necessary to utilize gait assessment tools. These tools give patients scores based on performance, and they allow a therapist to determine what, if any, progress has been made over the course of a therapy intervention. During testing,

---

Box 10-1
Stair Negotiation

Canes

1. Ascend by advancing the unaffected lower extremity up first, followed by the cane and then the affected lower extremity; alternatively, the patient can advance the cane and the affected lower extremity simultaneously. The patient should use a rail if available.

2. Descend by advancing the cane and then the affected lower extremity (or both simultaneously), followed by the unaffected lower extremity. The patient should use a rail if available.

Crutches, Nonweightbearing

1. Ascend by bearing weight on the crutches and stepping up with the unaffected lower extremity. Then lift the crutches to the next step, with the affected (NWB) lower extremity flexed at the knee and behind so it will not catch on the step.

2. Descend by advancing the crutches down, followed by the unaffected lower extremity. Keep the affected lower extremity with the knee extended out in front to avoid catching on the step.

Crutches, Partial Weightbearing

1. Ascend by bearing weight on the crutches and partially on affected lower extremity and advancing the unaffected lower extremity up to the next step. Then advance the crutches and the affected lower extremity.

2. Descend by advancing the crutches down a step followed by the affected lower extremity (or both simultaneously), followed by the unaffected lower extremity.

---

therapists should attempt to not place their hands on the patient. The results of the test are invalidated if the therapist must assist the patient, so testing should stop if the therapist intervenes. These tests have been determined to be valid, meaning they measure what they intend to measure, and are reliable, meaning the assessments are consistent. A therapist should be able to administer the same test on the same patient at 2 different times and achieve roughly the same score. These tests help determine a patient's need for therapy as well as document his or her progress; both of these factors are taken into consideration by health care payer sources when they determine whether they will pay for a patient's therapy. There are many such tests, but this book will only focus on a few of the most common tests seen in the clinic.

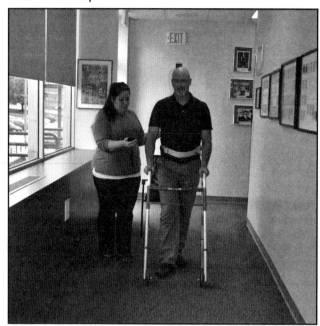

Figure 10-38. A patient performing the TUG.

Tinetti Test/Performance Oriented Mobility Assessment

The Tinetti test, sometimes known as the *Performance Oriented Mobility Assessment*, assesses patients' gait and motor function by using various everyday activities for the patient to perform.[9] The therapist then scores the patient on how well they are able to perform each task. The test is used often for patients who are weak or less functional, and it is often used for elderly patients. The patient can use an assistive device during the test, but points are deducted for using the device. Points are also deducted as the patient performs more poorly on the skills. The therapist needs an armless chair and room for gait. The patient is assessed on tasks such as sitting balance, sit to stand, turning 360 degrees, step length, foot clearance during gait, and gait path. The best score achievable is a 28 (the balance score is out of 16, and the gait score is out of 12).[9] A score of less than or equal to 18 indicates a high risk for falls.[9] A score of 19 to 23 is a moderate risk, and a score of greater than or equal to 24 is a low risk for falls.[9]

Timed Up and Go Test

The Timed Up and Go (TUG) test is used to assess a patient's mobility. Setup requires a stopwatch, a chair, and a marker for distance.[10] The therapist measures out 3 meters (approximately 10 feet) from a chair where the patient will sit. A patient can use an assistive device for this test without the score being affected. The therapist tells the patient, "when I say 'go,' stand up, walk to the marked location, turn around, return to the chair, and sit again." When the thera-

pist says "go," the timer starts, even if it takes the patient multiple attempts to stand. The therapist stops the timer once the patient returns to sitting in the chair. A time of greater than or equal to 12 seconds indicates the patient is at a higher risk for falls; a time of greater than 30 seconds indicates a very high risk for falls.[10] When observing the patient walk, you can also assess gait speed, balance, stride length, arm swing, or whether the patient uses his or her assistive device correctly. Figure 10-38 shows a patient performing the TUG.

Berg Balance Scale

The Berg Balance Scale assesses older patients' abilities to perform everyday tasks. Unlike the Tinetti test, the Berg Balance Scale does not allow the patient to use an assistive device. This means that patients participating in this test are generally a bit stronger and have better balance than those taking the Tinetti. The therapist must have a stopwatch, an armless and armed chair, a ruler, a footstool or step, and 15 feet to walk.[11] Like the Tinetti, points are deducted the more poorly the patient performs the skills. Patients are assessed on tasks such as sit to stand, standing balance, standing with eyes closed, picking up an object off the floor, alternately stepping on a footstool, turning 360 degrees, and standing on one leg, among others. The best score a patient can achieve is a 56.[11] A score of 0 to 20 indicates a high risk for falls; a 21 to 40 indicates a moderate risk; and a 41 to 56 indicates a low risk for falls.[11] An 8-point change in the score must occur to demonstrate a functional change or improvement for the patient.[11]

Dynamic Gait Index

Whereas the Berg Balance Scale assesses balance tasks in relatively stationary or static situations, the Dynamic Gait Index (DGI) assesses a patient's gait while performing dynamic tasks. The therapist needs to have a shoebox, 2 cones, 20 feet of walkway that is 15 feet wide, and stairs.[12] The patient can use an assistive device, but points are deducted if one is used. The patient is instructed to walk back and forth along the 20-foot walkway, but while doing so he or she must change gait speed, perform horizontal or vertical head turns, step over obstacles, and go up and down stairs. The best score is a 24, and if the patient receives less than or equal to a 19, the patient is at a higher risk for falls.[12] Anything higher than a 22 to 24 indicates the patient is relatively safe while ambulating.[12]

In some clinics you may run across another version of the DGI, called the *Functional Gait Assessment*. This test was fashioned after the DGI with the addition of 2 questions, and it was created to assess patients with vestibular problems.

SAFETY/RED FLAGS

As with transfers, there are several safety concerns or red flags you should be aware of to ensure the well-being of your patient when fitting for gait devices or performing gait training.

When measuring for fit of assistive devices, make sure your patient is safe when standing. Use a gait belt, or have the patient stand in the parallel bars. Have the patient sit when you are adjusting the device for height.

Improper fit of a device can cause pain, postural deviances, or injury. Make sure the assistive device fits the patient properly, and be sure to educate your patient in the use of the device to avoid injury.

Your patient should wear shoes, ideally, or at the least socks with nonslip tread on the soles. As with transfers, your patient should wear a gait belt during all gait training activities, no matter the patient's assist level. You should not grasp the patient's body in any way because you will likely injure the patient if the patient loses balance or falls.

Monitor your patient's vitals or any signs or symptoms of fatigue, dizziness, or loss of balance. As with transfers, patients who are diabetic may suffer from blood sugar drops, and those with blood pressure issues may have an orthostatic reaction to standing. Excessive activity or exercise may exacerbate heart or breathing conditions, so a patient may need more frequent rest breaks if heart rate increases beyond the expected norm or if breathing becomes too labored.

If the patient is connected to catheters, IVs, chest tubes, or other devices, you will need to determine how to handle these devices while performing gait training. At no time should machines or tubes become kinked, pulled, or removed in the process of gait training. Additionally, you may need to assist with carrying or handling this additional equipment while the patient walks. The more practice you have, the better you will become at this skill. You will see therapists hanging catheter bags from the walker or propping oxygen tanks on the IV pole. Your goal is to not disrupt the proper function of any of these items, but you also need to make sure they come along for the trip.

If the patient has a limitation on weightbearing, your responsibility is to ensure the patient maintains the proper status. That means the patient may need verbal as well as tactile cues, and if the patient is unable to maintain his or her weightbearing status, alternative activities may need to be performed. There are some tools to assist with maintaining weightbearing status, including boots that sense pressure and alert the patient if too much weight is being put on the limb.

You should be prepared for the possibility that your patient will lose his or her balance at some point during your session. That is why it is important to guard your

---

Box 10-2
Guarding Guidelines

- Consider patient's weight, height, and abilities, as well as your own.
- For sit to stand, position yourself to patient's weaker side and slightly behind patient.
- Use free hand on patient's shoulder.
- Hook hand under gait belt rather than over.
- During gait, position yourself to weaker side and slightly behind patient.
- If forward loss of balance occurs, pull patient back; if backward loss of balance occurs, push patient forward at pelvis and trunk; If loss of balance is to the side, either pull patient to you or use body to support patient.
- On stairs/curbs, position yourself behind when the patient is ascending and in front when the patient is descending with widened BOS and free hand on shoulder girdle.
- If loss of balance is unavoidable, use belt and your body to slow the descent.

---

patient during ambulation and stair activities. Consider the patient's weight and height, and acknowledge your own strength. Perhaps 2 persons are needed to guard the patient, depending on his or her abilities. When the patient goes from sitting to standing, it is best practice to stand on the side and slightly behind the patient on the weaker side. This is, of course, a different case than when the patient requires more assist and you must be positioned in front to facilitate the stand. When using the gait belt, hook your hand under it rather than over; this will better ensure that if the patient does fall, you do not lose your grip on the belt. Box 10-2 includes guidelines for guarding.

During gait, you can position your free hand over the patient's anterior shoulder to additionally assist with keeping the patient's balance. Be sure, however, to not pull too much at the shoulder or the gait belt; you still need to allow the patient to walk forward without feeling restricted. It is common for the therapist to position him- or herself to the side and slightly behind the patient, often on the patient's weaker side.

If the patient loses his or her balance forward, pull back on the gait belt, and use the other hand to pull the trunk up and back. If the patient loses balance backward, push forward at the pelvis and trunk. If the patient loses balance to the side away from you pull on the gait belt to bring him or her back toward your body, and if the loss of balance occurs toward you, use your body as a bolster (with a widened BOS).

The gait belt is meant to help a patient make minor adjustments if a small loss of balance occurs. However, if the patient truly loses his or her balance, your job is not to stop the fall. Rather, your goal is to slow down the descent. This may mean that you use the gait belt to pull the patient toward you and use your body as a means to slide the patient to the floor. Sometimes you can position the patient so he or she sits on your knee (while you have your legs anterior/posterior, with knees bent, and wide BOS) long enough for someone to help by getting a chair for the patient. More often, however, the patient will end up on the floor, but hopefully with less injury because you were able to slow down the fall.

As mentioned in the stair negotiation section, patients should wear gait belts during stair and curb training. You should position yourself behind the patient as they ascend the step or curb and in front of the patient as they descend the step or curb. You can use your free hand (the one not on the gait belt) to guard the patient at the shoulder girdle (either in front or behind) to control a minor loss of balance. You should straddle 2 steps (rather than have both feet parallel on one step below or behind the patient) to widen your BOS. Again, you may not be able to stop a fall; on stairs the patient may be able to sit down (either by you directing the patient backward or forward onto the step).

When preparing for ambulation with your patient, anticipate where you will go, and remove any obvious or especially challenging obstacles in order to have a safe and clear path (unless your goal is to have the patient work around obstacles).

DOCUMENTATION

When documenting assistive devices and gait, be sure to include the type of assistive device the patient uses, if you fit the patient for the device, the gait pattern you taught the patient to use with the device, the patient's weightbearing status, and the level of assist required. If stair training is performed, you must document the number of stairs, whether rails were used and on what side, the level of assist required, and the use of an assistive device if applicable.

S: Patient s/p Ⓡ CVA 3 weeks

O: Patient fitted for and educated on use of hemi-cane on Ⓡ. Patient used modified 4-point gait pattern with attempts to progress to modified 2-point, but patient had difficulty coordinating movements on this date. Patient educated on use of hemi-cane on stairs, as patient has 5 stairs to enter home and 12 stairs inside home to reach bedroom. Outside stairs have bilateral rails, but inside stairs have one rail on the right side ascending. Patient educated to use rails when possible and practiced stair negotiation with and without stairs. Patient's spouse will carry hemi-cane up stairs when patient is unable. Patient min Ⓐ on stairs with cues to advance Ⓛ foot up or down step. Tactile cues required 50% of the time for patient to shift weight when negotiating stairs.

S: Patient s/p Ⓛ femur fracture 2 weeks and is NWB on Ⓛ

O: Patient educated on use of axillary crutches to maintain NWB status. Patient educated on 3-point gait pattern; patient required verbal and tactile cues 80% of the time to maintain NWB status. Patient has no stairs to enter home but does have 12 stairs to basement. Stairs have one rail on Ⓛ side descending. Patient performed stair negotiation with use of crutches on Ⓡ and rail on Ⓛ, requiring mod Ⓐ to maintain balance. Patient had one LOB anteriorly during ascension of stairs requiring min A to correct. Patient educated to sit on stairs if feeling fatigued or LOB.

REVIEW QUESTIONS

1. Describe 2 pre-gait or developmental postures. What do these help patients strengthen or prepare for?
2. What are the parts of the stance phase? Swing phase?
3. Discuss the benefit of an SPC over crutches.
4. Your patient is seeing you after a bout of pneumonia. She is generally deconditioned and easily fatigued. She is 74 years old. What assistive device would you select for her? How would you fit it to her?
5. Your patient is PWB. What does this mean? What assistive devices are acceptable for him or her to use?
6. Describe how you would educate a patient to negotiate the stairs if he or she is PWB and using axillary crutches.
7. What gait/balance test is best for a patient with fair strength and balance, and who does not use an assistive device?
8. What are 5 safety concerns you should be aware of or follow when educating your patient on how to ambulate?

REFERENCES

1. Tilt table test. *American Heart Association.* http://www.heart.org/HEARTORG/Conditions/HeartAttack/DiagnosingaHeartAttack/Tilt-Table-Test_UCM_446441_Article.jsp#.WXjuIITyuUk. Updated July 31, 2015. Accessed September 12, 2018.
2. Mai Y, Lo W, Lin Q, et al. The effect of body weight supported treadmill training on gait recovery, proximal lower limb motor pattern, and balance in patients with subacute stroke. *BioMed Res Int.* 2015;2015:175719.
3. FreeStep SAS – supported ambulation system. *Biodex.* http://www.biodex.com/physical-medicine/products/supported-ambulation/freestep-sas. Accessed September 12, 2018.

4. SafeGait 360. *SafeGait*. http://safegait.com/360-balance-mobility-trainer/. Accessed November 7, 2018.

5. Hurrycane. *Hurrycane*. https://www.hurrycane.com/?AspxAutoDetectCookieSupport=1. Updated 2018. Accessed September 12, 2018.

6. PedAlert 100 and PedAlert 120 Operator's Manual. Planet LLC. *RehabMart*. http://www.rehabmart.com/pdfs/ped-alert_owners_manual.pdf. Published 1996. Accessed September 12, 2018.

7. Isakov E. Gait rehabilitation: a new biofeedback device for monitoring and enhancing weight-bearing over the affected lower limb. *Eura Medicophys*. 2007;43(1):21-26.

8. Thompson D. Stride analysis. *The University of Oklahoma Health Sciences Center*. https://ouhsc.edu/bserdac/dthompso/web/gait/knmatics/stride.htm. Updated April 24, 2002. Accessed November 7, 2018.

9. Tinetti ME, Williams TF, Mayewski R. Fall risk index for elderly patients based on number of chronic disabilities. *Am J Medicine*. 1986;80(3):429-434.

10. The Timed Up and Go (TUG) Test. *Centers for Disease Control and Prevention*. https://www.cdc.gov/steadi/pdf/TUG_Test-print.pdf. Published 2017. Accessed November 7, 2018.

11. Berg K, et al. Measuring balance in the elderly: validation of an instrument. *Can J Public Health*. 1992;83(supple 2):S7-S11.

12. Dynamic gait index. *Shirley Ryan Ability Lab*. https://www.sralab.org/rehabilitation-measures/dynamic-gait-index. Updated November 14, 2013. Accessed November 7, 2018.

Chapter 11

Activities of Daily Living

KEY TERMS Rehabilitation | Sign | Symptom

KEY ABBREVIATIONS ADL | BADL | FCE | IADL | MRADL

CHAPTER OBJECTIVES

1. Define and describe the different types of activities of daily living (ADL).
2. Describe examples of job related therapy interventions.
3. Understand the purpose of home assessments.
4. Be able to document a therapy intervention that includes ADL.

INTRODUCTION

In the world of physical therapy, clinicians often focus on helping a patient recover the ability to walk or to roll in bed. Physical Therapists think about gait patterns, assistive devices, and transfers. However, physical therapists need to consider the whole patient and that patient's needs, which includes more than the patient's ability to walk, push a wheelchair, or correctly use a cane.

For example, a patient with Parkinson's disease was on the inpatient rehabilitation floor to receive treatment after a fall. He was diagnosed with Parkinson's years ago, and although his symptoms had progressed slowly, he was now showing the classic signs of the disease: shuffling gait, forward head, flexed trunk, and decreased size of movements. The physical therapist had been working with him for some time on his gait, including taking bigger steps, stepping

on a rhythm or pattern, and controlling his difficulty with thresholds and visual distractions. His gait, bed mobility, and use of the Rollator walker were improving. However, he had another concern. He approached the physical therapist assistant with a question: how could he still be intimate with his wife despite his symptoms?

This was not so much an issue of muscle strength or range of motion (although these certainly factor into the question), but it was a functional task that he wanted and needed to perform as a part of his role in his marriage. The physical therapist assistant was surprised initially at the question, but she investigated and was able to return with information and reading material that could help him with his problem. The physical therapist assistant may also have considered either a referral to an occupational therapist, or, if the occupational therapist was already seeing the patient, alert the occupational therapist of this new concern.

Activities of daily living are the activities people may take for granted when they are healthy and functioning normally. This morning you woke up and brushed your teeth or ate your breakfast with no thought. You were able to put on your shoes and take a shower without difficulty. Patients who have had strokes, heart attacks, pneumonia, fractures, or who have progressive diseases like Parkinson's, however, are often unable to perform these basic tasks. The physical therapists' job is to treat the whole patient, and that includes ADL. Sometimes that means that the patient needs reeducation and practice, and although ADL training is not

Memolo J.
Procedures and Patient Care for the Physical Therapist Assistant
(pp 175-187). © 2019 SLACK Incorporated.

officially in the pysical therapist's scope of practice, physical therapists can often integrate physical therapy goals into ADL practice.

It is also worth noting that these situations offer ample opportunity for physical therapists and physical therapist assistants to work with occupational therapists and certified occupational therapy assistants. Interdisciplinary team meetings are fairly common in hospital, rehabilitation, and skilled nursing settings. A quick team meeting (including all the therapists/caregivers working with a specific patient) will allow the physical therapist assistant, for example, to communicate problems he or she observed with the patient regarding ADL practice. Even if the physical therapist assistant is not able to officially work on these skills with the patient, she can let the occupational therapist know that deficits exist and the patient needs assistance.

BASIC ACTIVITIES OF DAILY LIVING

Basic activities of daily living (BADL) include tasks familiar to physical therapist assistants. The list includes bed mobility, transfers, gait training, and wheelchair training; however, it also includes toileting, grooming, feeding, bathing, dressing, rest, and sleep.[1] Some clinicians include mobility-related activities of daily living (MRADL) into the instrumental activities of daily living (IADL) category, while others consider it a category of its own. Mobility-related activities of daily living include the BADL of grooming, dressing, toileting, feeding, and bathing, but consider the patients' restrictions resulting from mobility limitations (eg, wheelchair use or the use of assistive devices). Physical therapists assess whether the patient is unable to complete the MRADL, is at a heightened risk of morbidity or mortality in completing the MRADL, or is unable to complete the MRADL within a reasonable amount of time. While occupational therapists often take on the role as primary trainer in these latter tasks, including measuring patients for and assessing use and safety with wheelchairs, physical therapists and physical therapist assistants can also play a role. Physical therapists' and physical therapist assistants' scopes of practice include wheelchair measurements and assessments, as well as the selection, fitting, and training of assistive devices.

In the earlier example of the patient with Parkinson's disease inquiring about being intimate with his wife, one could categorize that as a BADL. Some people classify sex as the *forgotten ADL*, and it certainly is an aspect of a person's role in the home. The American Occupational Therapy Association states that sexuality is a "core characteristic" of being a human, and the *Occupational Therapy Practice Framework: Domain and Process* includes sexual activity as an ADL.[2]

As another example, nearly every time a certain physical therapist assistant entered a patient's room while working at a hospital, the patient in question needed to use the bathroom. The physical therapist assistant did not defer the task to the nursing staff because she was qualified to take the patient to the bathroom. The bonus was that the physical therapist assistant could work on the bed mobility, transfer, and gait or wheelchair training performed while getting the patient to the bathroom, all of which fall under the physical therapist assistant's scope of practice. Once in the bathroom, the patient often needed assistance with underwear or briefs and other articles of clothing. The patient sometimes was unable to stand from the toilet afterwards, or needed guarding and assistance while washing hands. While toileting or hygiene did not fall under the physical therapist assistant's scope of practice, she could still focus on and document the sit to stands or the static standing balance tasks, and at the same time she was helping the patient with these basic activities. The number of adaptive or assistive devices to assist with ADL is nearly endless, and occupational therapists and certified occupational therapy assistants are the best clinicians to match patients with the correct devices. Much thought about a patient's vision, cognition, strength, and duration of disability goes into assistive or adaptive device selection, especially because many of these items are not covered by insurance.[3]

Occupational therapists and certified occupational therapy assistants train specifically for this type of practice and education. They have learned adaptive techniques and have adaptive equipment to help patients with these tasks. For example, some patients have difficulty reaching over to put on socks. A handy sock aide allows the patient to pull the sock up and over the foot without bending. If a patient is unable to feed him- or herself because he or she cannot grip a fork, there are adaptive forks with widened and rubberized handles to allow the patient a better grip. There are reachers, plates, and adaptive steering wheels to allow patients with functional limitations to still perform daily activities and skills.

The goal, just as with gait training or bed mobility, is to teach the patient skills and have them practice said skills until they are proficient, with the hope and goal of the patient to become as independent as possible. This decreases the patient's burden of care for any caregiver and allows the patient the satisfaction of being independent in at least some areas of self-care.

INSTRUMENTAL ACTIVITIES OF DAILY LIVING

Instrumental activities of daily living include slightly more advanced skills from the basics of dressing, eating, and toileting. Some clinicians consider IADL as those that can be outsourced to others, and therefore are not as important as BADL. Instrumental activities of daily living include tasks such as cooking, completing household chores, driving, managing medications, managing finances, taking care of pets, caring for children, and skills generally considered a part of a person's role in the home and the community. For example, if a patient always picked up kids for carpooling to school, this would be considered an IADL. If a patient prided him- or herself on being the household chef, then the patient likely will want to return to cooking after his or her recovery.

In these examples and others, occupational therapists and certified occupational therapy assistants are often the default therapists to work with patients on these specific tasks. House cleaning tasks or pet care do not fall under a physical therapist's or physical therapist assistant's scope of practice. However, if the patient must be strong enough to lift the vacuum cleaner or the bag of pet food, physical therapists can work on strengthening, and if the patient needs good dynamic balance to bend over to pick up the dog dish or the trash, physical therapists can help the patient work on balance. If the patient needs to be able to transfer in and out of a car, physical therapists can help the patient work on that, and if the patient has questions or concerns regarding sexual activity or intimacy, perhaps the physical therapist can work with the patient on pelvic floor issues or patient positioning.

This is where physical therapists/physical therapist assistants and occupational therapists/certified occupational therapy assistants need to work together. Communication among the clinicians is key; if the occupational therapist determined that a patient needs to work on toileting, then what can the physical therapist assistant do to assist the patient in that task? If the patient has a goal that he or she will be able to walk 100 feet to the bus stop and catch the bus every day, what can the physical therapist assistant do to prepare the patient for this activity? When walking the patient to the kitchen to work on cooking tasks, an occupational therapist or certified occupational therapy assistant may observe that a patient has trouble with gait or his or her walker. The occupational therapist/certified occupational therapy assistant would then alert the physical therapist/physical therapist assistant that the patient is having trouble in this area. Communication between (and among) the disciplines is necessary for comprehensive patient care, and it is a 2-way street between the occupational and physical therapist. Occupational and physical therapy often work together in this way, and this greatly benefits the patient.

As mentioned before, one way that a patient can be assessed on performance of skills is via the Functional Independence Measure instrument. Physical therapy measurements include gait, transfers, and bed mobility (which fall under the category of ADL). Occupational therapists and certified occupational therapy assistants assess skills such as toileting, eating, grooming, dressing, and showering/bathing.[4] Physical therapists and physical therapist assistants sometimes do not score these areas because they may not feel comfortable making those assessments; however, the Functional Independence Measure instrument

Table 11-1
Examples of BADL and IADL

BADL	IADL
Walking	Managing finances
Feeding	Taking transportation
Dressing/grooming	Shopping and meal prep
Toileting	Housecleaning/home maintenance
Bathing	Communicating
Transferring	Managing medications

was created to be discipline-free, meaning any trained clinician can use it to measure disability.[5] If physical therapists and physical therapist assistants observe certain abilities or inabilities while working with the patient, they can communicate this information to the occupational therapists and certified occupational therapy assistants so the occupational therapist or certified occupational therapy assistant can assess the patient appropriately. Occupational therapists and certified occupational therapy assistants also use the Katz Index of Independence in Activities of Daily Living[6] and the Barthel Index of Activities of Daily Living[7] to assess patients' abilities; areas of assessment include continence of bowel/bladder, grooming, feeding, transferring, dressing, and bathing. Just like the aforementioned assessment tools that physical therapists and physical therapist assistants use for gait or balance (eg, the Berg Balance Scale or Dynamic Gait Index), these tools allow occupational therapists and certified occupational therapy assistants to assess ADL. This information can then be disseminated in the patient's chart as well as during interdisciplinary team meetings. Table 11-1 includes a list of BADL and IADL.

HOME ASSESSMENTS

The patient was ready to go home, or so he said. He had been on the rehabilitation unit for 6 weeks, and during that time, he had improved his gait, balance, and overall strength. The occupational therapist noted that the patient had improved in grooming and hygiene as well as dressing. However, before the staff could release him to go home, they had to perform a home assessment.

A home assessment is an opportunity for the therapy staff, often a physical therapist and occupational therapist or physical therapist assistant and certified occupational therapy assistant, to visit the patient's home with the patient prior to official discharge. It allows the therapy staff to see the patient's home and to observe any obstacles or challenges that may present themselves once the patient returns home.

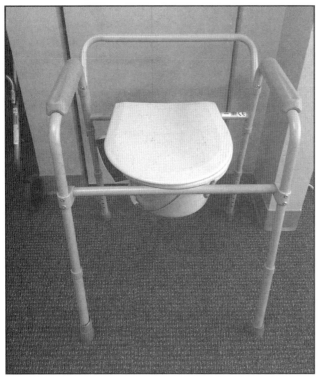

Figure 11-1. A portable commode.

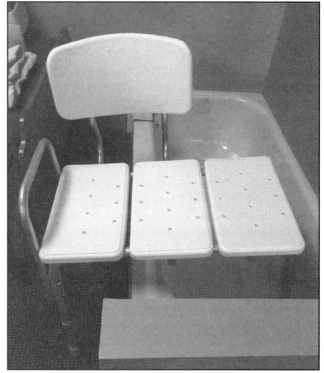

Figure 11-2. A bath chair.

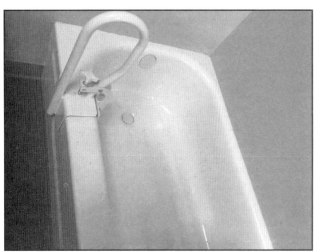

Figure 11-3. A grab bar.

Certain areas to consider are accessibility of the home. This will be covered in more detail in the last chapter regarding the Americans with Disabilities Act and accessibility, but it bears repeating. Per the Centers for Disease Control and Prevention, falls often result from home hazards such as broken or uneven steps, throw rugs, and clutter.[8] Falls cost over $31 billion (as of 2014), and they are the leading cause of fatal injury in older adults, so fall prevention is key.[9] As a result, the occupational therapist, certified occupational therapy assistant, physical therapist, or physical therapist assistant should ask questions and make observations that support fall prevention. Questions may include: Does the patient have stairs to enter? How many? Do the stairs have rails? Does the patient have stairs inside the home? Are the doorways wide enough to accommodate a wheelchair or walker? Other things to consider are floor rugs (tripping hazards); pets; furniture or the size of the area the patient can walk; and kitchen accessibility, such as the ability to reach items in the cabinets above or below. Bathrooms are assessed for safety; can the patient access the tub? Are there grab bars for the toilet or shower/tub? Does the patient need equipment, like a commode or shower chair, to be safe in the home? Refer to the appendix at the end of this chapter for a sample home assessment form. Figures 11-1, 11-2, and 11-3 show some home modification equipment such as a portable commode, a bath chair, and a grab bar that can be installed in a home to make it safer.

Sometimes therapists are not sure what they are getting into when they perform a home assessment. For example, there was once a home health physical therapist assistant who knocked on her patient's door. She had been warned by the supervising physical therapist that this patient was a hoarder. Sure enough, once inside the physical therapist assistant noted the narrow path, lined on either side with piles of clothes, old electronics and worst of all, dolls. Dolls were everywhere—even on shelves along the walls. The patient's home had paths all throughout the house; one led to the bathroom, another to the bedroom, another to the practically nonfunctioning kitchen. The path was narrow and not always clear; another complication was the small black cat that intermittently appeared and disappeared without warning.

When physical therapists, physical therapist assistants, occupational therapists, and certified occupational therapy assistants make these observations, they can then make recommendations to the patient or his or her caregiver(s) about any modifications or changes that should be made prior to the patient returning home. You would be surprised at how many patients balk at the idea of removing throw rugs or furniture. However, these things can present real safety hazards, and a bare floor is better than a patient ending up on the floor. The patient mentioned earlier was not willing to remove any of her clutter. Her son also tried to convince the patient to have a garage sale or donate to charity, but she would have none of it. Sometimes the therapist makes his or her recommendations and the patient does not follow them. However, you can at least document that you made the recommendations.

Some facilities have home assessment forms with check boxes or areas to write notes and comments. These can be filed in the patient's chart as evidence of the therapists' recommendations. Again, a patient may choose to go home or be at home without making any adjustments, but at least this way the therapy department has a record that recommendations were made. This could save you some hassle in the future if the patient suffers a fall or injury in the home.

Chapter 13 discusses the Americans with Disabilities Act and its role in accommodating people with disabilities in their community and work places. Home assessments are covered here again briefly, including what changes might be made to a home to make it safer for patients.

Chapter 10 also discussed balance and gait tests. These tests play an important role in home assessments because they point out areas of concern with a patient's functioning prior to being discharged. In the home setting, the physical therapist/occupational therapist and physical therapist assistant/certified occupational therapy assistant can consider the deficit notes in the Berg Balance Scale, Tinetti test, and Dynamic Gait Index and make recommendations based on those assessments. See the appendix at the end of this chapter for a sample home assessment form.

Job-Specific Work

One of the most common comments I hear from patients is "Occupational therapy? I'm retired; I don't need help with my job." The confusion is that occupational therapists and certified occupational therapy assistants only work with patients on job-related tasks; however, as discussed, a person's job may not just be something he or she gets paid for. A person's job also includes self-care and home and community roles.

That said, some patients do need to return to a job. If the patient is younger, the patient may need to return to a school environment.[10] Just as with ADL, the patient may face some challenges in navigating a school or work setting,

and both occupational and physical therapists can assist the patient in overcoming those challenges. Occupational therapy often works with the specific dynamics or requirements of returning to work. If the patient has a specific task to perform, such as typing on a computer or working a machine, the occupational therapist or certified occupational therapy assistant may work with the patient on this. Occupational therapists and certified occupational therapy assistants are specially trained to work with patients on skills like illness management, work conditioning, and environmental modification.[10] Physical therapy can, however, play a role in a patient returning to work or school. Again, physical therapists may work with the patient on aspects of strength, endurance, or balance. There was a patient who hoped to return to college, and so the physical therapist had her walk and walk and walk to improve her endurance in preparation for navigating a large college campus. Similarly, she also needed to be able to carry her books, and so strength was addressed. Another patient planned to return to her job as a waitress, which required walking short distances in the restaurant and standing for longer periods of time. She also had to be able to carry a tray with glasses and plates without dropping it. Together, she and the physical therapist worked on building up her standing endurance and gait to enhance her work performance while also practicing carrying a full tray to improve her balance.

Depending on a state's specific practice act, many physical therapist assistants can also participate in a Functional Capacity Evaluation (FCE). Per the Orthopaedic Section of the American Physical Therapy Association, an FCE is a series of tests that are used to determine a patient's ability for work, ADL, and other recreational activities.[11] The FCE was created to assist physicians, therapists, and patients in determining a patient's ability to return to work or what, if any, adaptive measures should be taken to allow a patient to return to work. It also allows for therapists to create rehabilitation plans to assist the patient in returning to work.

Functional Capacity Evaluations come in 2 forms: the General Purpose FCE, which applies to situations in which there is not a specific job or set of skills to target, and the Job-Specific FCE, which is designed to emphasize the skills and tasks specific to a particular job.[11]

Safety/Red Flags

One safety concern for patients when working on ADL is the use of a gait belt whenever the patient is being challenged physically. If the patient is working on endurance, strength, or balance, the patient needs a gait belt in case he or she loses balance.

Another concern includes the patient's physical ability to perform the tasks. Monitor the patient's vital signs during training to determine that the patient is able to tolerate the work involved. Some tasks may need frequent rest breaks, at least initially, in order for the patient to be safe. The patient may have orthostatic hypotension upon standing, or the patient may get shortness of breath with minimal activity. Your job is to monitor the patient to avoid these issues or to decrease exacerbation.

Some safety concerns are related to the tasks themselves. For example, if the patient plans to return to cooking once at home, the patient needs to be assessed for safety when using the oven or stove. Can he or she remember to turn off the stove or oven after cooking? Will he or she avoid touching the hot stovetop or accidentally leaving something flammable on the surface? Therapeutic education sometimes involves adaptation rather than full recovery; the patient may need to use a timer or a caregiver may need to monitor his or her cooking.

Home assessments are another safety concern. If the patient's home is not determined to be safe or appropriate for the patient, then changes or alternations can be recommended. Physical therapists cannot ultimately prevent a patient from going home against medical advice; however, if physical therapists educate their patients and strive to help them be as strong and prepared as they can be, physical therapists will have made a difference. The National Council on Aging also includes a list of evidence-based falls prevention programs, including Tai Chi, Fit & Strong!, and Stepping On.[12] Sometimes therapists make recommendations beyond the home and encourage patients to participate in these types of activities. These activities help with balance, and an added bonus is the patient gets an opportunity for socialization.

DOCUMENTATION

As mentioned earlier, a physical therapist's and physical therapist assistant's scope of practice does not include tasks such as toileting or hygiene. The scope of practice does, however, allow for sit to stands, gait, transfers, and balance. In your documentation, you will still note the tasks being performed, but your focus will be on the functional nature of your interventions and will always keep in mind the goals set by the supervising physical therapist in the plan of care.

S: Patient being seen for endurance and gait training after being hospitalized with pneumonia x 3 weeks.

O: Patient in bed when therapist arrived. Patient performed log roll to the right min Ⓐ with use of bed rail and supine to sit min Ⓐ. Lowered hospital bed and patient able to stand min Ⓐ with use of rail for support and gait belt. Patient ambulated in hospital room x 10 feet min Ⓐ and then reported need to urinate. Patient ambulated another 8 feet to bathroom and was unable to remove brief independently. Practiced static standing with one UE support on grab bar while therapist assisted with brief. Patient needed mod Ⓐ to stand from toilet but was able to pull up brief CGA after toileting. Patient was Ⓘ with hygiene. Patient

required min Ⓐ to stand statically at sink while washing hands. Patient then walked 14 feet in room to bedside chair, min Ⓐ.

REVIEW QUESTIONS

1. List 3 examples each of BADL and IADL.
2. Discuss what areas you may need to work on with a patient who plans to return to his or her job of teaching elementary school children.
3. What are 5 areas or things you should look for when performing a home assessment?
4. Your patient is in the hospital and you are treating her after back surgery. You are supposed to work on transfers, gait, and strength. Once the patient is up in bed, however, she verbalizes that she needs to use the bathroom. What ADL will she be working on in this process, and how can you still achieve the goals of your plan of care with this patient?
5. True or False: when your patient needs assistance getting dressed, you should get the occupational therapist because you cannot bill for this activity. Why is this true or false?
6. Your patient plans to return to work after having back surgery 4 weeks ago. What type of return-to-work assessment might you be able to perform (depending on the state practice act) and what does it assess?
7. What are MRADL and what role could you play in working on these?
8. List 3 safety concerns you should consider when working with patients related to ADL.

REFERENCES

1. Marger Picard M. Occupational therapy's role in sleep. *AOTA*. https://www.aota.org/About-Occupational-Therapy/Professionals/HW/Sleep.aspx. Updated 2017. Accessed September 12, 2018.
2. MacRae N. Sexuality and the role of occupational therapy. *AOTA*. https://www.aota.org/About-Occupational-Therapy/Professionals/RDP/Sexuality.aspx. Published 2013. Accessed September 12, 2018.
3. Medicare criteria for common equipment. *APA Medical Equipment*. http://apamedical.com/content/Medicare_criteria_for_common_equipment.pdf. Updated 2017. Accessed September 12, 2018.
4. Functional Independence Measure. *Shirley Ryan Ability Lab*. https://www.sralab.org/rehabilitation-measures/fimr-instrument-fim-fimr-trademark-uniform-data-system-fro-medical. Updated October 6, 2015. Accessed November 7, 2018.
5. IRF-PAI Training Manual. *Centers for Medicare & Medicaid Services*. https://www.cms.gov/Medicare/Medicare-Fee-for-Service-Payment/InpatientRehabFacPPS/downloads/irfpai-manualint.pdf. Revised January 16, 2002. Accessed September 12, 2018.

6. Shelkey M, Wallace M. Katz Index of Independence in Activities of Daily Living (ADL). *Try This: Best Practices in Nursing Care to Older Adults.* 2012;2:1-2.

7. Barthel activities of daily living (ADL) index. *Occas Pap R Coll Gen Pract.* 1993;(59):24.

8. Important facts about falls. *Centers for Disease Control and Prevention.* https://www.cdc.gov/homeandrecreationalsafety/falls/adultfalls.html. Updated February 10, 2017. Accessed September 12, 2018.

9. Falls prevention facts. *National Council on Aging.* https://www.ncoa.org/news/resources-for-reporters/get-the-facts/falls-prevention-facts/. Accessed September 12, 2018.

10. Dorsey J, Finch D, Ehrenfried H, Jaegers L. Work rehabilitation. *AOTA.* https://www.aota.org/about-occupational-therapy/professionals/wi/work-rehab.aspx. Updated 2017. Accessed September 12, 2018.

11. Occupational health physical therapy: evaluating functional capacity guidelines. *APTA Orthopaedic Section.* https://www.orthopt.org/uploads/content_files/OHSIG_Guidelines/OHSIG_guidelines_2/Occupational_Hlth_PT_Evaluating_Functional_Capacity_040610__2_.pdf. Published July 11, 2011. Accessed September 12, 2018.

12. Evidence-based falls prevention programs. *National Council on Aging.* https://www.ncoa.org/healthy-aging/falls-prevention/falls-prevention-programs-for-older-adults/. Accessed September 12, 2018.

APPENDIX

Home Assessment Form

General Information

Date _____

Patient name _____

Medical # _____

Persons present (including therapists) _____

Description of Home

Apartment	Floor level _____
Duplex	One level/upper level
Mobile Home	Singlewide/doublewide
Single Family Home	Split level/ranch/two story/three story

Parking

Type of Parking:

Private Driveway	Paved/grass/gravel
Garage	Attached/detached
	Manual door/automatic door
On-Street	Curb height
	Distance to primary entrance _____

Patient Vehicle:

Car	2-door/4-door
Van	Standard/modified
Truck	Running board/no running board
Other	

Mailbox

Location of mailbox _____

Is mailbox accessible to patient? Explain _____

Exterior Entrance

Most accessible entrance: Front/back/other

# of steps to enter _____

Railing? Yes/No

    Description of railing _____

Ramp present? Yes/No

    Appropriate slope? _____

Door width _____

Threshold height _____

Door handle: Knob/lever/other

Peephole present? Yes/No

Peephole accessible for patient? Yes/No

Lighting on steps and at doorway _____

Alternate exit information (steps, railing, lighting, door, etc) _____

_____

Living Area

Flooring: Plush carpet/short carpet/linoleum/hardwood/tile

Lighting _____

Adequate space for mobility between furniture? Yes/No

Where does patient typically sit? _____

Can patient sit/stand from furniture? Yes/No

Comments _____

_____

Bedroom Area

Door width _____

Flooring: Plush carpet/short carpet/linoleum/hardwood/tile

Lighting _____

Type of bed/mattress: Single/full/queen/king

Bed height _____

Is patient able to get into and out of bed? Yes/No

Does patient use bedside commode? Yes/No

What is closet/storage area like? _____

_____

Comments _____

_____

Bathroom

Door width _____

Flooring: Plush carpet/short carpet/linoleum/hardwood/tile

Lighting _____

Throw rugs? Yes/No Number _____

Are rugs a danger to patient? Yes/No

Space between fixtures:

      Tub/shower to Toilet _____

      Toilet to sink _____

      Sink to tub/shower _____

Is bathroom wheelchair accessible? Yes/No

Is bathroom walker/assistive device accessible? Yes/No

Toilet height _____

©SLACK Incorporated, 2019. Memolo, J. *Procedures and Patient Care for the Physical Therapist Assistant.* Thorofare, NJ: SLACK Incorporated; 2019.

Bathing:

    Tub   Height _____

                        R/L entrance _____

                        Faucet handle: Knob/lever

    Tub/shower   Height _____

                        R/L Entrance _____

                        Faucet handle: Knob/lever

                        Shower head: Wall mount/handheld

    Walk-in shower   Threshold height _____

                        Faucet handle: Knob/lever

                        Stall width _____

                        Stall depth _____

Sink:

    Pedestal/vanity/other

    Floor to sink height _____

    Sink depth _____

    Faucet handle: Knob/lever

    Storage above or below sink? _____

    Can the patient access the storage space? _____

What equipment, if any, does the patient have for the bathroom? _____

_____

Comments _____

_____

Kitchen

Entry width _____

©SLACK Incorporated, 2019. Memolo, J. *Procedures and Patient Care for the Physical Therapist Assistant*. Thorofare, NJ: SLACK Incorporated; 2019.

Flooring: Plush carpet/short carpet/linoleum/hardwood/tile

Are throw rugs present? Yes/No

Do they pose a danger to the patient? Yes/No

Lighting _____

Counter height _____

Stove/oven controls: Front/back

      Stove height _____

      Oven height _____

Can the patient access refrigerator? Yes/No

Sink faucet handles: Knob/lever/other

      Sink height _____

      Sink depth _____

      Does sink have cabinets below? Yes/No

Cabinet height

      Counter to first shelf _____

      Counter to second shelf _____

      Counter to third shelf _____

Is there a microwave? Yes/No

      Can the patient access the microwave? Yes/No

Comments _____

_____

Laundry

Will the patient be doing the laundry? Yes/No

Washer type _____

Dryer type _____

Comments _____

_____

Basement

Will the patient need to access the basement? Yes/No

How many stairs to the basement? _____

Rail present? Yes/No

Safety

Does the patient have a telephone? Yes/No

Are there working smoke detectors in the home? Yes/ No

Social Environment

List the other people living in the home or helping to care for the patient _____

_____

Barriers or Limitations

List all the architectural barriers, caregiver concerns, or patient safety concerns below:

_____
_____
_____
_____
_____
_____
_____

Recommendations

List all recommended modifications or equipment needs for the patient:

_____
_____
_____
_____
_____

Chapter 12

Emergencies

KEY TERMS Allergy | Anaphylaxis | Autonomic hyperreflexia (dysreflexia) | Contraindication | Indication | Orthostatic hypotension | Seizure | Shock | Syncope

KEY ABBREVIATIONS AED | CPR | SCI

CHAPTER OBJECTIVES

1. Identify the signs and symptoms of orthostatic hypotension, cardiac arrest, diabetes, and choking.
2. Understand the causes of autonomic hyperreflexia and how to treat or address it.
3. Understand when to modify or cease patient care interventions based on signs/symptoms noted.
4. Describe how one may prevent or avoid certain safety issues or injuries.
5. Understand when to administer cardiopulmonary resuscitation (CPR) per the American Heart Association recommendations.

INTRODUCTION

The patient sat comfortably in her chair while in the therapy gym and talked with the therapist, answering questions and making jokes. Suddenly, her words began to slur and she slid down in the chair; she lost consciousness. In that moment, the therapist first asked the patient's family members who were present to assist the patient to the floor safely. The therapist then pushed the staff emergency button. Within seconds, nursing and emergency staff rushed to the therapy gym and assisted the patient onto a gurney while monitoring the patient's vitals. The patient had suf-

fered a transient ischemic attack, which presents much like a stroke. The therapist's quick thinking and actions helped the patient receive rapid care, and the patient was back in therapy within 2 days.

In another example, there was a patient being seen by the home health physical therapist assistant. When the physical therapist assistant arrived, the patient was unable to answer the door, which was locked. The physical therapist assistant could hear the patient calling for help inside. The physical therapist assistant called 911, and the patient's door was opened to reveal she had fallen in her bathroom. She was weak but conscious, and the emergency medical technicians were able to transport the patient to the local hospital for assessment.

In home health, although this may happen in other settings too, patients may have medications prescribed by several different physicians, and each doctor may not carefully review or know about those medications. The physical therapist or physical therapist assistant is sometimes the one who, during a medication review, realizes that 2 or more medications interact with each other. Medication interactions can create emergency situations, so being vigilant with reviewing prescriptions with the patient is an important way you can help avoid a problem.

In some cases you will be in a hospital or clinical setting with emergency staff readily available. In other cases you may be the only primary caregiver present, and you will

189

Memolo J.
Procedures and Patient Care for the Physical Therapist Assistant
(pp 189-197). © 2019 SLACK Incorporated.

Box 12-1

Treatment of Allergic Reactions

Mild Reaction

1. Encourage the patient to be calm.
2. Identify the allergen, and remove the cause if able.
3. Apply a cool compress to patient's head or calamine lotion to relieve itch.
4. Observe the patient's vitals and reaction for worsening.
5. Obtain emergency services if needed.

Severe Reaction

1. Immediately contact emergency services.
2. Check the airway, and apply rescue breathing or CPR if necessary.
3. Assist the patient in ingesting or injecting emergency allergy medication.
4. Position the patient to prevent shock.

either need to call 911 or provide emergency treatment as you are able. Sometimes the patient or his or her caregiver is not sure how to handle an emergency situation. A home health physical therapist assistant made her semi-weekly visit to a 95-year-old woman who lived with her son. When she walked in the house, she discovered that the patient had fallen in the bathroom an hour earlier. She had broken her ankle in the process, but rather than calling 911 or transporting the patient to the hospital, the son chose to wait for the physical therapist assistant to arrive. Once the physical therapist assistant assessed the situation, she decided to call an ambulance because the patient could not safely be transferred to a car. In this and other cases, the patient and caregiver should be educated on how to handle anticipated emergency situations.

It is important to be able to recognize the signs and symptoms of common injuries and problems. Being able to recognize these signs and symptoms quickly will allow you to provide the correct emergency medical care or be able to know when or if you need to call emergency services.

SPECIFIC CONDITIONS

This list is not in any way comprehensive. A patient is never just the physical ailment for which you are seeing him or her; the patient is a culmination of his or her entire medical history, and no doubt he or she has other comorbidities. Rare is the patient who does not also have diabetes, high blood pressure, or respiratory problems. A good clinician keeps these things in mind when creating a plan for the patient, and the clinician should also monitor the patient's responses in order to prevent injury.

Allergies

Some of us may think of an allergy as relatively benign. I am allergic to cats; they make me sneeze, make my eyes itch, and sometimes I get wheezy. However, there is no risk of me dying from that allergy. Many allergies, however, are quite dangerous. People who have food allergies, such as to peanuts or strawberries, very well can die from their symptoms if not treated quickly. The best treatment in their cases is avoidance of the trigger. Other people have allergies to latex or certain antibiotics; while you are not prescribing medications, you may be the one to catch in a patient's chart an allergy that was not caught by a physician.

When a patient has an allergic reaction, his or her immune system is overreacting to a stimulus, called an *allergen*. The body releases histamine, and in extreme cases, anaphylaxis can result.[1] The initial reaction at first exposure may not be extreme, but repeated exposures can yield worsening symptoms. In the case of my cat allergy, the reaction may be sneezing or itching. For others, the symptoms can include difficulty breathing, a drop in blood pressure, or a loss of consciousness.[1]

If the patient is having a mild reaction, it is best to identify the allergen and remove it if possible; assist the patient in administering an antihistamine (eg, Benadryl [diphenhydramine]) or anti-itch cream (eg, calamine lotion); and observe the patient for any worsening signs or symptoms.[1] Anaphylaxis is a medical emergency. Immediately call a staff emergency or 911. If the patient is unable to breathe, rescue breathing should be initiated. If the patient has an emergency allergy medication, including an EpiPen (epinephrine), the patient should be encouraged to administer that drug immediately.[1] Even if signs and symptoms of the reaction dissipate with an EpiPen use, the patient should still go to the emergency room because symptoms may return. Box 12-1 includes instructions to treat mild and severe allergic reactions.[1]

Shock

A patient who has suffered a traumatic event or injury may go into shock. Shock is identified by a patient's pale, moist, and cool skin; shallow and irregular breathing; a rapid pulse; dilated pupils; sweating; nausea or dizziness; and syncope (fainting).[2] If you are able to determine and remove the cause of shock, do so. You need to monitor the patient's vital signs. If vitals indicate, call 911 or a staff emergency. The patient should be positioned in supine, ideally with the legs and feet elevated slightly. Of course, if you suspect the patient has a spinal cord injury (SCI), you should not reposition the patient in any way. Cover the patient with a blanket and do not let the patient eat or drink anything. Try to keep the patient still and quiet. If the patient is bleeding, apply pressure, and if the patient vomits, turn the patient to the side to prevent choking. Box 12-2 indicates the appropriate responses to treat shock.[2]

Lacerations

A laceration is a cut in a person's tissue. The biggest concern is blood loss, so the primary response should be to decrease the bleeding and prevent shock. To treat, you should ideally have clean hands and gloves. You may need to elevate the bleeding body part to decrease the swelling, and you should apply direct pressure to the wound. The patient should try to avoid using the extremity or body part in question. If the bleeding is excessive, you may need to call 911 or a staff emergency. You should follow infection control procedures while treating a laceration. Box 12-3 provides information on treating lacerations.

Choking

Treatment of choking is somewhat determined by the age of the patient and whether the patient is conscious or unconscious. The Heimlich maneuver is the most commonly used method to remove an object blocking the airway. The main goal is to open or maintain the patient's airway and normal breathing; in some cases the object cannot be removed, so rescue breathing may need to be performed.

If the patient is conscious and older than 1 year, first determine that the patient is unable to talk or breathe. If the patient is indeed choking, first call 911 or a staff emergency (or have someone else do so) in case the object cannot be dislodged. If the patient is still unable to breathe, administer 5 abdominal thrusts via the Heimlich maneuver.[3] Stand behind the person and wrap your arms around the abdomen. Make a fist with one hand and cover it with the other hand. Position your hands just above the patient's navel and make a quick, upward thrust. If the object is still not dislodged, repeat the Heimlich maneuver until either the object is dislodged or the patient loses consciousness (Figure 12-1).[3]

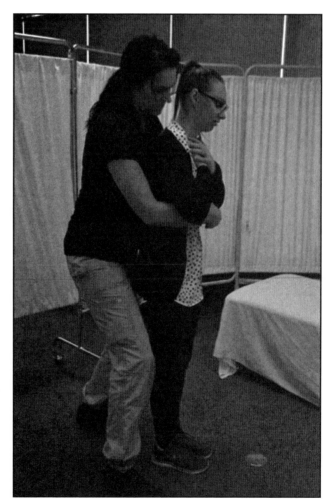

Figure 12-1. The Heimlich maneuver.

Box 12-4

Treatment of Autonomic Hyperreflexia (Dysreflexia)

1. Place the patient in a seated or semirecumbent position; do not place the patient in supine.
2. If able to identify and remove the noxious stimulus, do so.
3. Monitor the patient's vitals frequently.
4. Contact emergency services if necessary.

If the patient is unconscious, place the patient in supine, and if you see the object blocking the airway, remove it. A blind finger sweep is not recommended because it can push the item further into the airway. If the object remains lodged in place, tilt the head back and open the mouth; apply ventilation first. You can attempt abdominal thrusts with 2 hands, or, if necessary, perform chest compressions for CPR.[3] You would continue this until the object is dislodged and the patient is stable or until medical support arrives.

If the person choking is an infant (younger than 1 year old), turn the baby over and apply 5 back blows between the shoulder blades with the heel of your hand.[4] Then turn the baby over, and give 5 chest thrusts in the center of the infant's chest (below the nipple line). Continue this process of 5 back blows and 5 chest thrusts until the infant expels the object or the infant becomes unconscious.[4]

If the baby is unconscious, place the baby in supine. If you see the object blocking the airway, remove it. Otherwise, tilt the head back, and provide rescue breaths. Then apply 30 chest compressions using your first and second fingers in the center of the chest.[4] Look for the object again before resuming rescue breaths. Repeat until emergency help arrives.

The American Red Cross occasionally changes their recommendations, and you should be aware of any updates. As a part of your job, you will be required to obtain and maintain certification in Basic Life Support for Healthcare Providers, which will ensure you are up to date on the American Red Cross' recommendations.

Orthostatic Hypotension

Orthostatic hypotension, or postural hypotension, is a sudden drop in blood pressure as a result of postural changes.[5] When a person goes from lying down to sitting or from sitting to standing, the body may not be able to pump blood up toward the brain fast enough. The resulting symptoms are dizziness, nausea, blurry vision, or even syncope.

Sometimes this happens because a patient is dehydrated, and it is common in patients who have been supine or sitting for prolonged periods and who are not used to sitting up or standing. Other causes can include heart problems (eg, issues with valves), heart failure, or endocrine problems (eg, diabetes).

If a patient demonstrates the signs or symptoms of orthostatic hypotension, your job is to help prevent injury. If the symptoms are mild, the patient may be able to sit up or stand up for a few moments, and the blood pressure will right itself. However, if the patient complains of increasing dizziness, nausea, or starts to have vision changes, you may need to assist the patient back to sitting or supine. Sometimes wrapping the patient's lower extremities or applying an abdominal binder can keep blood moving upward toward the brain and minimize these symptoms. Patients who have severe issues with orthostatic hypotension may need to use a tilt table to acclimate to being upright.

Autonomic Hyperreflexia (Dysreflexia)

Autonomic hyperreflexia (also known as *dysreflexia*) is a life-threatening event that must be addressed as soon as symptoms are noted. It is affiliated with patients who have had SCIs, and it results from an imbalance in the body systems that control blood pressure.[6] A noxious stimulus causes the muscles around blood vessels to contract, which increases blood pressure.[6] A person with an SCI lacks the additional body systems that act as checks and balances on this reaction, so blood pressure can rise dangerously high.

Symptoms include raised blood pressure, headache, flushed face, sweating above the level of the SCI, nausea, slow pulse, goose bumps (piloerection) below the level of injury, and cold or clammy skin below the level of injury.[6]

The quickest way to resolve this issue is to remove the noxious stimulus. As the patient may not be able to actually feel the stimulus due to the SCI, your job is to act as a detective. Common causes include bladder issues, such as a urinary tract infection, a blocked catheter, or an overfilled catheter bag; bowel issues, such as constipation, hemorrhoids, or infection; an irritant below the level of injury (an object in a shoe, a cut, or an abrasion), pressure injuries, tight or restrictive clothing, or ingrown toenails; or issues such as menstrual cramps, labor, gastric ulcers, or fractures.[6] Physical therapists cannot address some of these issues; however, if you notice a kinked catheter tube or socks that are too tight, you can remedy that immediately. You should also monitor the patient's vital signs.

Whether you can remove the noxious stimulus or not, you should call 911 or a staff emergency. The patient will need to be monitored even after the episode has been resolved to ensure the patient is safe. Prevention is the best treatment; make sure the patient has frequent pressure relief, adheres to a bowel and bladder program, and maintains a good diet and fluid intake. Box 12-4 lists the appropriate responses for autonomic hyperreflexia.

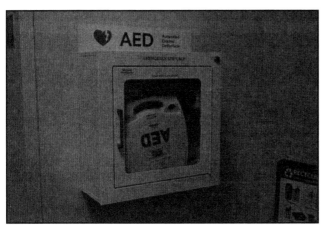

Figure 12-2. An AED.

Box 12-5
FAST Acronym

- F: Face. Ask the person to smile and observe if one side droops.

- A: Arms. Ask the person to raise both arms and observe if one arm drifts downward.

- S: Speech. Ask the person to repeat a simple phrase and observe if speech is slurred/strange.

- T: Time. If you observe any of these signs, call 911 immediately.

Cardiac Arrest

Cardiac arrest occurs when the heart abruptly stops functioning. The person experiencing this may or may not have a diagnosis of heart disease, and death can occur quickly if it is not addressed. Cardiac arrest is not the same as a heart attack; however, a heart attack can cause cardiac arrest.

Signs and symptoms include a sudden loss of responsiveness and abnormal or no breathing.[7] If the patient demonstrates these signs, first call 911 or ask someone else to do so. If the patient is not breathing or only gasping, administer CPR. Cardiopulmonary resuscitation requires that you push down at a rate of 100 to 120 compressions per minute in the center of the chest to a depth of approximately 2 inches, allowing the chest to recoil after each compression. The compression-ventilation ratio should be 30 to 2, and rescue breaths should be 1 breath every 6 seconds.[3] You may need to use an automated external defibrillator (AED) if one is accessible; follow the instructions the machine provides. The AED will assess the patient and determine if a shock is necessary (Figure 12-2). The American Heart Association asserts that hands only CPR can be just as effective as CPR with breathing.[8] As with choking, recommendations for CPR change occasionally; maintaining your certification in Basic Life Support for Healthcare Providers will ensure you are up to date on the most recent recommendations.

Stroke: Cerebrovascular Accident and Transient Ischemic Attack

If you think of a heart attack as a lack of blood flow to the heart, a stroke (cerebrovascular accident) is a brain attack that results from a lack of blood flow to the brain. This can come from an ischemic event, in which blood is restricted by a clot, or it can be a hemorrhagic event, in which blood hemorrhages into the brain. Either way, oxygen supply is depleted, and the longer oxygen is absent, the more brain cells die. As these brain cells die, so do their corresponding actions and memories suffer.

A transient ischemic attack is when blood flow is temporarily stopped from accessing a part of the brain. It mimics stroke symptoms, but those symptoms are also temporary, disappearing typically within 24 hours.

Signs and symptoms can be recalled using the FAST acronym (Box 12-5).[9] Does the person's face droop on one side? Does one arm not move the same as the other? Does the person's speech seem slurred or impaired? If so, time is of the essence, and you should call 911 immediately. The sooner the patient can be seen in the emergency department, the more likely he or she is to survive and recover.

Diabetes

Diabetes can come in a few different forms. Type 1 is diagnosed in children and young adults, whereas type 2 presents itself in adulthood. Patients who are pregnant can have gestational diabetes. When a patient has diabetes, his or her blood sugar must be monitored regularly. If a patient has too low or too high blood sugar, the patient can have symptoms that are dangerous. Therapists must be especially attentive to patients with diabetes because exercise can cause a drop in blood sugar. Patients who are hypoglycemic (ie, low blood sugar) may demonstrate fatigue, anxiety, sweating, hunger, irritability, and shakiness.[10] Worsening signs and symptoms include confusion, visual changes, and loss of consciousness.[10] Patients who are hyperglycemic (ie, high blood sugar) will show frequent urination, blurred vision, fatigue, and headache.[11] Worsening signs and symptoms include nausea, vomiting, shortness of breath, weakness, and coma.[11] If your patient shows signs or symptoms of low blood sugar, have the patient stop activity. If the patient can check his or her blood sugar, have him or her do so. If the readings are low, the patient should ingest some form of sugar. Juice or candy are quick routes to increase blood sugar readings. If the patient demonstrates severe signs or symptoms, alert the nursing staff so they may better assess and monitor the patient. The patient may need some education on how to maintain blood sugar at normal levels. If the patient shows signs or symptoms of

Box 12-6

Treatment of Burns

1. Remove the agent causing the burn if able.

2. Cut away or remove clothing from the area around the burn.

3. Remove jewelry if it will not cause injury to area.

4. Apply clean, sterile dressing or towel loosely over the wound; can be moist if more comfortable for the patient. Do not apply creams or ointments to the wound.

5. Use water to wash the wound if the burns are caused by chemicals, but take care to not wash the uninjured skin with the chemical.

6. Observe the respiratory rate, consciousness, etc; alert emergency services if the patient shows signs of shock or worsening of condition.

Box 12-7

Treatment of Seizures

1. Place the patient in safe position.

2. Do not attempt to restrain the patient.

3. Contact emergency services if warranted.

4. Monitor the respiratory rate and quality of the respirations.

5. Do not place anything in the patient's mouth, including fingers, wooden or metal objects, etc.

6. Turn the patient's head to one side after a seizure in case the patient vomits.

7. Allow the patient to rest; cover with a blanket for modesty and warmth.

8. If the cause of seizure is unknown, the patient will need to be evaluated by physician.

hyperglycemia, the patient will need emergency assistance. The patient may need an injection of insulin to restore normal blood sugar readings.

Burns

If a patient suffers a burn, your goal is to get the patient immediate medical attention and prevent shock in the meantime. Minor burns may not require emergency assistance; however, you should aid the patient in avoiding infection. If the burn is localized, hold the burn under cool (not cold) water for 10 to 15 minutes.[12] If blisters form, do not break them. An over the counter pain reliever may be all the patient needs for small burns. If the burn is from a chemical, follow the safety data sheets recommended procedures for cleaning the area. Clothing or jewelry may need to be removed from the burned area. You may also apply a clean dressing or towel (moist or dry) to the area. For small burns, it can be appropriate to apply aloe vera, but if the burn is extensive, avoid application of salves or ointments.[12] If the burn is significant, call 911. If the patient is not breathing, initiate CPR. Elevate the burned area(s) and stay with the patient until emergency assistance arrives. Box 12-6 denotes the treatment for burns.[12]

Seizures

A seizure is when the electrical activity in the brain surges or changes.[13] It affects how a person acts and can cause the person to become unconscious. Some patients know when a seizure is coming; they experience an aura or some other sign.[13] There was once a patient who sneezed 6 times before a seizure happened; he knew that if he sneezed 6 times, he needed to get on the floor because a seizure was coming. Some seizures are quiet and the patient may seem to stare off into space. The patient may lose awareness of what is happening or feel confused.[13] The patient may see flashing lights, be unable to hear, or have numbness

or tingling. The patient may have tense muscles, tremors, decrease of muscle tone, drooling, difficulty talking, or convulsions.[13] If your patient has a seizure, make sure the patient is safe on the floor, and turn the patient to the side to assist with breathing. Remove glasses, and loosen shirts or ties that might be constricting. If the seizure lasts longer than five minutes, call 911.[14] Stay with the person until the seizure is over or until emergency assistance arrives. Do not try to stop the patient from moving, do not put anything in the patient's mouth, and do not offer food or water until the patient is fully conscious and alert. Box 12-7 indicates how to treat seizures.[14]

Falls

Falls are common in elderly patients, but anyone can fall. Changes in vision; vestibular function; episodes of syncope or seizures; medications; use of assistive devices; and environmental factors, such as cluttered rooms, uneven sidewalks, snowy or icy streets, slippery tubs, or stairs without handrails can contribute to falls. Treatment for falls includes prevention of shock and attention to abrasions or cuts if they occur. If the patient falls and you suspect a fracture, additional actions may be needed. Table 12-1 lists the various risk factors for falls, both human and environmental.[15]

Fractures

If a patient suffers a fracture (or suspected fracture), your goal is to protect the fracture site while preventing shock, controlling bleeding (if any), reducing pain, and seeking medical attention. If the patient is unable to ambulate or otherwise be transported to the emergency department or physician, you may need to call 911. Encourage the patient to avoid movement of the fractured area, and, if possible, elevate the area. If the fracture is open, apply a dressing or towel to control the bleeding. If the fracture is a spinal fracture, do not move the patient and immediately call 911.

Table 12-1 Risk Factors for Falls	
Human Factors	Environmental Factors
Advanced age (greater than 65 years old)	Uneven flooring
Impaired vision/hearing	Thresholds
Impaired balance/coordination	Throw or area rugs
Use of assistive device	Obstacles (eg, furniture, electrical cords, books, toys)
Medications	Pets
History of falls	Wet, icy, or slippery surfaces
Episodes of seizures or syncope	Steps, especially without rails
	No grab bars in bathrooms
	No anti-slip surface in tub
	Insufficient lighting

Heat Exhaustion

If a patient shows the signs and symptoms of heat exhaustion, including heavy sweating, faintness, dizziness, rapid pulse, nausea, or muscle cramps, it is important to cool the patient and offer hydration.[16] The patient should rest, and if signs of shock appear, you should treat the patient accordingly. Heat exhaustion is not as immediately life-threatening as heat stroke, but it can evolve into heat stroke if not addressed. Heat exhaustion results from overheating by being exposed to high temperatures, high humidity, and strenuous activity.[16] Box 12-8 lists how to treat heat exhaustion.

Heat Stroke

Heat stroke also results from the body overheating, usually due to exposure to high temperatures for a prolonged period of time. If your body temperature rises above 104°F, you could suffer a heat stroke.[17]

Heat stroke is life-threatening, so first aid should be immediately administered if the signs or symptoms are present. These include a high body temperature over 104°F, an altered mental state or behavior, nausea, vomiting, flushed skin, rapid breathing, a racing pulse, a headache, and changes in sweating.[17] If these signs and symptoms are observed, you should seek emergency aid immediately by calling 911. In the meantime, place the patient in a semireclining position, ideally in the shade. Remove outer clothing and monitor vitals. Apply cold, wet compresses to the body, especially wrists, ankles, groin, axilla, and lateral neck. The patient should not drink anything if he or she is not alert or is vomiting. The patient may seizure, in which case you should follow the seizure protocol. Box 12-9 lists how to treat heat stroke.[17]

Box 12-8
Treatment of Heat Exhaustion

1. Place the patient in a comfortable position in a shady or ventilated area.

2. Loosen or remove the patient's outer clothing.

3. Monitor the vital signs.

4. Apply a cold sponge/compress to the forehead or neck.

5. Offer water or electrolyte solution to rehydrate (if the patient is conscious).

6. Observe the patient for signs of shock or heat stroke; contact emergency services immediately if the patient shows no signs of improving (loss of consciousness, refusal of liquids, vomiting, etc).

7. Have the patient rest for the remainder of the day.

SAFETY/RED FLAGS

As already mentioned, the clinician needs to keep in mind the patient's health history and be mindful of any signs or symptoms that display distress or injury. The therapist may need to adjust or decrease the intensity of the activity, or the activity may need to be changed altogether. The patient may need frequent rest breaks. The therapist should monitor the patient's vital signs, especially if the patient has cardiac or respiratory issues. Some health conditions or the medications or treatments the patient is receiving for certain health conditions present as contraindications or precautions for treatment, so you should be aware of the medications the patient is taking and should know the patient's basic past medical history. A therapist

Box 12-9

Treatment of Heat Stroke

1. Seek emergency care immediately.

2. Place the patient in semireclining position in a shady or ventilated area.

3. Remove the patient's outer clothing.

4. Monitor the pulse and respiratory rate.

5. Cool the patient with large amounts of cool/cold water or a cold, wet compresses/towels/sheets. Apply to the groin, axilla, lateral neck, wrists, and ankles to cool rapidly.

6. Do not give the patient anything to drink if he or she is either not alert or vomiting.

7. Apply seizure precautions if the patient has a seizure.

should be aware of this in order to avoid inadvertently injuring the patient. In cases that the patient is not demonstrating recovery, the nursing staff or emergency staff may need to be contacted. If the therapist is having the patient perform activities that are challenging or difficult, the patient should wear a gait belt. If a patient loses consciousness or begins to fall, you may not be able to prevent it; however, you may be able to slow the descent and prevent significant injury.

DOCUMENTATION

When documenting a medical emergency in your note, you will need to include the signs or symptoms you observed, the vital signs you measured (and when you checked those vital signs), and what you did to address the situation. This may be something as simple as positioning the patient safely and then calling a staff emergency or code, or it could include more involved actions such as performing CPR or applying pressure to slow down bleeding. As with all documentation, your note should reflect what you did during your session.

S: Patient being seen by home health for recovery from pneumonia s/p 6 weeks. Patient c/o rapid fatigue with minimal activity and increase of pain to 6/10 in Ⓑ knees.

O: Patient performed 3 sit to stand with min Ⓐ. Patient c/o dizziness with sit to stand attempts. Patient's blood pressure in sitting 128/88 mmHg; upon standing blood pressure dropped to 98/82 mmHg. Had patient stand statically x 5 minutes to see if dizziness decreased. Blood pressure after 5 minutes of standing 104/86 mmHg with patient reporting lessening symptoms of dizziness.

S: Patient being seen by therapy for wound care on Ⓡ greater trochanter secondary to SCI and pressure.

O: Patient wound dressing and packing removed. Wound measurements this date 2.3 cm x 1.4 cm x 1.4 cm with tunneling noted at the 3-o'clock position x 1.8 cm. Wound irrigated and packing placed inside wound. Patient c/o headache and nausea during treatment. Therapist took blood pressure at 192/98 mmHg. Possible noxious stimulus of patient positioning during wound care; repositioned patient and called staff emergency. Nursing staff and physician arrived quickly and took over, monitoring blood pressure. Vitals stabilized after repositioning patient, blood pressure 128/78 mmHg. Wound care completed with no other issues.

REVIEW QUESTIONS

1. What are the signs/symptoms of cardiac arrest?

2. Your patient who had an SCI demonstrates piloerection below the level of injury, sweating above the level of injury, and high blood pressure. What is the possible diagnosis and how should you address it?

3. Your patient is a 45-year-old male with type 2 diabetes. During therapy you notice he starts to get shaky, sweaty, and fatigued. What is the possible cause of this and how should you address it?

4. Describe how one might prevent or avoid certain safety issues or injuries during a therapy session.

5. What is the protocol for when a patient is choking?

6. What should you *not* do when a patient is having a seizure?

7. Describe the method for preventing/treating shock in a patient.

8. Your patient begins demonstrating difficulty breathing, and you learn that he or she has a severe peanut allergy. What should you do?

9. Describe the functioning of patients with type 2 diabetes using the *International Classification of Functioning, Disability and Health*.

REFERENCES

1. Allergies: symptoms and causes. *Mayo Clinic*. http://www.mayoclinic.org/diseases-conditions/allergies/symptoms-causes/dxc-20270197. Updated January 6, 2018. Accessed September 13, 2018.

2. Shock: first aid. *Mayo Clinic*. http://www.mayoclinic.org/first-aid/first-aid-shock/basics/art-20056620. Updated July 27, 2017. Accessed September 13, 2018.

3. American Heart Association. *Basic Life Support Provider Manual*. South Deerfield, MA: Chenning Bete Company; 2016.

4. Pediatric first aid/CRP/AED ready reference. *American Red Cross*. https://www.redcross.org/images/MEDIA_CustomProductCatalog/m4240175_Pediatric_ready_reference.pdf. Published 2011. Accessed September 13, 2018.

5. Orthostatic hypotension (postural hypotension): symptoms and causes. *Mayo Clinic*. http://www.mayoclinic.org/diseases-conditions/orthostatic-hypotension/symptoms-causes/dxc-20324950. Updated July 11, 2017. Accessed September 13, 2018.

6. Autonomic dysreflexia. *United Spinal Association*. https://www.unitedspinal.org/resource-center/askus/?pg=kb.page&id=248. Accessed September 13, 2018.

7. Cardiac arrest. *American Heart Association*. http://www.heart.org/HEARTORG/Conditions/More/CardiacArrest/Cardiac-Arrest_UCM_002081_SubHomePage.jsp. Updated March 31, 2017. Accessed September 13, 2018.

8. Hands-only CPR. *American Heart Association*. http://cpr.heart.org/AHAECC/CPRAndECC/Programs/HandsOnlyCPR/UCM_473196_Hands-Only-CPR.jsp. Updated 2018. Accessed September 13, 2018.

9. Act FAST. *The National Stroke Association*. http://support.stroke.org/acute_site/having-stroke/. Published 2014. Accessed June 20, 2017.

10. Hypoglycemia in diabetes. *Mayo Clinic*. http://www.mayoclinic.org/diseases-conditions/hypoglycemia/basics/symptoms/con-20021103. Updated 2018. Accessed September 13, 2018.

11. Hyperglycemia in diabetes. *Mayo Clinic*. http://www.mayoclinic.org/diseases-conditions/hyperglycemia/basics/symptoms/con-20034795. Updated July 26, 2018. Accessed September 13, 2018.

12. Burns: first aid. *Mayo Clinic*. http://www.mayoclinic.org/first-aid/first-aid-burns/basics/art-20056649. Updated January 30, 2018. Accessed September 13, 2018.

13. Schachter SC, Shafer PO, Sirven JI. What happens during a seizure? *Epilepsy Foundation*. http://www.epilepsy.com/learn/epilepsy-101/what-happens-during-seizure. Published March 19, 2014. Accessed September 13, 2018.

14. Seizure first aid. *Centers for Disease Control and Prevention*. https://www.cdc.gov/epilepsy/basics/first-aid.htm. Updated April 23, 2018. Accessed September 13, 2018.

15. Important facts about falls. *Centers for Disease Control and Prevention*. https://www.cdc.gov/homeandrecreationalsafety/falls/adultfalls.html. Updated February 10, 2017. Accessed September 13, 2018.

16. Heat exhaustion. *Mayo Clinic*. http://www.mayoclinic.org/diseases-conditions/heat-exhaustion/basics/definition/con-20033366. Updated December 14, 2017. Accessed September 13, 2018.

17. Heatstroke. *Mayo Clinic*. http://www.mayoclinic.org/diseases-conditions/heat-stroke/home/ovc-20346531. Updated August 15, 2017. Accessed September 13, 2018.

Chapter 13

Americans With Disabilities Act

CHAPTER OBJECTIVES

1. Describe the Americans with Disabilities Act (ADA) and its purpose.
2. Describe an environmental assessment and the physical therapist's role in this assessment.
3. List the specific requirements for a wheelchair-accessible home.

INTRODUCTION

The ADA was signed in 1990. Prior to that, in 1968, The Fair Housing Act and the Architectural Barriers Act served as an early step toward requiring public buildings to be accessible to people with disabilities and that people with disabilities seeking housing could not be rejected solely based on the fact that they were disabled.[1,2] Additionally, landlords were required to make reasonable accommodations for tenants with disabilities. These acts were updated in 1988.[1,2] Section 504 of the 1973 Rehabilitation Act banned discrimination based on disabilities of recipients of federal funds.[3] In 1975, the Individuals with Disabilities Education Act required public schools to make themselves available to all children, including those with disabilities, within the least restrictive environment available.[4] Students requiring special education are provided this also. This law

was reauthorized in 2004, and an amendment, the Every Student Succeeds Act, was added in 2015.[5]

It was not until the ADA, however, that many of these concepts were brought together into one law. Much like the Civil Rights Act of 1964, the ADA was meant to serve as a law recognizing persons with disabilities as minority groups who deserve equal opportunity. The ADA was amended in 2008, and individual titles have been revised to account for changes in technology.[6] Title II and III were revised in 2010 and again in 2016, particularly to accommodate the change of the term *disability* and the requirement of public services to provide auxiliary aids such as closed captioning.[6] The ADA is comprised of 5 titles: the first addresses employment, the second addresses accessibility to state and local government services or programs, the third addresses public accommodations (eg, for theaters, doctors' offices, or schools, as well as office buildings), the fourth addresses telecommunications, and the fifth addresses miscellaneous provisions.[6]

AMERICANS WITH DISABILITIES ACT DEFINED

As mentioned previously, the ADA has 5 titles, and the first 4 receive the most attention. Each addresses a different component of accessibility and equal opportunity for people with disabilities.

Memolo J.
Procedures and Patient Care for the Physical Therapist Assistant
(pp 199-205). © 2019 SLACK Incorporated.

Box 13-1

Removal of Barriers

- Install ramps.
- Make curb cutouts in sidewalks/entrances.
- Reposition shelves.
- Rearrange tables, chairs, vending machines, and other furniture.
- Reposition telephones.
- Add raised markings on elevator buttons.
- Install flashing alarm lights.
- Widen doorways.
- Install offset hinges to widen doorways.
- Eliminate turnstiles or provide alternate paths.
- Install accessible door hardware.
- Install grab bars in toilet stalls.
- Rearrange toilet partitions to increase space.
- Insulate plumbing under sinks.
- Install full length bathroom mirror.
- Reposition paper towel dispenser in bathroom.
- Increase accessible parking spaces.
- Install accessible paper cup dispenser at water fountain.
- Remove high pile carpeting.

Title I, which addresses employment, prevents employers (eg, private, state or local government, labor unions) from discriminating against those with a disability when it comes to hiring, firing, promotions, pay, and training.[6,7] A potential employer cannot pass on hiring a person solely based on his or her disability, and the employer must make reasonable accommodations so the person can perform at optimal ability. Reasonable accommodations include modifications to the job or work environment, including modification of work schedule, furniture, restrooms, or assistive devices. Employees must request accommodations, however, and employers have the right to select from several options the accommodation(s) that requires the least burden or cost. An employer is not required to give preference to someone with a disability; the employer is allowed to select the candidate for a job who can best perform that job.

Title II protects individuals with disabilities from discrimination in programs, activities, and services of public entities (eg, public transportation and communication).[6,7] A state or local government cannot exclude or create exclusionary criteria that would prevent people with disabilities from participating in public programs or activities, and reasonable modifications must be made to avoid discrimination.

Title III states that public and private locations, such as restaurants, hotels, stores, theaters, office buildings, museums, and libraries, must be accessible to those with disabilities.[6,7] Churches and private clubs are excluded from this law, and alterations or changes to locations must not present as an undue burden. If the owner or leasee is not able to make changes readily, alternate methods of access or service must be provided. Changes include curb cutouts, telephone accessibility, raised toilet seats, wider bathroom stalls, grab bars in bathrooms, removal of carpet, and alternate door access if the only door is a revolving door. New facilities are built with these accommodations in mind, including handicap parking spaces and lower water fountains.

Title IV addresses telecommunications and stipulates that businesses offering telephone services offer telecommunication devices for those who are hearing impaired or deaf, and Title V stipulates that any public television service announcement funded in part or whole by the federal government should include closed captioning.[6,7]

COMPLIANCE

Any place of business should have an ADA compliance policy in place. Potential employers, managers, or administrators should be familiar with the ADA rules/regulations and may need to speak with human resources or legal counsel to be knowledgeable and compliant. It is a good idea to be generally knowledgeable, but if the manager or employer is made aware of a specific case, additional time and effort should be spent to avoid breaking the rules. In the terms of employment, a manager should make a specific job description that lists all the requirements to avoid confusion or trouble, including how much weight a person must lift or how long a person must stand, as well as special skills or training required. A manager or employer should be able and willing to make any reasonable accommodations, and other employees or staff may need to be educated on how to provide accommodations. Staff might need to be educated or trained on how to communicate and interact with persons with disabilities in order to provide a safe, fair, and comfortable working environment.[7] Employers and managers must remember that it is not appropriate to ask a person about potential disabilities, health status, drug use, or psychiatric history. This includes in-person communication as well as on any employment forms.

If an employer or manager is seeking information on how to determine if a location is compliant (or what needs to be changed in order to be compliant), he or she can consult the ADA Checklist for Existing Facilities, which offers a fillable Word document that goes through all areas that need to be accessible per the ADA (www.adachecklist.org/checklist.html).[8] An employer can and will be held liable for any barriers not removed, unless it places an undue burden or expense on the employer. Box 13-1 includes a list of barriers that can be removed to comply with Title III of the ADA.

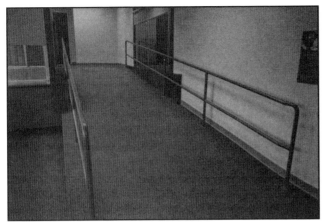

Figure 13-1. Ramp.

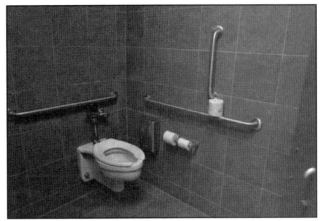

Figure 13-2. Grab bars in a bathroom.

If a person feels that he or she has been discriminated against, he or she can file a complaint online, via fax, or via mail. Complaints are sent to the Department of Justice, the Disability Rights Section.[9] The complainant includes information about him- or herself as well as the acts of discrimination. Reviews can take up to 3 months. Mediation might be the recommended route of addressing the complaint, especially if it is in regard to issues like barrier removal, communication, or modification of policies or procedures. Alternatively, the complaint can be opened for investigation, and an investigator or attorney will be assigned to the complainant. This could result in a settlement or lawsuit, depending on the situation.[9]

ENVIRONMENTAL ASSESSMENTS

Chapter 11 discussed performing home assessments to better prepare patients and caregivers for the patient to return home safely. Cosmetic or easy changes such as removing throw rugs and adding grabs bars are one set of recommendations; adding heftier items such as stair lifts and ramps are another.

This chapter refers to environmental assessments as those occurring not just in the home (and more specific to certain disabilities or equipment) but also in the outside world, such as the grocery store or library. The 2010 ADA Standards for Accessible Design includes detailed specifications for accessible components, such as drinking fountains, signs, parking spaces, door knobs, curbs, and ramps.[10]

Universal design, as described by Ron Mace when he worked at North Carolina State University (Raleigh, North Carolina), is not so much accommodating to a person's disability but designing a place with certain disabilities in mind.[11] Per North Carolina State University's Center for Universal Design, there are 7 principles of universal design. These include equitable use, flexibility in use, simple and intuitive use, perceptible information, tolerance for error, low physical effort, and size and space for approach and use.[11] Examples may include lever-type doorknobs, wider doorways and halls, relocated light switches and outlets, recessed areas under sinks and cabinets, lower countertops and cabinets, and flat threshold entries to showers. Some of these concepts can be added to a home or building after it has been built, and, in many cases, must be according to the ADA; however, some places are built with these modifications already made.

Environmental assessments often require the health care provider, such as a physical therapist, physical therapist assistant, and/or occupational therapist, to visit the location(s) in question. Measurements can be taken to determine if accessibility is an issue. For example, a ramp should not rise greater than a 1:12 ratio (so no more than 1 inch of rise for every 12 inches of vertical length) and a ramp should be 36 to 48 inches wide to accommodate wheelchairs and assistive devices.[10] The surface must be slip resistant, and the ramp should also have one or more landings (Figure 13-1).[10] Doorways must be at least 32 inches wide, but a wider doorway may be needed if the patient uses a bariatric device.[10] Hallways, too, should be at least 32 inches wide.[10] Toilets should be between 16 inches and 19 inches from the floor, and grab bars should be installed horizontally 33 to 36 inches from the floor and installed in the floor or wall stud for stability (Figure 13-2).[10] Table 13-1 includes a more detailed list of wheelchair-accessible specifications for a person's home.[10] Going through a person's home or workplace and noting these measurements will give the patient and therapist a clear idea of what needs work.

Table 13-1
Wheelchair-Accessible Measurements at Home

Feature	Specifications
Doorways	Minimum 32 inches, 36 inches recommended
Hallways	Minimum 32 inches, 36 inches recommended
Threshold	No greater than ¼ inch to ½ inch
Outlets	18 inches from floor
Light switches	No greater than 48 inches from floor and can be operated with one hand (rocker-type)
Door handles	Operable with one hand (lever, push) and no greater than 48 inches and no less than 34 inches from floor
Ramps	1:12 ratio; 36 inches wide; slip resistant; landing at top/bottom of ramp and if ramp changes directions
Windows	Easily operable with one hand (vertical sliding or crank) and 36 inches from floor
Countertops	No greater than 36 inches from floor (allowing also for knee clearance, at least 27 inches)
Sinks	No greater than 34 inches from floor, pipe insulated with at least 8 inches clearance for knees (depth); faucets operable without grasping, pinching, or twisting of wrist
Cabinets	Positioned so patient can reach (20- to 44-inch reach range); countertop could allow knee clearance or greater than 4 inches toe kick to allow closer access
Toilets	Flushable with one hand (lever style); no greater than 19 inches and no less than 17 inches from floor; at least 60 inches from side wall and 56 inches from rear wall clearance to access
Showers	Regular: 36 x 36 inches with fixed seat, handheld shower head Roll-in: 30/36 x 60 inches with handheld shower head and threshold no greater than ½ inch; shower control operable with one hand (lever)
Bathtubs	Fixed seat, nonslip floor, 30 x 60 inches
Grab bars	No greater than 36 inches and no less than 33 inches from floor; horizontal installation, installed in stud or other sturdy manner
Closets	Rods at accessible height, opening accessible for wheelchair (door at least 32 inches wide and roll-in style preferable)

Box 13-2
Assessment of the Workplace

- Parking: location, size, condition, surface type, as well as availability of parking
- Entry: number of steps, rails, ramp, lighting, door width, type of door opening/closing, threshold
- Sidewalk: type of surface, condition, width
- Access to work station/office
- Door and hallway widths
- Bathroom access: doors, stalls, sinks, toilets, grab bars
- Water fountains or vending access
- Escalators/elevator access
- Access to cafeteria or eating facilities
- Access to supplies, cabinets, work surfaces/spaces

These assessments and recommendations can be made in writing to the patient, his or her caregivers, and/or his or her employer. This document may include measurements, photographs, diagrams, and plans to make the home or workplace more accessible. Box 13-2 includes areas to consider when performing a workplace assessment. Figures 13-3 and 13-4 include pictures of workplace accommodations, including lower water fountains and accessible bathrooms. The patient may need a contractor or other assistance to have these modifications made; in many cities or towns there are contractors who make these modifications at a decreased cost for people with lower or fixed incomes.

When it comes to the community, the patient may need information or education on how to best adapt to community environments. The physical therapist assistant or other health care provider can go out in the community with the patient to practice frequent activities or go to locations the patient might frequently visit. For example, a patient had

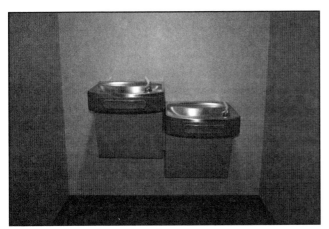

Figure 13-3. Lowered water fountains.

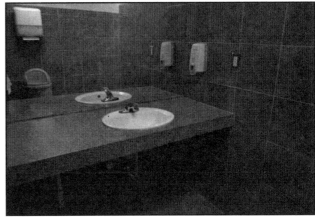

Figure 13-4. Accessible bathrooms.

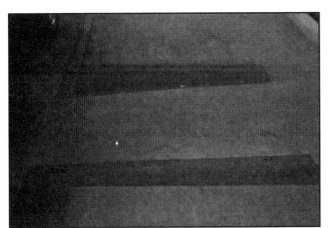

Figure 13-5. Curb cutouts.

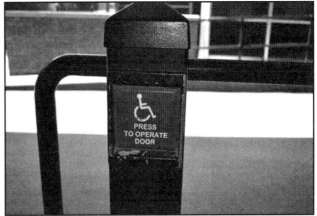

Figure 13-6. Accessible doors (automatic open).

incurred a traumatic brain injury 8 weeks previously and was now on a rehabilitation unit. She was almost ready to go home, but before she left, the therapists wanted to make sure she was ready to be out in the community. As a means of assessing her ability to function in the community, the therapists took her to a local grocery store to buy some food. For the patient, this outing was fun. She was able to leave the hospital setting for a little while and buy snacks. However, in preparation she had to make a list, and once in the store, she had to find the items on the list with little assistance. She had to get the grocery cart, navigate the aisles, and make the monetary transaction while interacting with the grocery store staff appropriately. After shopping, she had to walk to the nearest bus stop and indicate what bus she would take to get home. While this outing did not require measurements of doorways and ramps, it did assess the patient's ability to function in the community safely.

Aspects considered in a community outing may include public transportation stops; frequently navigated curbs, sidewalks, and crosswalks; grocery store doorways or entryways, as well as business bathrooms or elevators; and favorite recreational areas such as gyms, libraries, or sporting arenas.[10] Figures 13-5, 13-6, and 13-7 include pictures of curb cutouts, accessible doors, and handicap parking spaces as examples of community facility changes. Likely, most of these places have some kind of accommodations made for persons with disabilities; however, your patient may need education on what to look for and how to navigate these options. Box 13-3 includes areas to look at for a community assessment.

Environmental (and home) assessments may require multiple trips to gain a full understanding of what the patient might need, both in terms of architectural modifications as well as education and psychological adaptation. Having the patient's family, friends, or caregivers present can also be helpful. The therapist should bring a tape measure, a flashlight, paper (possibly graph paper if diagrams are needed), a camera, and some kind of assessment form (if available) to properly collect all the needed data.

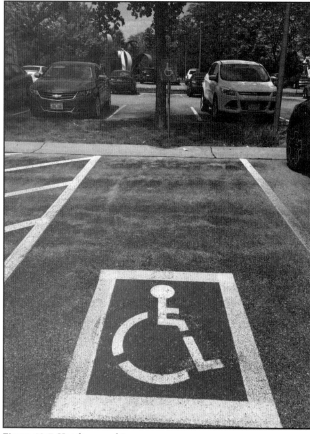

Figure 13-7. Handicap parking spaces.

DOCUMENTATION

When documenting how the patient interacts with home, work, or community settings, you should include the measurements you take and the barriers you observe. In addition, you can include what steps you took to address those barriers, such as removing dangerous furniture or training the patient to negotiate certain environmental situations. You can note the progress the patient makes toward returning to his or her home, work, and community.

S: Patient being seen for therapy due to Ⓑ LE amputation below the knees, s/p 1 month. Physician states patient is medically stable.

O: Patient has been on rehab floor x 4 weeks and is almost ready to return home, having achieved all STG and LTG on PT POC. Patient, PT, OT, and patient's spouse visited patient's workplace this date. Patient in wheelchair d/t prosthetics not fitting properly. Measured office entry doorway, bathroom accessibility, and work space accessibility. Measurements and pictures noted in environmental assessment document, see attached.

Box 13-3
Assessment of Community

- Type of transportation and access/location
- Sidewalks, curb cutouts, crosswalks
- Parking for restaurants, stores, public facilities (libraries, courthouse, etc), banks, grocery stores, theaters, etc
- Entry to buildings: door widths, door opening/closing, thresholds
- Access to telephones, bathrooms, water fountains, elevators, emergency exits, and counter services inside buildings
- Access to recreational areas/facilities

REVIEW QUESTIONS

1. What are the 5 Titles of the ADA and what does each Title address?
2. What is an environmental assessment and what is the physical therapist's role?
3. What are some of the specific requirements or measurements for a wheelchair-accessible home?
4. Access the ADA Checklist for Existing Facilities. Now go out into the community to a place of business, a school, a library, a store, etc. Walk through the parking lots, curbs, doorways, bathrooms, offices, aisles, water fountains, and other areas. How easy or hard would it be to get around if you were in a wheelchair or used a walker? If you took measurements, what did you note? What modifications did you think could be made to make the location more accessible?
5. What are at least 3 things a manager or employer could do to be better prepared to employ or interact with persons with disabilities?
6. You have a patient who is blind who needs an environmental assessment of his workplace. What are some areas you may pay attention to or note in your assessment (both inside and outside)?
7. Your patient is going home in a wheelchair. How would you prepare the patient for going home, and what areas should be assessed in your pre-discharge visit?
8. Your patient is going home and will use a front-wheeled walker inside and outside the home after suffering a stroke affecting his right side. The house has 2 steps to enter without a rail; 12 stairs inside the home to the basement with a rail on the right, which the patient must access in case of a tornado and to do laundry; and a half bath on the main floor with a narrow (26 inches) entryway. The garage is detached, but the garage door is automatic. What recommendations might you make to assist this patient with his transition home (both exterior and interior)?

REFERENCES

1. Fair housing act. A guide to disability rights laws. *United States Department of Justice, Civil Rights Division*. https://www.ada.gov/cguide.htm. Published July 2009. Updated March 2017. Accessed September 14, 2018.

2. Architectural barriers act. A guide to disability rights laws. *United States Department of Justice, Civil Rights Division*. https://www.ada.gov/cguide.htm. Published July 2009. Updated March 2017. Accessed September 14, 2018.

3. A guide to disability rights laws. *United States Department of Justice, Civil Rights Division*. https://www.ada.gov/cguide.htm#anchor65610. Published July 2009. Updated March 2017. Accessed September 14, 2018.

4. Individuals with disabilities education act. A guide to disability rights laws. *United States Department of Justice, Civil Rights Division*. https://www.ada.gov/cguide.htm. Published July 2009. Updated March 2017. Accessed September 14, 2018.

5. About IDEA. *IDEA: Individuals With Disabilities Education Act*. https://sites.ed.gov/idea/about-idea/. Accessed September 14, 2018.

6. Introduction to the ADA. *United States Department of Justice, Civil Rights Division*. https://www.ada.gov/ada_intro.htm. Accessed September 14, 2018.

7. Americans with disabilities act questions and answers. *United States Department of Justice, Civil Rights Division*. https://www.ada.gov/hiv/ada_q&a_aids.htm. Accessed November 7, 2018.

8. ADA checklist for existing facilities. *New England ADA Center*. http://adachecklist.org/checklist.html. Updated 2017. Accessed September 14, 2018.

9. How to file an ADA complaint with the US Department of Justice. *United States Department of Justice, Civil Rights Division*. https://www.ada.gov/filing_complaint.htm. Accessed September 14, 2018.

10. 2010 ADA standards for accessible design. *United States Department of Justice, Civil Rights Division*. https://www.ada.gov/regs2010/2010ADAStandards/2010ADAstandards.htm#Bars. Published September 15, 2010. Updated December 7, 2012. Accessed September 14, 2018.

11. Connell BR, Jones M, Mace R, et al. The principles of universal design. *NC State University, The Center for Universal Design*. https://projects.ncsu.edu/www/ncsu/design/sod5/cud/about_ud/udprinciplestext.htm. Published April 1, 1997. Accessed September 14, 2018.

Glossary

A

Accessible: the design of products, devices, services, or environments for people with disabilities; can be direct or indirect.

Acute: the first 24 to 48 hours after an injury due to a traumatic event such as a car accident or sporting event.

Adapt: to become adjusted to new conditions or to make suitable for a new purpose; to modify.

Airborne: any disease caused by pathogens that can be transmitted through the air, through breathing, coughing, sneezing, raising dust, spraying liquids, flushing toilets, or any activity that generates aerosol particles or droplets.

Allergy: hypersensitivity of the immune system to something in the environment, such as dust, animals, or food, that usually causes no problem in the average population.

Ambulation: to walk about or move from place to place.

Americans with Disabilities Act: a civil rights law that prohibits discrimination against individuals with disabilities in areas of public life (jobs, schools, transportation, and public/private places open to the general public).

Anaphylaxis: serious allergic reaction that is rapid in onset and may cause death; includes swelling, shortness of breath, vomiting, and low blood pressure.

Apnea: the suspension of breathing, or no movement of the muscles of inhalation; sleep apnea occurs when an individual is sleeping.

Ascend: to go upward or rise.

Autonomic hyperreflexia (dysreflexia): Syndrome in which there is a sudden onset of excessively elevated blood pressure; most common in patients with spinal cord injuries at T6 or above. It occurs with a noxious stimulus, such as tight clothing or a full bladder, below the level of injury, causing a dangerous elevation of blood pressure. It is a medical emergency, and if possible, the noxious stimulus should be removed and 911 should be called.

B

Bilateral: having or relating to 2 sides; affecting both sides.

Blanch: to make white or pale by extracting color (blood).

Body mechanics: exercises designed to improve posture, coordination, and stamina.

Bradycardia: slow heart rate, less than 60 beats per minute in adults (at rest).

Bridging: a close-chained exercise performed in supine, in which the patient lifts hips and buttocks off the surface of the bed/mat.

C

Chronic: persisting for a long time or constantly recurring.

Communication: the imparting or exchanging of information or news.

Memolo J.
Procedures and Patient Care for the Physical Therapist Assistant
(pp 207-212). © 2019 SLACK Incorporated.

Comorbidities: the simultaneous presence of 2 chronic diseases or conditions in a patient.

Concentric: shortening a muscle as it acts against a resistive force (such as a weight), bringing origin and insertion closer together.

Contact: form of isolation in which anyone entering the patient's room and having direct contact with the patient should wear personal protective equipment (PPE), such as gloves and a gown; includes diseases such as methicillin-resistant *Staphylococcus aureus* and *Clostridium difficile.*

Contractures: permanent shortening of a muscle or joint in response to prolonged hypertonic spasticity or positioning.

Contraindication: specific situation in which a drug, procedure, or surgery should not be used because it may be harmful to the patient.

Contralateral: relating to or denoting the side of the body opposite to that on which a particular structure or condition occurs.

D

Dermatomes: area of skin supplied by a single spinal nerve relaying sensation to the brain.

Descend: to move or fall downward.

Diaphoresis: sweating, especially to an unusual degree; sometimes as a symptom of disease or drug.

Diastolic: bottom number of a blood pressure reading; denotes pressure in the arteries when the heart rests between beats; typically less than 80 mmHg.

Disability: defined by ADA as "physical or mental impairment that substantially limits one or more major life activities, a person who has a history or record of such an impairment, or a person who is perceived by others as having such an impairment."[1]

Documentation: method by which the physical therapist or physical therapist assistant records the intervention(s) provided in a therapy session; a means of communication among the physical therapist, physical therapist assistant, and other health care providers; a means to support insurance payment and need for therapy.

Droplet: isolation used for diseases that are spread in tiny droplets caused by coughing or sneezing, such as Influenza and pertussis; health care workers should wear PPE such as gown and gloves, as well as a mask or respirator.

Dyspnea: difficult or labored breathing.

E

Eccentric: muscle contraction that involves the lengthening of the muscle while under a load or resistance (eg, lowering yourself down slowly when sitting).

Edema: swelling caused by excess fluid trapped in the body's tissues; can be the result of medications, disease processes, or pregnancy.

Ergonomics: the study of people's efficiency in their working environment.

Erythema: superficial reddening of the skin as a result of injury or irritation.

Evaluation/assessment: initial assessment of a patient performed by the supervising physical therapist in which the patient's baseline functions are recorded; used to create a plan of care for the patient, which the physical therapist and physical therapist assistant follow.

Exudate: a mass of cells and fluid that has seeped out of blood vessels, especially with inflammation.

F

Febrile/pyrexic: having or showing the symptoms of a fever.

Flaccid: a part of the body that is soft and hanging loosely or limply; lacking muscle tone.

Flat back: decreased lumbar lordosis.

Fowler's position: standard patient position in a hospital bed; the patient is positioned with the head and trunk elevated between 45 and 60 degrees.

Friction: the action of one surface or object rubbing against another.

Frontal plane: coronal plane; vertical plane that divides the body in to ventral and dorsal (belly and back) sections.

G

Gait belt: device used by therapists and caregivers to more safely transfer or ambulate with patients who have problems with strength and/or balance; typically worn around patient's waist at umbilicus.

Genu recurvatum: hyperextension of knees.

Genu valgum: knock-knees.

Genu varum: bowlegged.

Granulation: new vascular tissue in granular form; new connective tissue and microscopic blood vessels that form on a wound during the healing process.

Gravity: the pull on an object toward the center of the Earth.

H

Handicap: results when an individual with an impairment cannot fulfill a normal life role.

Hemiplegia: paralysis of one side of the body.

Hook lying: patient is positioned in supine with bilateral knees flexed and feet flat on the floor or bed.

Hypertension: high blood pressure.

Hyperthermia/hyperpyrexia: elevated body temperature due to failed thermoregulation that occurs when a body produces or absorbs more heat than it dissipates; can become a medical emergency.

Hypotension: low blood pressure.

Hypothermia: low body temperature due to losing heat faster than the body can produce it; can become a medical emergency.

I

Impairment: any loss or abnormality of psychological, physiological, or anatomical structure or function.

Indication: a symptom that suggests certain medical treatment is necessary.

Inflammatory phase: occurs right after an injury; controls bleeding and prevents infection; signs/symptoms include redness, heat, swelling, and pain.

Informed consent: permission granted in the knowledge of possible consequences (when a health care practitioner gives information about risks and benefits prior to performing a procedure).

Ipsilateral: belonging to or occurring on the same side of the body.

Isolation: precautions used to help stop/prevent the spread of germs from one person to another—to protect patients, families, visitors, and health care practitioners—through the use of PPE.

Irregular: arrhythmia/dysrhythmia; rhythms and beats can be irregular; any change from the normal sequence of electrical impulses in the heart.

K

Korotkoff sounds: blood flow sounds that health care providers observe when taking blood pressure; these 5 sounds (or lack of sounds) represent changes in the blood flow when occluded and reopened with a sphygmomanometer.

Kyphosis: posterior curvature of spine (seen in thoracic and sacral spine).

Kyphosis-Lordosis: increased kyphosis and lordosis.

L

Local(ized): restricted to a particular place or location.

Lofstrands: forearm crutches; crutches with cuffs that partially or fully encompass the forearms along with having hand grips for the patient to hold; these work together to support the patient's body weight or contribute to balance.

Lordosis: anterior curvature of spine (seen in cervical and lumbar spine).

M

Medical asepsis: the state of being free from disease causing microorganisms; concerned with restricting/eliminating the spread of microorganisms throughout a facility or from person to person.

Micturate: to urinate.

Mobility: "the ability to move or be moved freely and easily."[2]

Modality: a type of electrical, thermal, or mechanical energy that causes physiological changes in the body; used to relieve pain, improve circulation, decrease swelling, reduce muscle spasm, improve muscle function, or deliver medication in conjunction with other procedures.

N

Necrosis: the death of most or all of the cells in an organ or tissue due to disease, injury, or a failure of blood supply.

Nosocomial: a disease acquired in or originating from a hospital.

O

Orthopnea: shortness of breath occurring when lying flat (recumbent).

Orthostatic hypotension: postural hypotension; form of low blood pressure that occurs when a person sits up from lying down or stands from sitting.

Ostomy: surgically created opening in the body for the discharge of bodily waste.

P

Paralysis: the loss of the ability to move (and sometimes the loss of sensation) in part or most of the body, often as a result of injury, illness, or poison.

Paresis: condition of muscular weakness caused by nerve damage or disease; partial paralysis.

Pelvic tilt: can be anterior (increased lordosis) or posterior (decreased lordosis).

Pneumatic: a tire designed to provide flexible cover with an impermeable lining to contain and restrain compressed air; can withstand the cutting and abrasive wear of road contact and protects the tire against puncture and air loss.

Pes planus: flat foot.

Plan of care: plan created by the supervising physical therapist after conducting the initial evaluation/assessment, which sets goals for the patient (short term and long term) and lists general interventions to be used, as well as proposed duration and frequency of interventions and anticipated discharge plans.

Popliteal space/fossa: the space behind the knee at the back of the knee joint.

Pressure injury: localized skin or tissue damage as a result of pressure, shear, and/or friction over a bony prominence, such as sacrum, calcaneus, or olecranon; also known as *decubitus ulcer* or *pressure ulcer*.

Primary intention: first intention healing; healing via surgical intervention, such as stitches or staples, for wounds whose edges can be approximated or have little tissue loss.

Proliferative phase: epithelialization, fibroplasia, and angiogenesis occur during this phase, and a scar begins to form.

Prone: positioning flat on the stomach.

Pyogenic: involving or relating to the production of pus.

Q

Qualified individual with a disability: a person who meets legitimate skill experience, education, or other requirements of an employment position that he or she holds or seeks, and who can perform the essential functions of the position with or without reasonable accommodation.

Quad cane: a cane with 4 feet in touch with the ground, which can be wide or narrow in width.

R

Reasonable accommodation: assistance or changes to a position or workplace that will enable an employee to do his or her job despite having a disability; under the Americans with Disabilities Act, employers are required to provide this to qualified individuals with a disability unless doing so would create undue hardship.

Reasonable modification: a structural change made to an existing premises occupied by a person with a disability in order to afford the person the full enjoyment of the premises.

Rehabilitation: to restore to a condition of good health, ability to work, etc.

Remodeling phase: maturation phase; when collagen is remodeled from type III to type I and wound fully closes. The scar becomes less thick, smaller, and stronger; can take up to 2 years after initial injury to complete.

Restraint: a measure or condition that keeps someone or something under control; a physician's order is needed to use restraints.

Rollator: wheeled walker; 3- or 4-wheeled walker, often with a seat or basket and hand brakes; used by patients with fair balance and cognition.

S

Sagittal plane: median or longitudinal plane; divides body into left and right sides.

Scoliosis: laterally curved spine.

Secondary intention: healing of a wound whose edges cannot be approximated or there has been extensive tissue loss; done via wound packing, administration of bandaging, use of modalities, etc.

Seizure: sudden uncontrolled electrical activity in the brain, which may produce a physical convulsion, physical signs, thought disturbances, or a combination of symptoms.

Semi-Fowler's position: Patient positioning in a hospital bed, in which the head and trunk are elevated between 15 and 45 degrees (30 degrees is most common).

Semipneumatic: tires made of solid rubber with a hollow air pocket through the center; lack the bounce or cushion of pneumatic tires.

Septic: infected with bacteria; when referring to septic shock, it is a serious medical condition resulting from sepsis leading to low blood pressure and abnormalities in cellular metabolism.

Shear: force acting on a substance in a direction perpendicular to the substance, such as sliding a patient across a bed.

Shock: life-threatening medical condition of low blood perfusion to tissues resulting in cellular injury and inadequate tissue function.

Sidelying: positioning the patient on his or her side in bed or on a mat.

Sign: any objective evidence of disease or injury (can be detected by someone other than the individual affected by the disease).

Slough: yellow, devitalized tissue that can be thick, stringy, or adherent to tissue bed; should be debrided to allow for healthy granulation tissue to grow.

Sphygmomanometer: instrument by which blood pressure is measured consisting of a cuff applied to the arm, connected to a scale and bulb to inflate the cuff.

Staging: method of assessing pressure injuries according to severity.

State Practice Act: constitutes the law governing physical therapy practice within a state, including continuing education and prohibited procedures.

Stoma: surgically created opening on the surface of the abdomen to divert the flow of feces or urine.

Supine: when a patient is positioned on his or her back.

Surgical asepsis: exclusion of all microorganisms before they can enter an open wound or contaminate a sterile field during surgery; includes sterilization of instruments and washing hands, as well as wearing sterile gown/gloves/mask.

Sway back: very pronounced increased lumbar lordosis with forward head.

Symptom: subjective evidence of disease or injury, such as pain.

Syncope: temporary loss of consciousness usually related to insufficient blood flow to the brain; fainting or passing out.

Systemic: illness or disorder that affects the entire body.

Systolic: top number in a blood pressure reading representing the amount of pressure in the arteries during a contraction of the heart muscle; typically less than 120 mmHg.

T

Tachycardia: abnormally rapid heart rate.

Tachypnea: abnormally rapid breathing.

Thready: pulse that is weak, difficult to feel, or easily obliterated with slight pressure.

Trendelenburg position: body is supine and feet are higher than the head by 15 to 30 degrees; reverse Trendelenburg is when head is 15 to 30 degrees higher than the feet.

U

Undue burden/hardship: action requiring significant difficulty or expense for employer to make reasonable accommodations.

Unilateral: occurring on one side.

Universal design: "the design of products and environments to be usable by all people, to the greatest extent possible, without the need for adaptation or specialized design."[3]

V

Valsalva maneuver: moderately forceful attempted exhalation against a closed airway; often seen in patients performing strenuous activity such as lifting a heavy object or performing a difficult exercise.

W

Walker: two- or four-footed device used for patients with decreased strength or balance; can have no wheels, two front wheels, or skis on front/back legs.

REFERENCES

1. A guide to disability rights laws. *United States Department of Justice, Civil Rights Division.* https://www.ada.gov/cguide.htm. Published July 2009. Updated March 2017. Accessed November 7, 2018.

2. Mobility. *English Oxford Living Dictionaries.* https://en.oxforddictionaries.com/definition/mobility. Accessed September 14, 2018.

3. Connell BR, Jones M, Mace R, et al. The principles of universal design. *NC State University, The Center for Universal Design.* https://projects.ncsu.edu/www/ncsu/design/sod5/cud/about_ud/udprinciplestext.htm. Published April 1, 1997. Accessed September 14, 2018.

Appendix
Key Abbreviations

A

ADA	Americans with Disabilities Act
ADL	activities of daily living
AED	automated external defibrillator
AHA	American Heart Association
APTA	American Physical Therapy Association
AROM	active range of motion
ASIS	anterior superior iliac spine

B

Ⓑ	bilateral
BADL	basic activities of daily living
BOS	base of support
BP	blood pressure
Bpm	beats per minute
BWST	body weight supported treadmill

C

C	Celsius
CAPTE	The Commission on Accreditation in Physical Therapy Education
CDC	Centers for Disease Control and Prevention
C difficile	Clostridium difficile
CGA	contact guard assist
CHF	congestive heart failure
COG	center of gravity
COPD	chronic obstructive pulmonary disease
COTA	certified occupational therapy assistant
CPAP	continuous positive airway pressure ventilators
CPR	cardiopulmonary resuscitation
CVA	cerebrovascular accident
CVC	central venous catheter

Memolo J.
Procedures and Patient Care for the Physical Therapist Assistant
(pp 213-216). © 2019 SLACK Incorporated.

D

Ⓓ	dependent
DGI	Dynamic Gait Index
DM	diabetes mellitus
DTPI	deep tissue pressure injury
DVT	deep vein thrombosis

E

ECG	electrocardiogram
EMT	emergency medical technician
EOB	edge of bed
ER/ED	emergency room/emergency department

F

F	Fahrenheit
FIM	Functional Independence Measure
FWB	full weightbearing
FWW	front-wheeled walker

G

| G tube | gastric tube |

H

HAI	health care-associated infection
Hct	hematocrit
Hgb	hemoglobin
HIPPA	Health Insurance Portability and Accountability Act
HOB	head of bed
HR	heart rate

I

Ⓘ	independent
IADL	instrumental activities of daily living
ICF	*International Classification of Functioning, Disability and Health*
ICP	intracranial pressure monitor
ICU	intensive care unit
ID	identification
INR	international normalized ratio
IV	intravenous

L

| Ⓛ | left |
| LBQC | large-based quad cane |

M

max Ⓐ	maximal assist
MI	myocardial infarction
min Ⓐ	minimal assist
MHP	moist hot pack
mod Ⓐ	moderate assist
mmHg	millimeters of mercury
MRADL	mobility-related activities of daily living
MRSA	methicillin-resistant *Staphylococcus aureus*

N

NG tube	nasogastric tube
NICU	neonatal intensive care unit
NPUAP	National Pressure Ulcer Advisory Panel
NWB	nonweightbearing

O

OCR	Office for Civil Rights
ORIF	open reduction internal fixator/fixation
OSHA	Occupational Safety and Health Administration
OT	occupational therapist

P

PCA	patient controlled analgesia
PEG tube	percutaneous endoscopic gastrostomy tube
PICO	Patient, Intervention, Comparison, Outcome
POC	plan of care
POS	point of service
PPE	personal protective equipment
PROM	passive range of motion
PSIS	posterior superior iliac spine
PT	physical therapist
PTA	physical therapist assistant
PWB	partial weightbearing

R

Ⓡ	right
RBC	red blood cell
ROM	range of motion
RR	respiratory rate
RW	rollator walker

S

ⓢ	supervision
SBA	standby assist
SBQC	small-based quad cane
SCI	spinal cord injury
SDS	safety data sheets
SLP	speech-language pathologist
SOAP	Subjective, Objective, Assessment, Plan
SOB	shortness of breath
SPC	single-point cane
s/p	status post

T

TDWB/TTWB	touch down weightbearing/toe touch weightbearing
THA	total hip arthroplasty
TUG	Timed Up and Go

U

UTI	urinary tract infection

V

VGL	vertical gravity line
VRE	vancomycin-resistant *Enterococcus*

W

WBAT	weightbearing as tolerated
WBC	white blood cell
w/c	wheelchair
WHO	World Health Organization

Index